Color Atlas of
Life Before Birth
Normal Fetal Development

Library of Congress Catalog Card Number: 83-060616
International Standard Book Number: 0-8151-3119-4

Printed by Royal Smeets Offset b.v., Weert, Netherlands

Color Atlas of Life Before Birth
Normal Fetal Development

Marjorie A. England
Senior Lecturer in Anatomy
Medical Sciences
University of Leicester

Year Book Medical Publishers Inc
35 East Wacker Drive, Chicago

The *Humane Fœtus* tho no bigger then a *Green Pea*,
yet is furnifhed with all its parts.
Antonj van Leeuwenhoek, 1683

Contents

To
Olga A. Smith, B.A., M.S., (M.S. Hon.)
Lawrence University, Wisconsin, U.S.A.
An inspiring teacher

Acknowledgements

This book has only been possible because of the goodwill and generosity of several people and their institutions. In particular, Professor R.E.M. Bowden, Royal Free Hospital School of Medicine (R.F.H.S.M.), Professor R.M.H. McMinn, Royal College of Surgeons of England (R.C.S.E.), Dr R.M. Ransom, Consultant Pathologist, Watford General Hospital, Dr T. El-Sayed, Consultant Radiologist, Watford General Hospital, and Dr G. Slavin, Consultant Pathologist, Northwich Park Hospital, provided access to personal collections of material or ones prepared for their institutions by many workers through several generations. I am very grateful for this privilege.

I am also grateful to Professor T.W.A. Glenister, Charing Cross Hospital Medical School (C.C.H.M.S.) and to the Anatomy Department for allowing me to photograph some of the specimens in their collection.

I am indebted to Professor I. Craft, Royal Free Hospital for the photographs of *in vitro* fertilization.

Professor F.R. Johnson, London Hospital School of Medicine (L.H.S.M.) allowed me to photograph several specimens from his department.

Professor R.E. Coupland, University of Nottingham, also allowed me to photograph specimens from his departmental collection.

Professor F. Walker, University of Leicester, also gave permission to photograph material.

Dr D. Dooley, lately Her Majesty's Inspector of Anatomy, provided an alizarin red specimen.

Professor H. Nishimura, Professor Emeritus of Anatomy, Kyoto University, kindly provided the photographs of the somite embryos.

I am also grateful for the assistance and advice received from Dr A.J. Palfrey, Charing Cross Hospital Medical School, Dr A. Gulamhusein, University of Leicester, Dr I. Zadawi, Leicester General Hospital, Dr S.A. Ayettey and Dr M.E. Ward, Department of Anatomy, University of Ghana, and Mr R. Watts, Chief Technician, Charing Cross Hospital Medical School, who also allowed me to use his photographs of the radio-opaque studies of fetal circulation. Dr E.C. Blenkinsopp, Consultant Pathologist, Watford General Hospital, Dr A.M.C. Burgess, London Hospital Medical School, Dr J. Wakely, University of Leicester, Dr T. Boulos and Dr C. Tagoe, University of Leicester, Mr G. Bottomley, Chief Technician, University of Leicester, all made specimens available.

Assistance was also received from Miss E. Allen, Hunterian Museum, and Mr B.M. Logan, Department of Anatomy, Royal College of Surgeons of England, Miss M. Hudson, Charing Cross Hospital Medical School, Mr F. Young, Chief Technician, Nottingham University, Mrs S. Barraclough, Watford General Hospital, Mr R.C. Preston, Miss A. Cole, Mr C.G. Brooks, Mr H.J. Kowalski, Mr G.M. Lee, Mr. I. Paterson, and Mr G.L.C. McTurk, University of Leicester, and Mr J.E. Cartledge, Leicester General Hospital.

Dr C. Ockleford read the section on the developing fetal membranes and placenta; his constructive advice is gratefully acknowledged. Professor R. Wheeler Haines, Medical College, Baghdad, and Dr J. Wakely, University of Leicester, read the finished text and made suggestions for alterations and clarification. Professor J.L. Emery, University of Sheffield, commented upon the photographs. I am very grateful for their kindness in assuming this task though I accept full responsibility for any remaining errors or omissions.

I should like to thank Professor F. Beck for his interest and encouragement during the writing of this book.

Dr J.M. England, Consultant Hematologist, Watford General Hospital kindly assisted and encouraged me throughout the writing of this book.

I am also grateful to W.B. Saunders Co., Philadelphia, U.S.A. for permission to reproduce the figures provided by Professor H. Nishimura, Kyoto University which were published in *The Developing Human (Clinically Oriented Embryology)* by Keith L. Moore (1973).

A very especial acknowledgement is made to Mr K. Garfield, Chief Technician, Central Photographic Unit, University of Leicester, who was responsible for many of the photographs in this book. His encouragement and work have contributed greatly.

Preface

This Atlas is intended to illustrate some aspects of normal human development *in utero*. The descriptions accompanying the photographs serve as a link between them and as an *aide memoire* of embryology. The reader would be well advised also to consult the textbooks listed in Suggestions for Further Reading.

All the illustrations contained in this book are from human specimens, many of which were prepared over 40 years ago. A number of specimens had previously been mis-sexed; it is hoped the illustrations in this book will help prevent such confusion in the future. It must also be remembered that, although embryos of identical lengths are comparable, each organ is individual in its rate of growth and differentiation. For example, the arm primordia in one embryo of 12 mm crown–rump length may be only present as buds whilst in another they may already have differentiated into arm, forearm and hand sections.

Some of the specimens appear poorly dissected, but when compared with the head of a pin (p.125) the difficulties with dissection become apparent. Many of the smallest specimens were dissected with cactus spines mounted on handles as conventional instruments were too large. Some early specimens have crystals of fixative on their surface which were impossible to remove without damaging the specimen.

It was not intended to label every structure present on a specimen, but rather to label structures of interest and orientation for the reader. Photographs illustrating several points may be used on more than one occasion.

It is hoped this book will assist students of medicine, nursing, and the allied fields to visualize the structures which hereto have been largely illustrated by line drawings.

Terminology

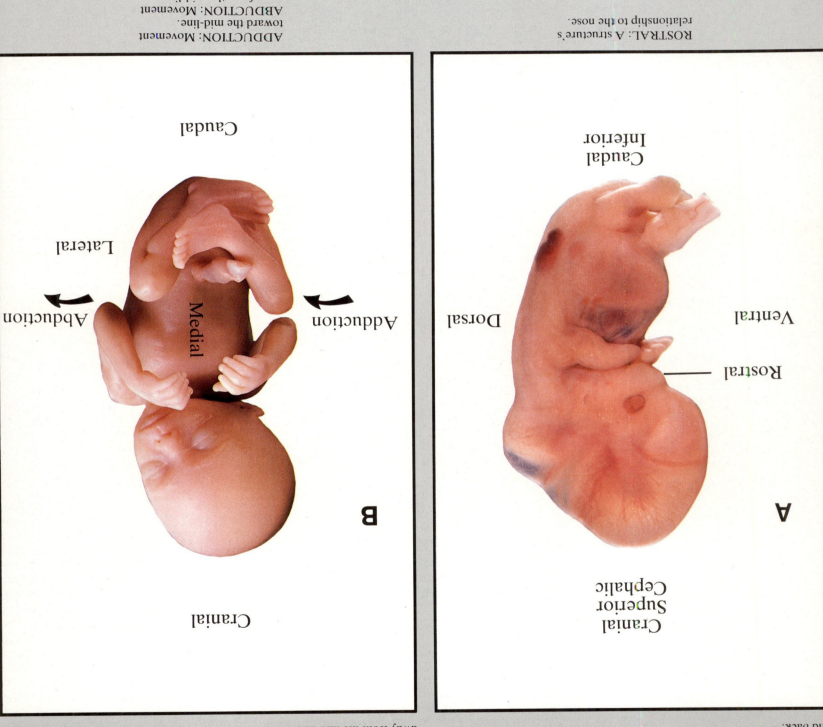

ROSTRAL. A structure's relationship to the nose.

Cranial
Superior
Cephalic

Dorsal — Rostral — Ventral

Caudal
Inferior

A. Terminology used to indicate top, bottom, front, and back.

ADDUCTION: Movement toward the mid-line.

ABDUCTION: Movement away from the mid-line.

Caudal

Lateral

Abduction — Medial — Adduction

Cranial

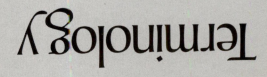

B. Terminology used to indicate movement toward and away from the mid-line.

Planes of Section

An embryo or fetus is usually sectioned in the following planes:

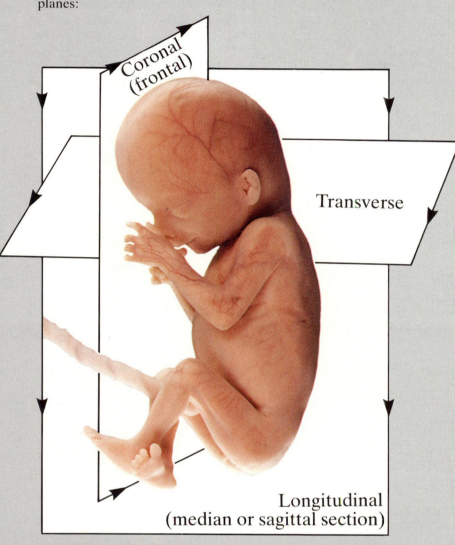

Coronal (frontal)

Transverse

Longitudinal (median or sagittal section)

The arrows indicate the direction of the plane of section.

●   Early embryos are flexed and it is possible in one transverse section to cross both the head and heart regions.

Gestational Age

An estimate of gestational age can be made by measuring the embryo or fetus. Various methods of measurement have been developed each with its own limitations and inaccuracies. Crown–rump and crown–heel lengths are the commonest measurements; this book uses crown–rump (CR) length in mm. Crown–heel (CH) lengths are difficult to measure because the legs are often flexed in different positions.

Most methods based on measurements are inaccurate because the specimens can be changed by stretching in handling or shrinking in fixation.

A series of developing external and internal features of an embryo is a more accurate measure of maturity. Streeter presented a series of Horizons I–XXIII, which he used to age embryos until Day 47. These descriptions are based on a *true age* stretching from fertilization at time 0 to term at Week 38 (Day 266). Recent research has necessitated some slight alterations of Streeter's original tables. The reader is advised to consult Iffy *et al.* (1967), O'Rahilly (1973), and Gasser (1975). This Atlas uses Streeter's original tables.

Most clinicians do not know the fertilization date; the only date available to them is the first day of the last menstrual period. They use this date to assign a *menstrual age* stretching from time 0, which is usually 14 days before fertilization, to term at Week 40 (9.2 calendar months).

In this book descriptions of early development are based on the fertilization date and expressed as true ages in hours, days or weeks and as Horizons. For the very late fetuses the dates are often based on the last menstrual period and expressed as menstrual ages in calendar months. Readers should be aware that other workers have used lunar months (4 weeks) rather than calendar months; term is 10 lunar months from the first day of the last menstrual period.

References

Iffy, L., Shepard, T.H., Jakobovits, A., Lemire, R.J. & Kerner, P. (1967) *Acta Anat.* **66**, 178–186.

O'Rahilly, R. (1973) Carnegie Institution of Washington Publications 631.

Gasser, R. (1975) *Atlas of Human Embryos.* Hagerstown, Harper & Row.

Streeter, G.L. (1942) Carnegie Institution of Washington Publications **30**, 211–245.

Streeter, G.L. (1948) Carnegie Institution of Washington Publications **32**, 133–203.

A summary of different methods of describing human prenatal development and the method used in this Atlas

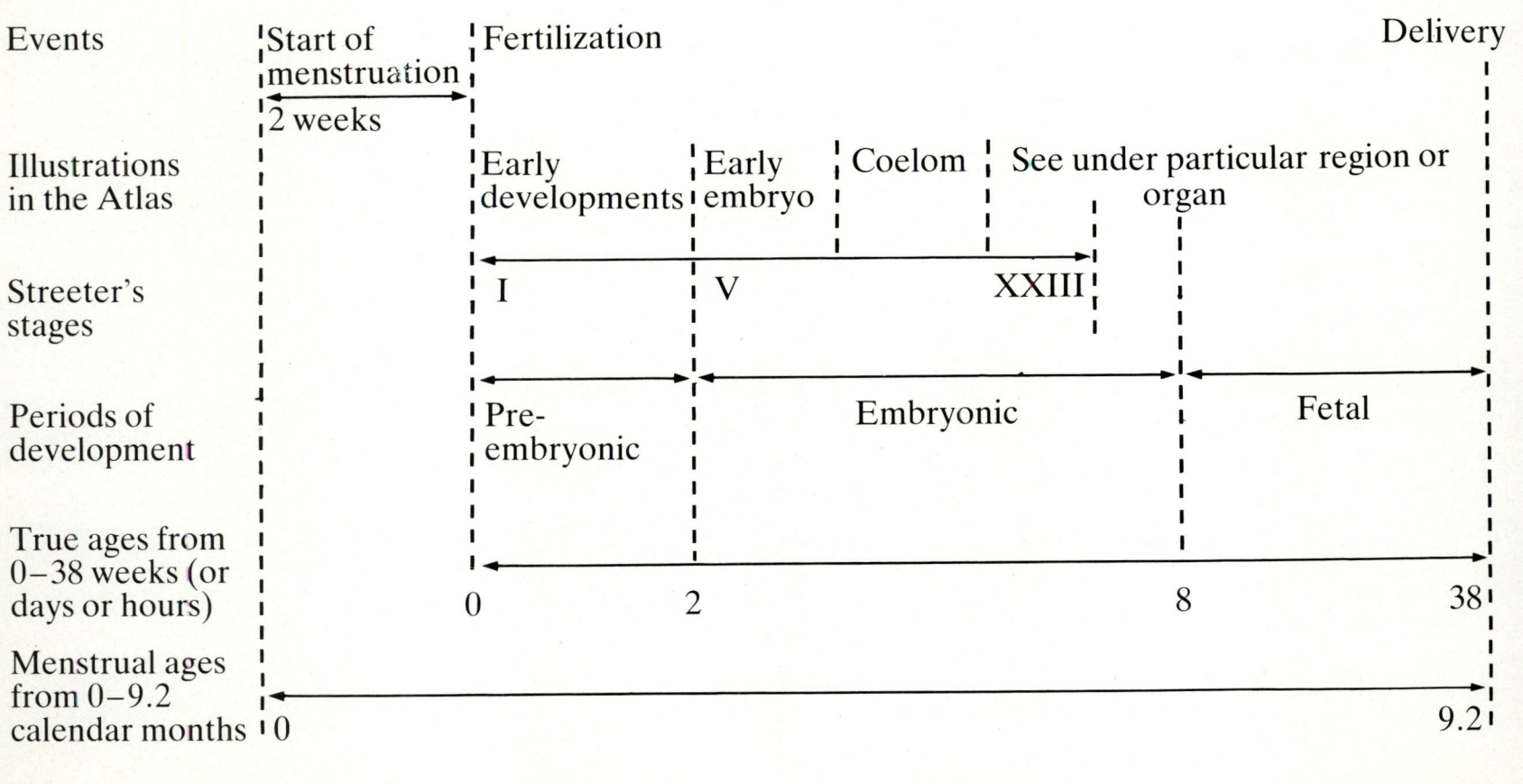

A

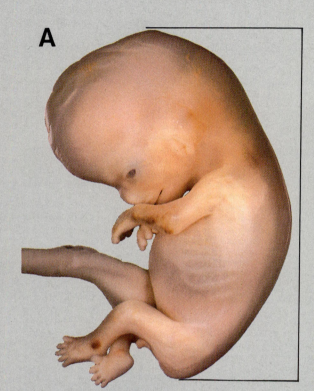

A. Crown–rump (CR) measurement from the crown of the head to the rump of the embryo or fetus.

Crown–Rump

B

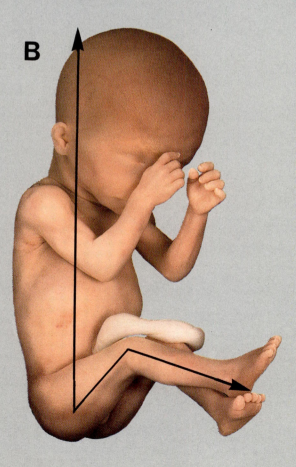

B. Crown–heel (CH) measurement from the crown of the head to the heel of the fetus. (Standing height.)

Crown–Heel

Normal Series of Development

The pre-embryonic period

Horizons I–III   Fertilization to the fourth day. These stages include the single cell fertilized ovum (oocyte), the segmenting ovum, and the free morula.

Horizon IV   Day 4–7. The avillous morula implants in the uterus.

Horizon V   Day 7–12. The implanted blastocyst is embedded more deeply in the uterine endometrium. The amniotic and exocoelomic cavities are present. This stage is usually subdivided on the basis of trophoblastic development.

Horizons VI–VIII   Day 13–19. The chorionic villi branch, the yolk sac is present and so are the primitive streak and knot (Hensen's). Toward the end of the period the neural plate and folds appear. This completes the presomite period.

Horizons IX and X   Day 20–23. Embryo: 1.5–2.0 mmCR. The somites form, the neural folds and notochord elongate and the head and tail folds are apparent. The cloacal membrane and hindgut differentiate.

Horizons XI and XII   Day 24–27. Embryo: 4 mmCR. The head and tail folds are distinct, the neural groove closes and the primary brain vesicles form. The optic vesicles and lens form, the otic vesicles are present and the brain bends at the midbrain flexure.

Limb buds are present. The primordia of liver, pancreas, lungs, thyroid gland, mesonephric tubules and heart appear. The two heart tubes are fused in the mid-line and contractions commence.

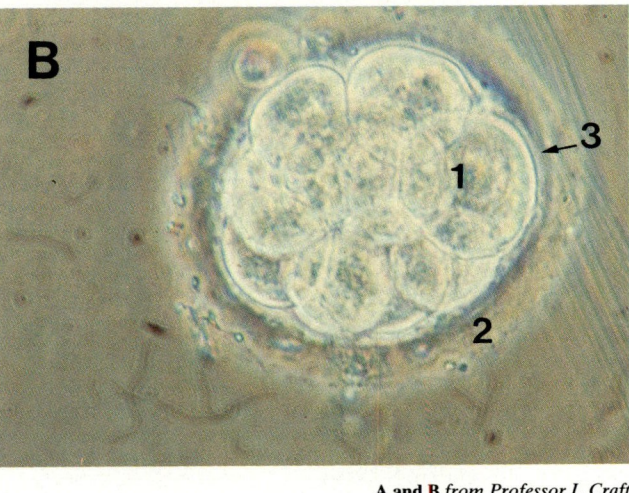

A. Horizon I. The immature ovum with one polar body after maturation *in vitro* for 48 hours. (×530)

1. ovum
2. polar body
3. zona pellucida

B. Horizon II. The nine cell embryo after maturation *in vitro* for 72 hours. (×530)

1. cell (blastomere)
2. corona radiata
3. zona pellucida

A and B *from Professor I. Craft*

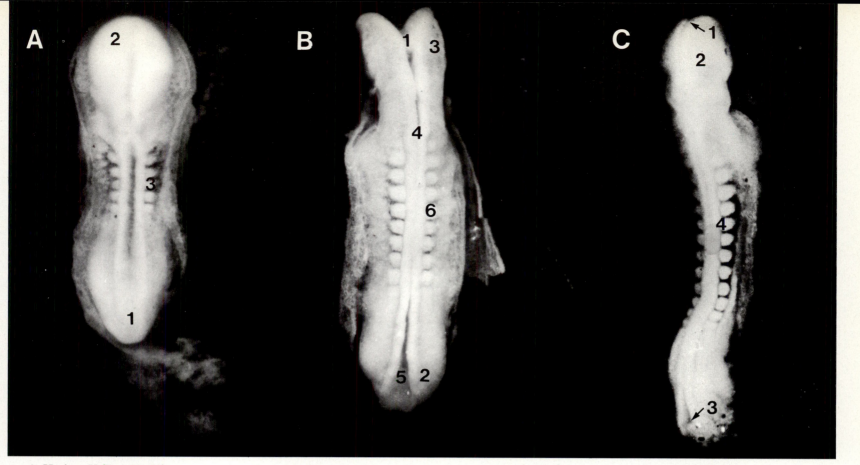

A. Horizon X (Day 22–23). The cephalic and caudal ends of the embryo can be distinguished at this stage, as well as right and left sides.

1. caudal
2. cephalic
3. somites

B. Horizon X (Day 22–23). The neural tube is fusing opposite the somites. The anterior and posterior neuropores remain widely opened.

1. anterior neuropore
2. caudal
3. cephalic
4. neural tube
5. posterior neuropore
6. somites

*Figures **A–C** from Professor H. Nishimura*

C. Horizon XI (Day 24–25). The anterior neuropore is closing while the posterior neuropore remains open.

1. anterior neuropore
2. brain
3. posterior neuropore
4. somites

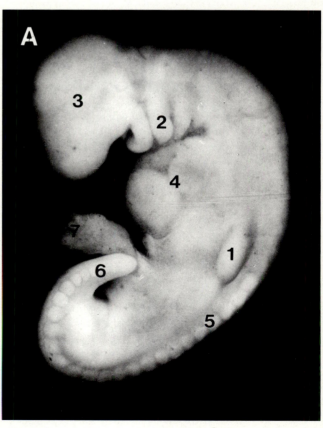

A. Horizon XII (Day 26–27). The arm bud is just appearing. 3.5 mm CR (×10)

From Dr E.C. Blenkinsopp

1. branchial arch
2. embryonic membranes
3. forebrain prominence
4. heart bulge
5. tail

A. Horizon XIII (Day 28). The embryo is flexed in a 'C' shape. The head, tail and arm bud are easily distinguished. Four branchial arches are present and the heart bulges prominently.

1. arm
2. branchial arches
3. head
4. heart bulge
5. somites
6. tail
7. umbilical stalk

From Professor H. Nishimura

The embryonic period

Horizon XIII Day 27–29. Embryo: 4–5 mmCR. Four branchial arches are present. The otic invagination is now closed. The lens vesicle is present but not indented. The leg bud is beginning to appear and a definite ridge is present between the arm and leg. The heart bulges from the body.

Horizon XIV Day 28–30. Embryo: 6–7 mmCR. The optic lens invaginates. The primary bronchi of the lungs are present. The arm buds have elongated, the leg buds appear as short fins. The metanephric bud and cap are present.

Horizon XV Day 31–32. Embryo: 7–8 mmCR. The cerebral hemispheres are enlarging and the corpora striata are definite. The lens vesicles are closed. The olfactory placodes are beginning to sink into the face.

The arm buds have divided into a hand segment and arm–shoulder segment. The leg buds are beginning their regional divisions. In the gut the primary intestinal loop is present and a definite ileocecal junction identifiable.

Horizon XVI Day 32–34. Embryo: 9–10 mmCR. On the face the nostrils have overhanging borders. The eyes have a dark tinge from early retinal pigment. Auricular hillocks are apparent.

The hand has differentiated into a carpal and digital region. The leg bud can be differentiated into thigh, leg and foot. Somites above the arm are smoothed over, while below the arm are still distinct. A gut mesentery is present.

Horizon XVII Day 34–36. Embryo: 11–13 mmCR. The head is relatively larger. The main body axis is straighter than earlier stages. Somites are clearly visible in the lumbosacral region.

On the face the olfactory pits have moved toward one another and the nostrils are directed ventrally. The nasofrontal grooves are present. On the ear the auricular hillocks are present and the branchial groove between the first and second arches is forming the external auditory meatus.

The hand plate has digital rays, and the leg a digital plate.

In the heart the aortic trunk and pulmonary trunk separate and there is complete separation between the right and left atrioventricular canals.

In the gut the appendix is present, the dorsal and ventral pancreas have fused but their ducts remain separate.

The midgut herniates into the umbilical cord.

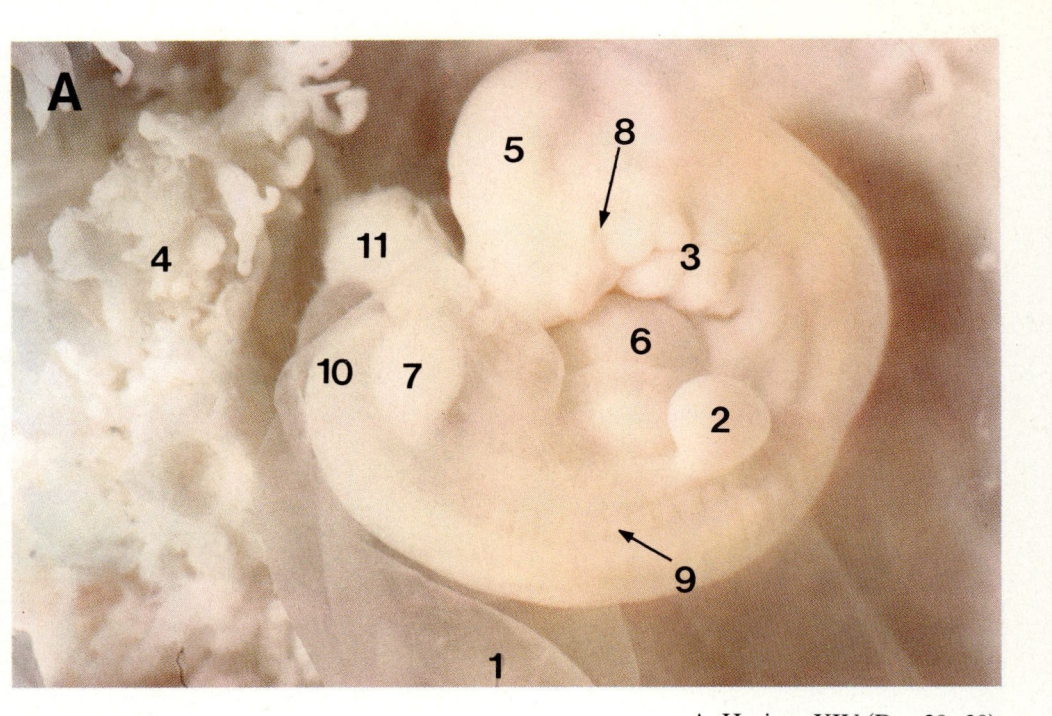

From C.C.H.M.S.

A. Horizon XIV (Day 28–30). The leg bud is present. 6 mmCR (×13)

1. amnion
2. arm bud
3. branchial arches
4. chorion
5. head
6. heart bulge
7. leg bud
8. lens invagination
9. somites
10. tail
11. umbilical cord

Horizon XVIII Day 36–38. Embryo: 14–16 mmCR. The paramesonephric (Müllerian) ducts are present. The cervical flexure and pontine flexure are present. The elbow is present, and the digital rays of the hand notched. Toe rays are present on the foot.

Eyelid folds are forming. The pigmented retina is covered by scleral masses. The tip of the nose is present (in profile). The auricular hillocks are fusing to form the external ear and the inner ear has one to three semi-circular ducts.

The secondary bronchi of the lungs are branched. There is a long ureter, and the renal pelvis is branching to form calyces. In the heart the aortic and pulmonary valves are distinct.

A. Horizon XVII (Day 34–36). The embryo attached by the umbilical cord to the early membranes. 12mmCR (×5.9)

1. arm bud
2. branchial arches
3. early membranes
4. eye
5. genital tubercle
6. heart bulge
7. leg bud
8. tail
9. umbilical cord

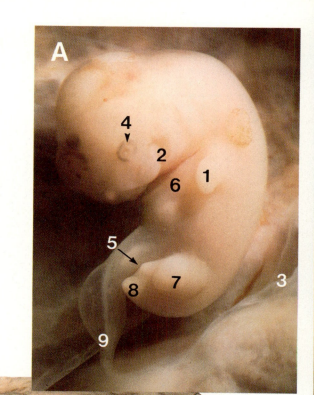

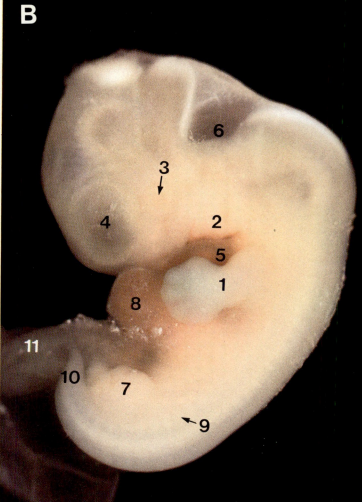

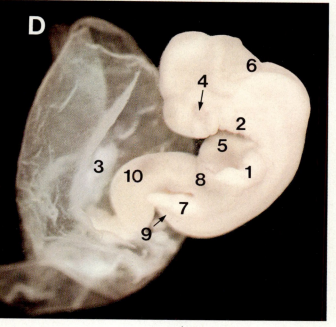

From R.C.S.E.

C. Horizon XVII (Day 34–36). The embryo *in situ* in the uterus. 12.6mmCR (×2)

1. chorion
2. embryo
3. uterus

From R.C.S.E.

B. Horizon XVII (Day 34–36). The hand plates have developed and the digital rays are present. 12mmCR (×9.4)

1. arm bud (with hand plate and digital ridges)
2. branchial arches
3. eye
4. forebrain
5. heart bulge
6. hindbrain
7. leg bud
8. liver bulge
9. somites
10. tail
11. umbilical cord

D. Horizon XVIII (Day 36–38). The diamond-shaped hindbrain is clearly visible and the arm bud has an elbow. 14mmCR (×4)

1. arm bud
2. branchial arches
3. embryonic membrane
4. eye
5. heart bulge
6. hindbrain
7. leg bud
8. liver bulge
9. tail
10. umbilical cord

Horizon XIX　Day 38–40. Embryo: 17–20mmCR. The trunk region is elongating and straightening. The arms and legs extend straight forward. Toe (digital) rays (ridges) are evident, but notches (grooves) have not yet appeared.

Horizon XX　Day 40–42. Embryo: 21–23mmCR. The arms are longer, and bend at the elbows and curve slightly over the heart. The hands are far apart and tend to reach the lateral margins of the nose.

The superficial vascular plexus appears in the temporofrontal region of the scalp.

Horizon XXI　Day 42–44. Embryo: 22–24mmCR. The superficial scalp plexus has spread further toward the vertex of the head. The hands are flexed at the wrist and meet over the heart bulge.

The fingers are longer and the tips are slightly swollen where touch pads are developing. The feet are approaching the mid-line and may meet.

Horizon XXII　Day 44–46. Embryo: 25–27mmCR. The eyelids have almost covered the eyes. The external ear is well advanced in form. The hands extend further in front of the body.

Horizon XXIII　Day 46–48. Embryo: 28–30mmCR. The head is in a more erect position and the neck more developed. The limbs are longer and are more differentiated.

Horizon series　True ages in days from fertilization cannot be given further as the Horizon series end here.

Week 7　Using ultrasound, the first movements are apparent.

A. Horizon XX (Day 40–42). The arms curve over the heart bulge and the toe rays are present on the foot. 20mmCR (×6.7)

1. arm
2. ear
3. elbow
4. eye
5. forebrain
6. heart bulge
7. hindbrain
8. liver bulge
9. midbrain
10. midgut herniation
11. mouth
12. notched hand plate
13. umbilical cord

C. Horizon XXII (Day 44–46). 27mmCR (×3.6)

D. Horizon XXII (Day 44–46). 27mmCR (×3.6)

B. Horizon XXII (Day 44–46). The toes have formed and the feet approach the mid-line. 25mmCR (×3.6)

1. arm
2. ear
3. elbow
4. eye
5. foot
6. forebrain bulge
7. hand
8. knee
9. liver bulge
10. midbrain bulge
11. mouth
12. nose
13. ribs
14. tail
15. toes
16. umbilical cord

18

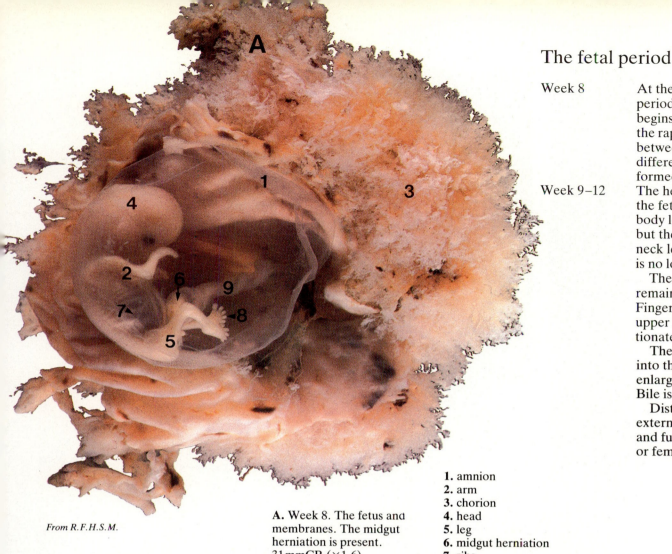

From R.F.H.S.M.

The fetal period

Week 8

At the end of Week 8 the embryonic period is complete and the fetal period begins. This period is characterized by the rapid growth of the fetus (especially between Week 9–20) and the further differentiation of the organs and tissues formed in the embryonic period.

Week 9–12

The head at Week 9 is almost half of the fetus. With the rapid growth the body length (CR) doubles by Week 12, but the head grows more slowly. The neck lengthens and extends so the chin is no longer contacting the body.

The eyelids meet, fuse, and the eyes remain closed until Week 25. Fingernails appear on the digits. The upper limb becomes disproportionately large.

The midgut, which was herniated into the umbilical cord, returns to the enlarged abdominal cavity (Week 10). Bile is secreted.

Distinguishing features of the external genitalia appear in Week 9, and fully differentiate into male (♂) or female (♀) by Week 12.

A. Week 8. The fetus and membranes. The midgut herniation is present. 31 mmCR (×1.6)

1. amnion
2. arm
3. chorion
4. head
5. leg
6. midgut herniation
7. ribs
8. toes
9. umbilical cord

B. Week 9. The head is almost half the fetal length. As the head extends and the chin is raised from the thorax the neck develops. The eyelids have fused. 44 mmCR (×2.2)

C. Week 9. The fingernails appear about this time. 46 mmCR (×2.1)

D. Week 9. The external genitalia are differentiating. 50 mmCR (×1.9)
Note: This fetus has been stretched in handling.

1. brain
2. ear
3. external genitalia at indifferent stage
4. eye
5. ribs
6. tail
7. umbilical cord

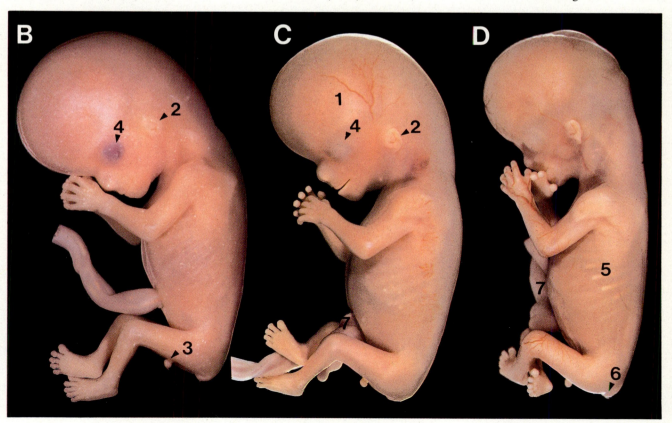

B. Week 12. The fetus and membranes, 85 mmCR ♂
(×1.8)

1. ear
2. eye
3. placenta
4. umbilical cord

E. Week 10. The fetus has doubled in length since Week 7 and the midgut herniation returns into the enlarged abdomen. 60 mmCR ♂
(×1.7)

1. arm
2. brain
3. ear
4. eye
5. knee
6. mouth
7. toes
8. umbilical cord

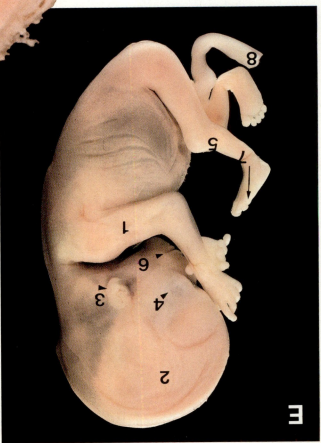

A. Week 12. The ear has moved from the neck on to the head. The eyes have moved to the front of the face. 82 mmCR ♀ (×0.8)

1. arm
2. ear
3. eye
4. foot
5. plastic specimen grip
6. umbilical cord

From R.F.H.S.M.

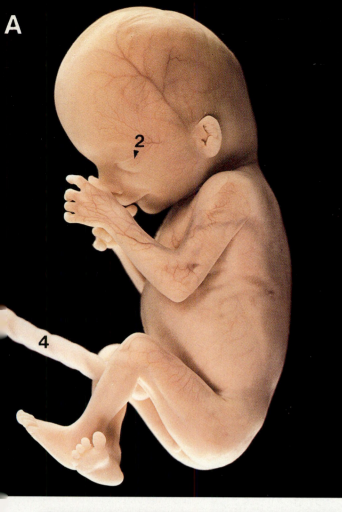

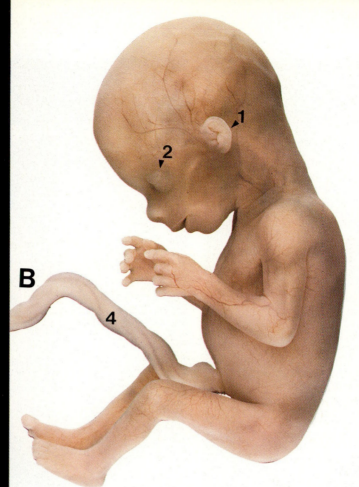

B. Week 13. The fetus may
suck its thumb from this stage.
97 mm CR ♂ (×1.4)

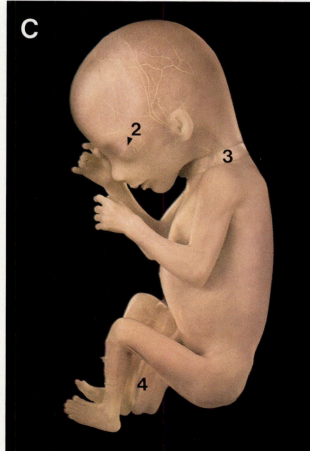

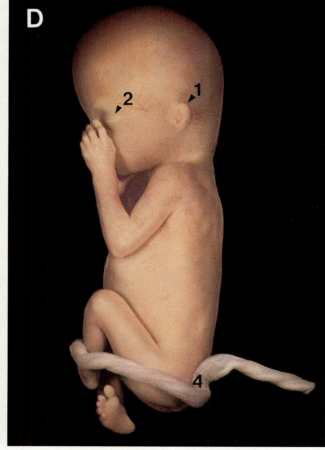

C. Week 13. 98 mm CR ♀
(×1.1)

From R.F.H.S.M.

D. Week 14. 105 mm CR ♀
(×1)

Week 13–16

Rapid growth continues. On the erect
head the eyes have moved on to the
front of the face but are still widely
separated. The external ear is
differentiating and has moved on to the
side of the head from the upper neck.

Ossification is progressing rapidly.
The skeleton is clearly outlined on X-
rays of the fetus. Lanugo hairs cover
the body.

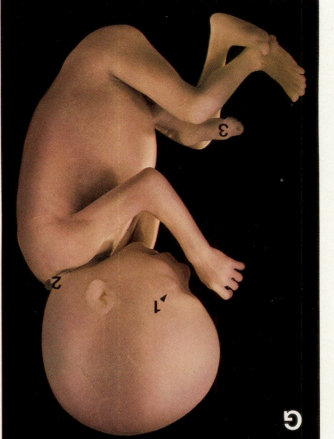

G. Week 14. Fine lanugo hairs are present on the head. The attachment of the umbilical cord is low on the abdomen.
110mmCR ♂ (×1)

F and G from R.F.H.S.M.

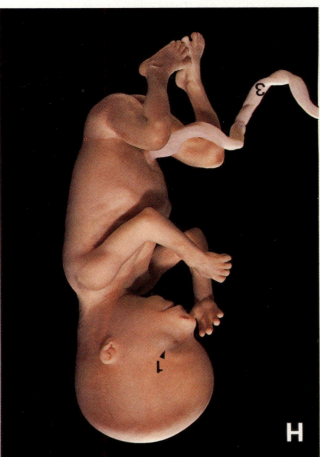

H. Week 14. 120mmCR ♂ (×0.8)

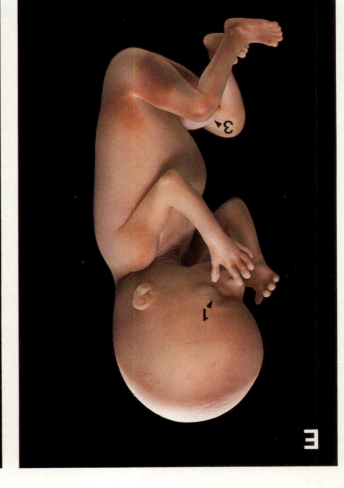

E. Week 14. The nails are well formed. 106mmCR ♀ (×0.9)

1. eye
2. plastic specimen grip
3. umbilical cord

F. Week 14. The lower limb is longer than the upper limb at this stage of development. Note the umbilical cord looped around the neck. 106mmCR ♂ (×0.9)

I. Week 14. 120 mmCR ♂
(×0.9)

1. ear
2. eye
3. umbilical cord

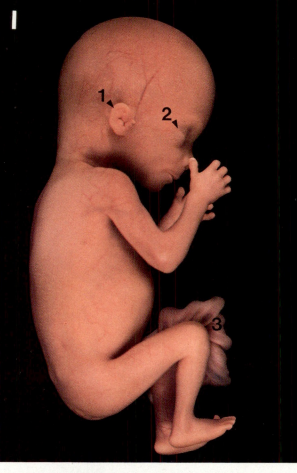

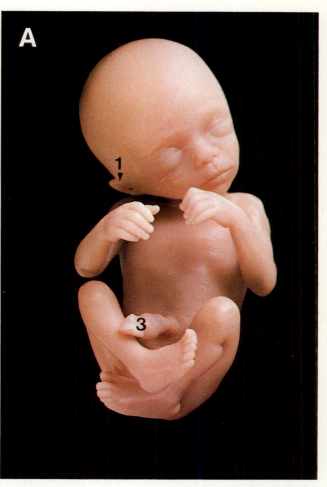

A. Week 15. Brown fat begins
to form in this month.
130 mmCR ♀ (×0.8)

B. Week 16. 133 mmCR ♀
(×0.7)

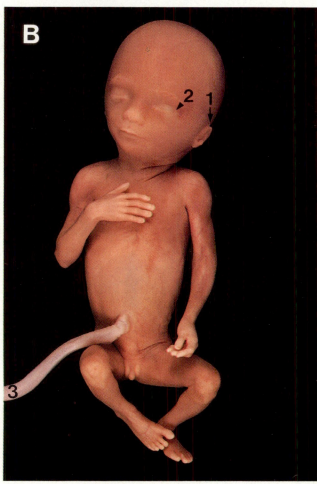

C. Week 16. 140 mmCR ♀
(×0.8)

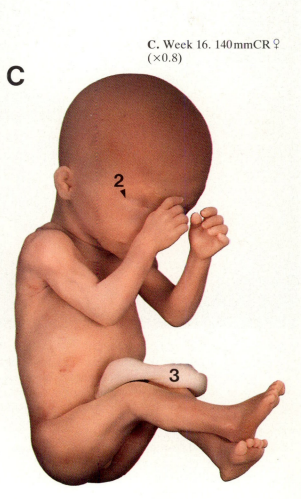

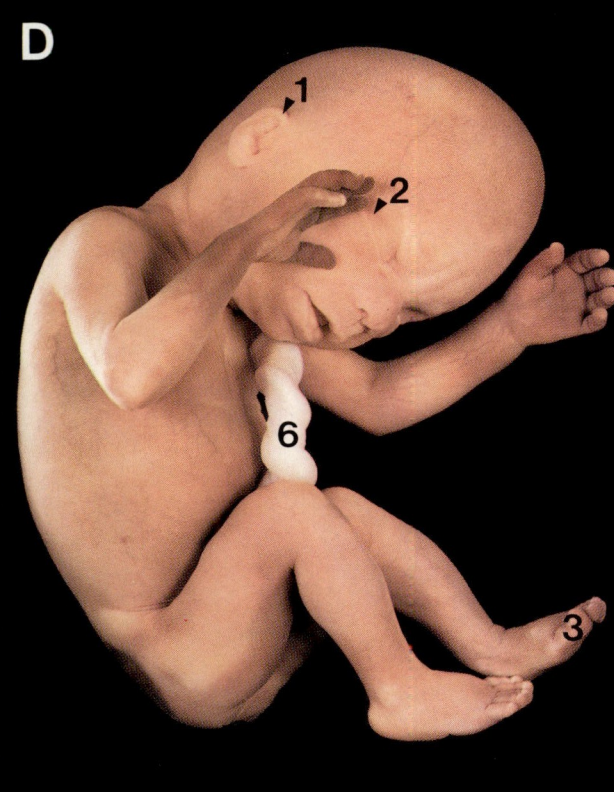

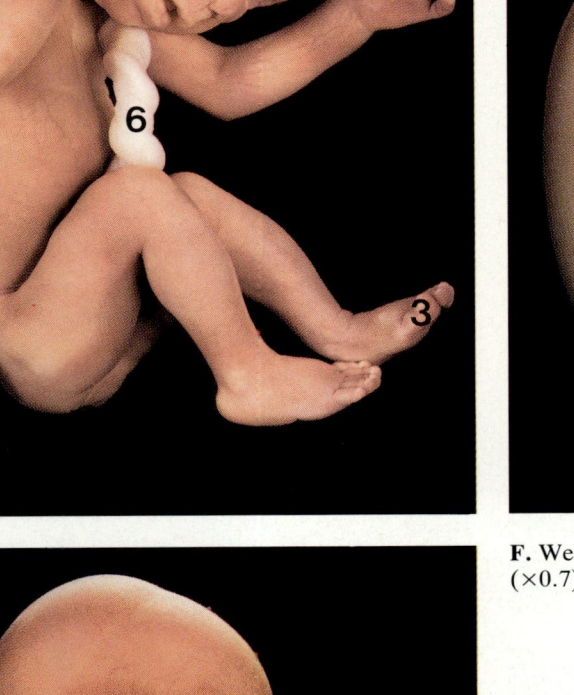

D. Week 17. Parts of the leg reach their relative proportions in this month. 141 mmCR ♀ (×0.7)

1. ear
2. eye
3. foot
4. mouth
5. plastic specimen grip
6. umbilical cord

E. Week 17. (Fetal movements are present which the mother can consciously feel in the abdomen.) 144 mmCR ♀ (×0.7)

F. Week 18. 152 mmCR ♂ (×0.7)

G. Week 18. The sebaceous glands become active and *vernix caseosa* forms to protect the skin from the amniotic fluid. 152 mmCR ♂ (×0.8)

H. Week 18. 153 mmCR ♂ (×0.6)

Week 17–20 The rapid growth rate slows down. The relative proportions of the parts of the lower limb are reached. Sebaceous glands become active and *vernix caseosa* forms to cover and protect the skin from the macerating amniotic fluid.

Myelination of the spinal cord begins.

Brown fat forms. The mother becomes conscious of fetal movements (quickening).

From R.F.H.S.M.

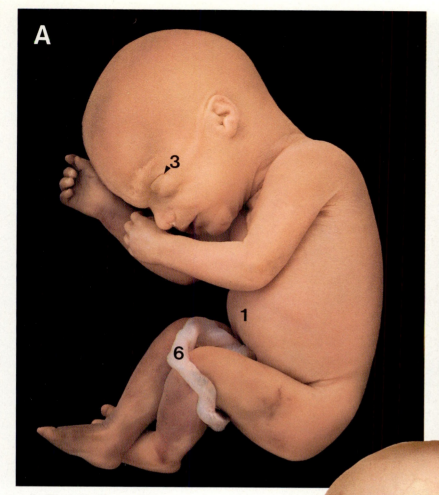

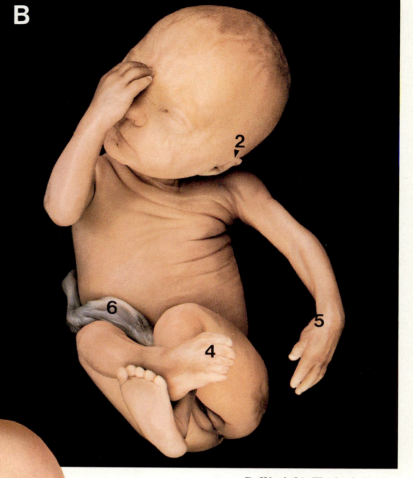

A. Week 20. The eyelids and eyebrows are very well developed as are the fingernails. 185 mm CR ♀ (×0.7)

1. abdomen
2. ear
3. eye
4. foot
5. hand
6. umbilical cord

B. Week 21. The body is beginning to become plump. 200 mm CR ♀ (×0.6)

C. Week 21. 200 mm CR ♂ (×0.7)

From C.C.H.M.S.

C

Week 21–25   The eyelids and eyebrows are well developed. The lanugo darkens and there is more *vernix caseosa*. The skin may be very wrinkled due to the lack of subcutaneous fat and a relative increase in the growth of the skin. Fingernails are present.

The face and body generally assume the appearance of the infant at birth. Fetuses born from Week 25 onwards are usually viable.

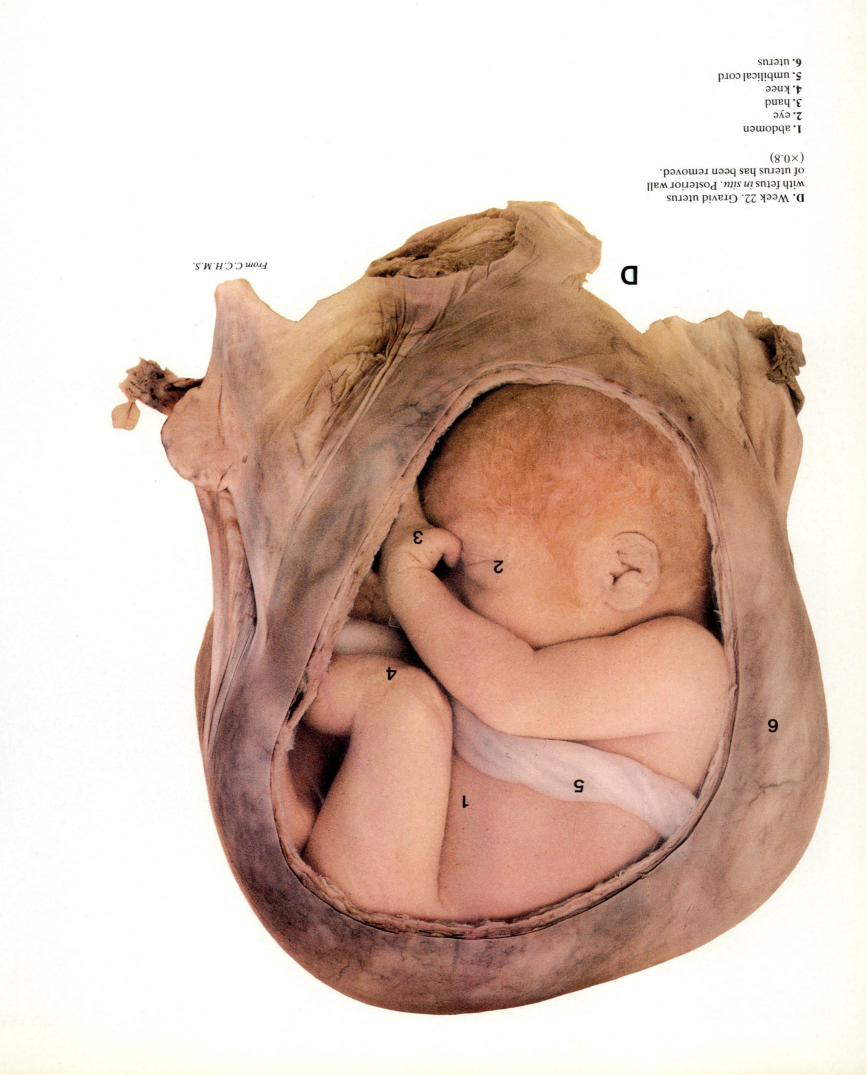

D. Week 22. Gravid uterus
with fetus *in situ*. Posterior wall
of uterus has been removed.
(×0.8)

1. abdomen
2. eye
3. hand
4. knee
5. umbilical cord
6. uterus

From C.C.H.M.S.

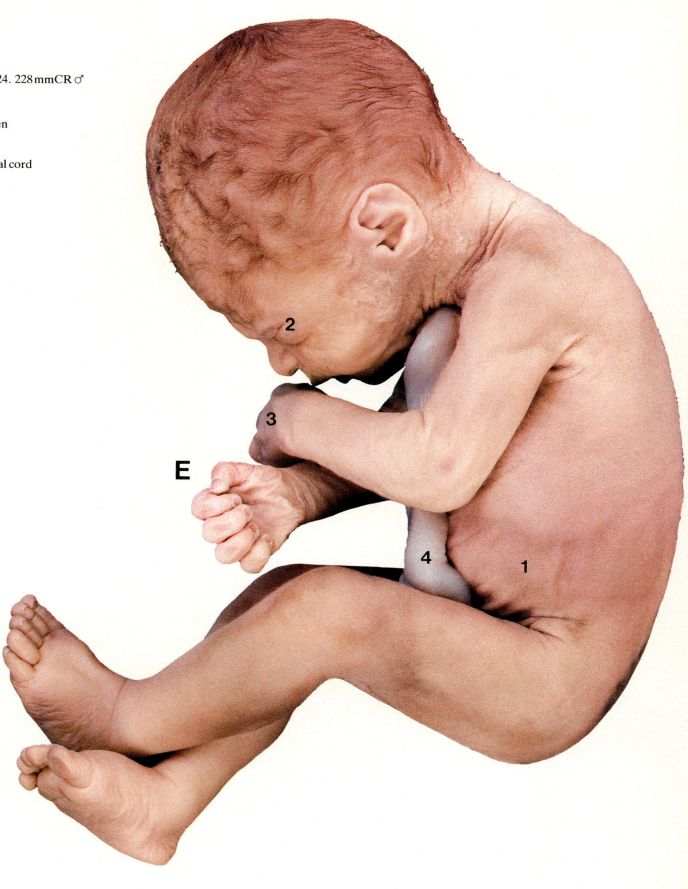

E. Week 24. 228 mmCR ♂
(×0.9)

1. abdomen
2. eye
3. hand
4. umbilical cord

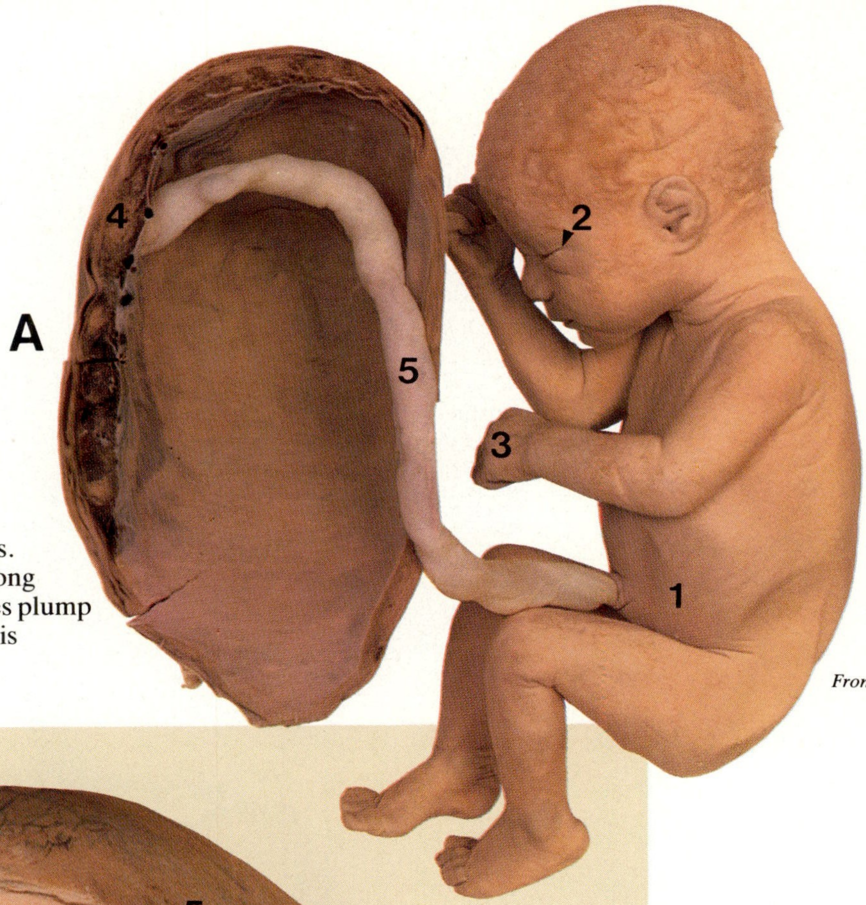

A. Week 26. A section of the anterior wall of the uterus to show the attachment of the fetus to the placenta. 250mmCR (×0.4)

1. abdomen
2. eye
3. hand
4. placenta
5. umbilical cord

Week 26–29   The eyes are open again and the eyebrows and eyelashes are well developed. The pupillary membrane disappears. The scalp hairs are becoming long and the body generally becomes plump and round as subcutaneous fat is deposited.

From C.C.H.M.S.

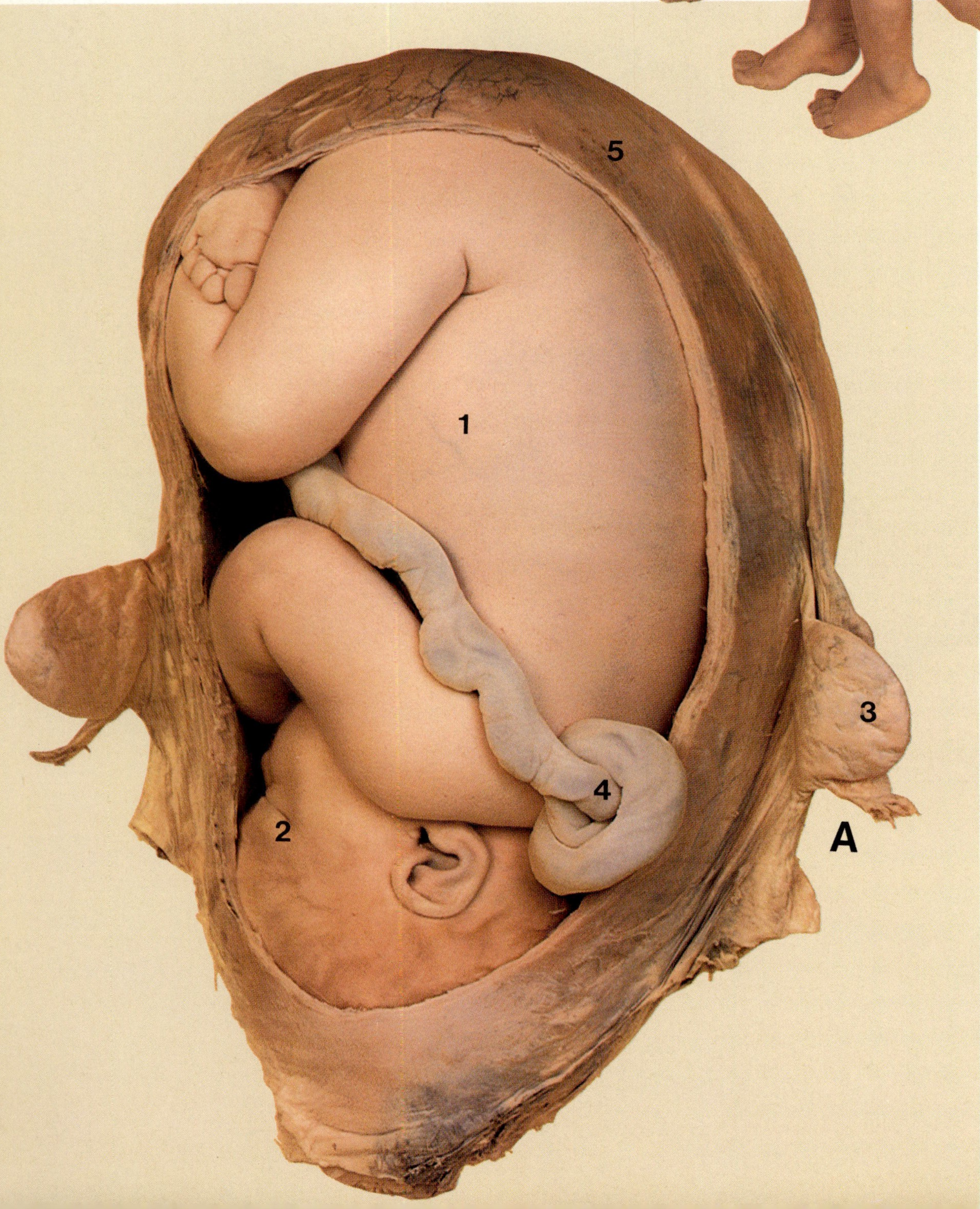

A. Week 28. The fetus *in situ* with a 'true' knot in the umbilical cord. The testes are descending into the scrotum. (×0.5)

1. abdomen
2. eye
3. maternal ovary
4. umbilical cord with knot
5. uterus

From C.C.H.M.S.

Week 30–34   The body is becoming plumper and the skin is pink. Toenails are present and the testes are descending. The fingernails have reached the tips of the fingers.

Week 35–38   The body is plump. The toenails have reached the tips of the toes. Almost all the lanugo hairs have been shed and the skin is covered with *vernix caseosa*. The umbilicus is central in the abdomen. The testes have descended into the scrotum, but the ovaries are still above the level of the pelvic brim and do not reach their final position by birth. Brain myelination begins.

During the final weeks, approximately 14 g of fat a day is laid down. The neonate weighs about 3400 g and is about 360 mmCR.

The male infant normally weighs more than the female infant at birth.

● Clinicians divide pregnancy into three parts or trimesters (each three calendar months). Natural abortions usually occur during the first trimester.

● Prematurely born male infants normally have undescended testes.

A. Week 38. A full-term gravid uterus, one half of which has been removed to demonstrate the fetus.

The body is round and plump. The lanugo hairs have almost completely disappeared and the skin is covered with *vernix caseosa*. The umbilicus is central in the abdomen. It is not unusual to find scratches on the face from the long fingernails. (×0.5)

1. abdomen
2. arm
3. buttock
4. maternal ovary
5. umbilical cord
6. uterus

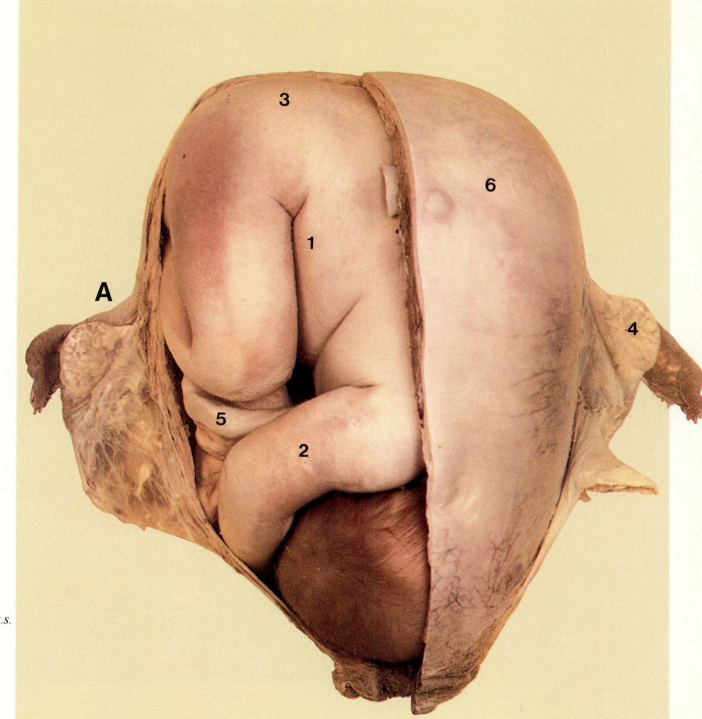

From C.C.H.M.S.

Ultrasound

Development *in utero* is assessed very accurately by using ultrasound methods to scan the maternal abdomen. The membranes are detectable at Week 6 and the embryo from Week 7. The embryo or fetus can be measured and its viability confirmed by heart movements. Multiple conceptions can be recognized as can the placental positions in the second trimester.

During the first trimester the CR length is measured giving an estimate of age which is accurate to within one or two days. From Week 12 flexion makes the CR measurement more unreliable and the bi-parietal diameter of the head is used instead. The date of delivery can be predicted to within seven days if the bi-parietal diameter is measured prior to Week 24. Later in pregnancy (Week 34–38) the bi-parietal measurement becomes inaccurate.

Several developmental abnormalities can be detected by ultrasound, e.g. spina bifida both open and closed, anencephaly, etc. X-rays are a very accurate method of assessment but they are only rarely used now because of the effects of radiation on the developing fetus, e.g. leukemia later in life.

A. Longitudinal scan of a Week 12 fetus.

1. abdomen
2. anterior abdominal wall (maternal)
3. face
4. limb
5. skull

A and B. Longitudinal scan of a Week 14 fetus.

A. The fetus facing the chorionic plate.

1. anterior abdominal wall (maternal)
2. bladder (maternal)
3. chorionic plate
4. closed spinal cord
5. heart (fetal)
6. limb
7. placenta
8. ribs
9. skull

B. The closed spinal canal.

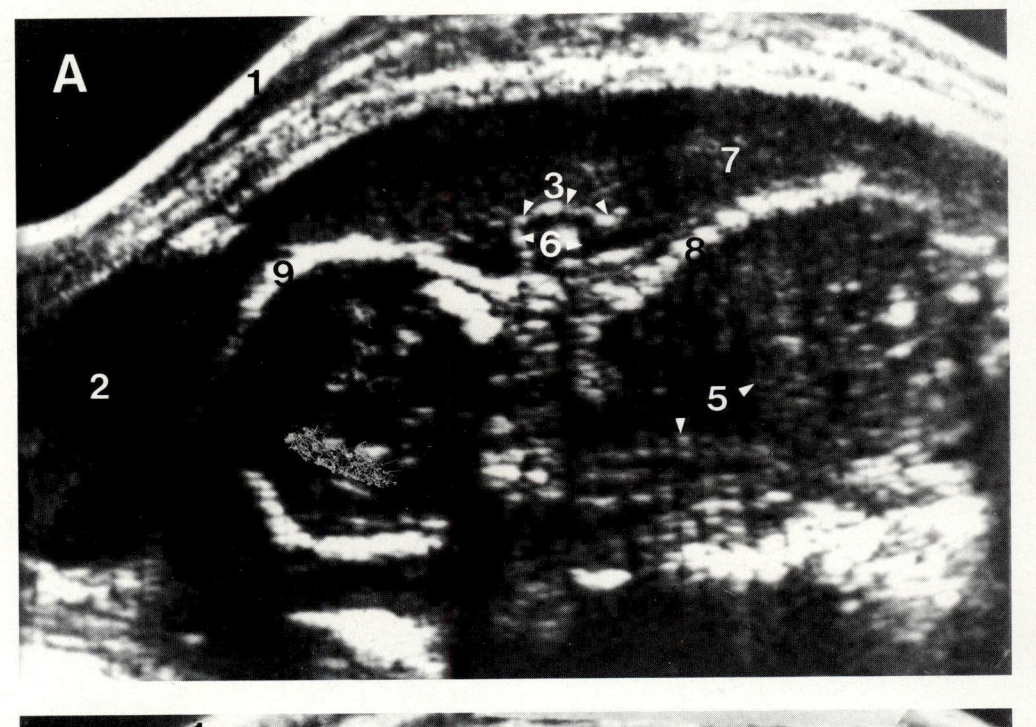

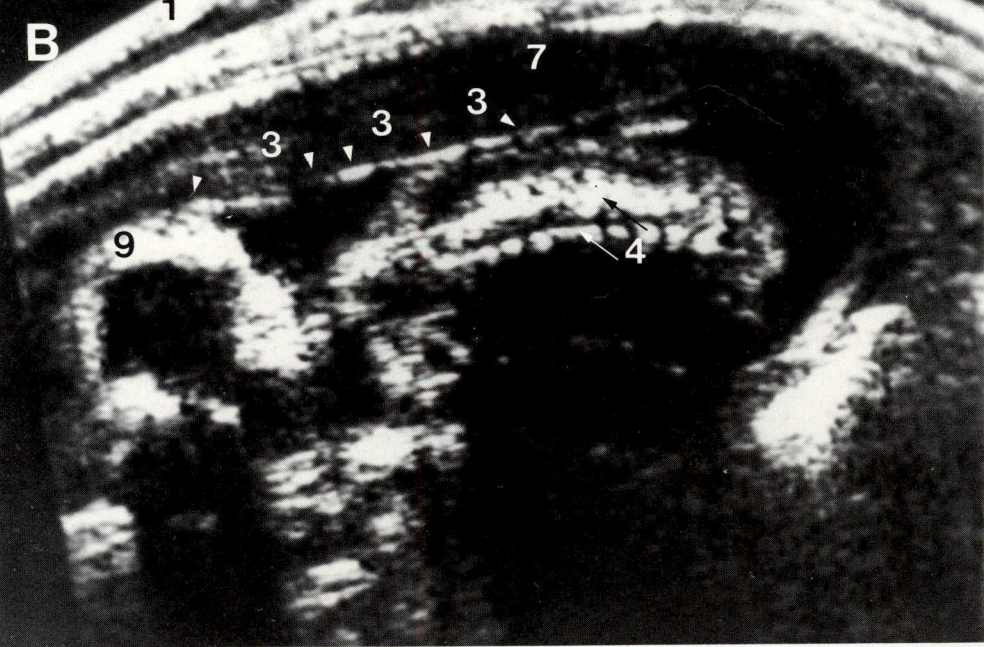

All ultrasound photographs from Dr T. El-Sayed

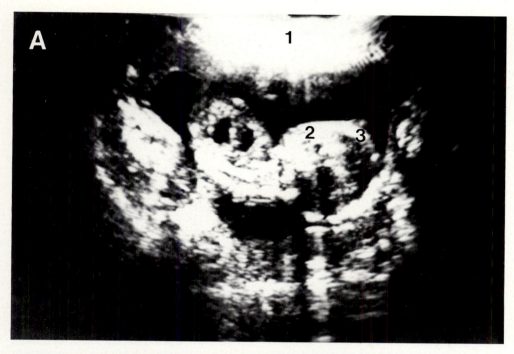

A. Longitudinal scan of a Week 14.5 fetus.

1. anterior abdominal wall (maternal)
2. face
3. skull

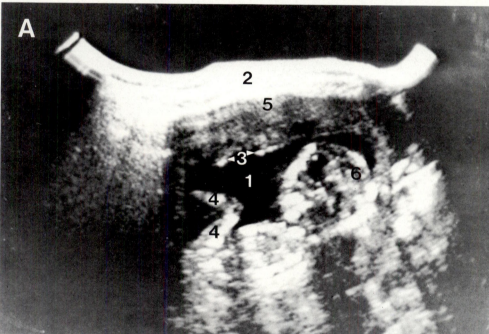

A. Longitudinal scan of a Week 15.5 fetus.

1. amniotic fluid
2. anterior abdominal wall (maternal)
3. chorionic plate
4. limb
5. placenta (anterior)
6. skull

A and B. Longitudinal and transverse scans of a Week 15.5 fetus.
A. The fetus by longitudinal scan.

1. amniotic fluid
2. anterior abdominal wall (maternal)
3. bladder (maternal)
4. chorionic plate
5. falx cerebri
6. fundus of the stomach
7. lateral ventricle
8. placenta
9. rib
10. skull
11. spine

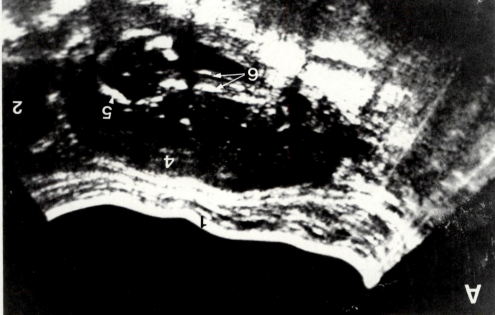

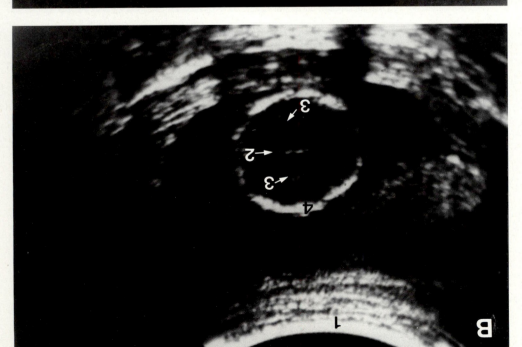

A–C. The same Week 16 fetus
in several different positions.

1. anterior abdominal wall
   (maternal)
2. bladder (maternal)
3. falx cerebri
4. placenta
5. skull
6. spine

B. The fetal skull by transverse
scan.

1. anterior abdominal wall
   (maternal)
2. falx cerebri
3. lateral ventricle
4. skull

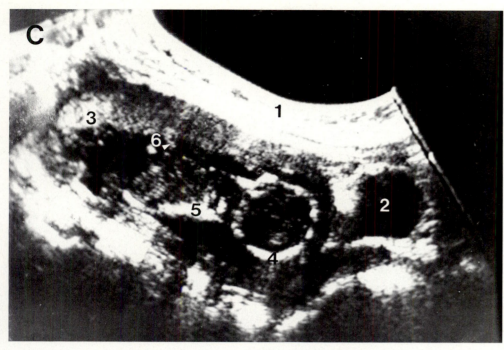

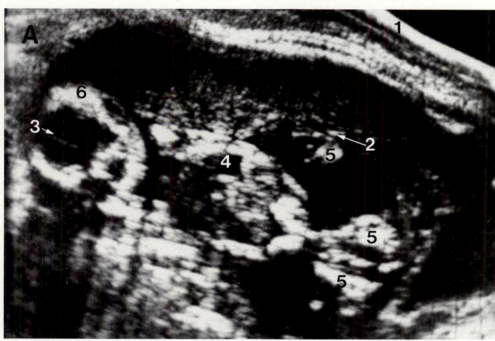

1. anterior abdominal wall
   (maternal)
2. bladder (maternal)
3. placenta (fundal)
4. skull
5. spine
6. umbilical cord

A. Longitudinal scan of Week 20.5 twins. Initially one fetus was scanned. Subsequently a second fetus was diagnosed.

1. anterior abdominal wall
   (maternal)
2. chorionic plate
3. falx cerebri
4. fundus of stomach
5. limb
6. skull

B. Transverse scan of the same Week 20.5 fetus reveals a twin.

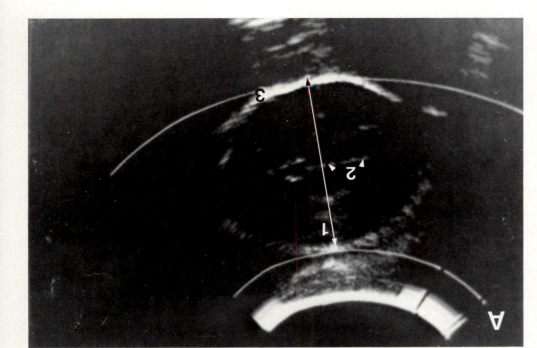

A. Transverse scan of the
Week 33 fetal skull.
1. bi-parietal diameter
2. falx cerebri
3. skull

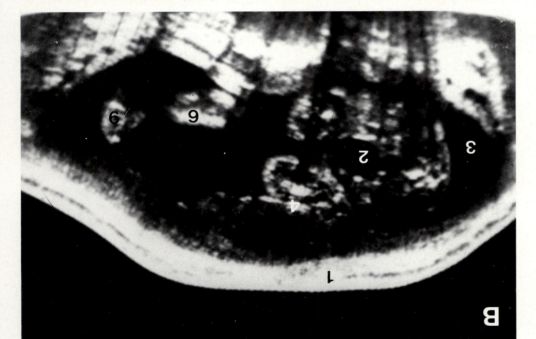

B. The fetal bladder.

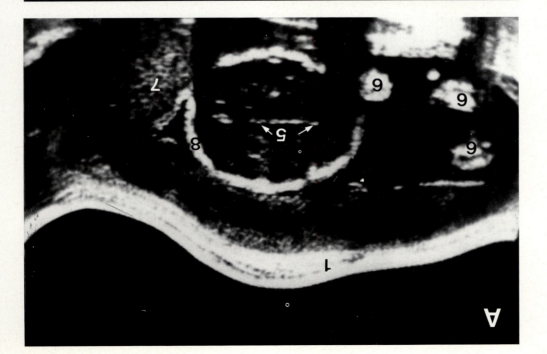

9. toes
8. skull
7. placenta previa
6. limbs
5. falx cerebri
4. chorionic plate
3. bladder (maternal)
2. bladder (fetal)
1. anterior abdominal wall
(maternal)
A. The fetal head and limbs.
Week 23 fetus.
A and B. Transverse scan of a

Early Development

A. Horizon I. The immature ovum with one polar body after maturation *in vitro* for 48 hours. (×530)

1. ovum
2. polar body
3. zona pellucida

B. Horizon II. The nine cell embryo after maturation *in vitro* for 72 hours. (×530)

1. cell (blastomere)
2. corona radiata
3. zona pellucida

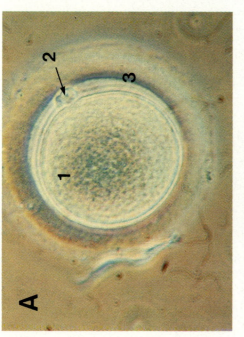

A

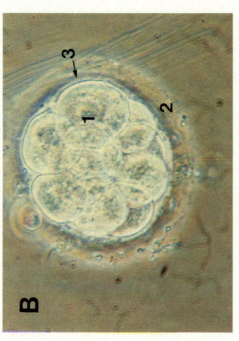

B

A and B from Professor I. Craft

Development of the embryo begins at Horizon I when a sperm fertilizes an ovum (oocyte) and together they form a zygote. As the zygote travels down the uterine (Fallopian) tube it divides (cleavage) into two blastomeres at about 30 hours after fertilization. The cells continue to divide until a ball or morula of 16 or more cells is present. The morula enters the uterus, and at Day 4 fluid from the uterine cavity enters the morula and the cells rearrange themselves to form the blastocyst. Some of the cells form a single layered hollow ball called the trophoblast which will form part of the placenta. Other cells form the inner cell mass attached to one pole of the trophoblast. The blastocyst is enclosed in an acellular layer, the zona pellucida.

The blastocyst lies free in the uterine cavity for about two days, then loses its zona pellucida at Day 4 to 5 and attaches to the maternal endometrium Day 5 to 6. The trophoblast cells invade the endometrium and gradually differentiate into two layers; cytotrophoblast and syncytiotrophoblast (outermost layer).

As the embryo differentiates, endoderm forms at about Day 7 from cells of the inner cell mass which are closest to the blastocyst cavity. Small spaces appear in the remaining inner cell mass which coalesce to form the amniotic cavity (see Amnion).

The remaining cells of the inner cell mass form the ectoderm and mesoderm layers during Week 3. The embryo is then a bilaminar embryonic disc with the amnion above and the blastocyst cavity below. Cytotrophoblast cells delaminate and form an inner exocoelomic lining (Heuser's membrane) to the blastocyst so enclosing the primary yolk sac. Further trophoblastic cells delaminate to form extra-embryonic mesoderm around the amnion and yolk sac. The extra-embryonic mesoderm increases and spaces appear in it which coalesce to form the extra-embryonic coelom. This coelom surrounds the amnion and yolk stalk except at the connecting (body or umbilical) stalk. As the extra-embryonic coelom develops, the secondary yolk sac forms below the embryonic endoderm. The extra-embryonic mesoderm is also split into two layers; somatic (somatopleuric) mesoderm lining the trophoblast and amnion and splanchnic (splanchnopleuric) mesoderm lining the yolk sac.

Together the extra-embryonic somatic mesoderm and trophoblast form the chorion, while the cavity is the extra-embryonic coelom.

Early Embryo

The embryo is a bilaminar disc with a localized thickening of the endoderm called the prochordal plate at the future site of the mouth. The embryo at Day 15 (Horizon VI) has reached the primitive streak stage, the streak having a primitive knot or node at its cephalic end with a primitive pit. Recent studies have reported the primitive streak appearing by Day 12–14 and to be the sole source of the extra-embryonic mesoderm of the chorion, chorionic villi and body stalk. The primitive streak gives the first indication of the cephalic, caudal, dorsal, ventral, right and left sides of the embryo.

By Day 16 ectoderm cells which have migrated toward the primitive streak invaginate to form intra-embryonic mesoderm cells. Some of these cells cranial to the knot form the notochordal process, while other mesoderm cells migrate between the ectoderm and endoderm layers until they reach the margins of the disc and become continuous with the amniotic and yolk sac mesoderm. Some of these cells form the cardiogenic area. By the middle of Week 3 mesoderm cells are present throughout the embryo except in the region of the prochordal plate, the cloacal membrane, and notochordal process. Mesoderm cells are produced actively until the end of Week 4. The primitive streak becomes relatively diminished in size as the notochord increases in length. The primitive pit extends into the notochordal process to form the notochordal canal. The notochordal process fuses with the underlying endoderm layer and where fusion occurs degeneration takes place and the notochordal canal becomes continuous with the yolk sac. The roof or notochordal plate upfolds to form the notochord itself and the endoderm again forms a continuous layer ventral to the notochord. For a short period the amniotic cavity and yolk sac are continuous through the neurenteric canal which is completely obliterated as the notochord forms fully.

Whilst the notochord is developing the overlying ectoderm forms neuroectoderm which will give rise to the central nervous system. The neuroectoderm has a neural groove and neural folds which fuse by the end of Week 3 and form the neural tube. The neural crest cells form from some of the more lateral neuroectoderm cells which are not incorporated into the neural tube.

As the notochord and neural tube form the mesoderm adjacent to the mid-line forms paraxial mesoderm which is continuous laterally with intermediate mesoderm and through that with the lateral mesoderm, the yolk sac and amniotic mesoderm.

At about Day 20 the paraxial mesoderm divides into paired blocks of somites. The first 38 pairs of somites are formed between Day 20–30 but eventually 42–44 pairs are formed. Each block has a cavity or myocoele which quickly disappears. The ventromedial part (sclerotome) of each somite will differentiate into cartilage, bones and ligaments. The dorsolateral part (dermomyotome) will give rise to skeletal muscles and the dermal layer of the skin.

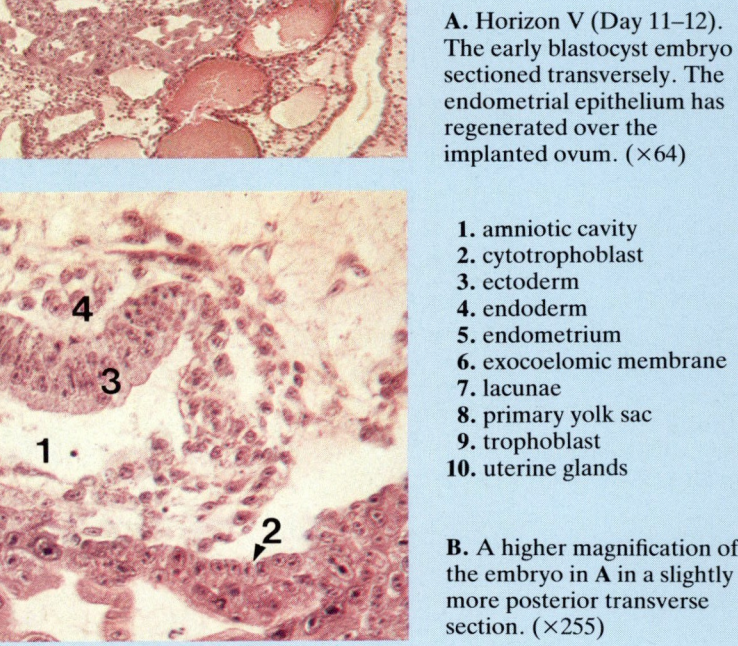

A. Horizon V (Day 11–12). The early blastocyst embryo sectioned transversely. The endometrial epithelium has regenerated over the implanted ovum. (×64)

1. amniotic cavity
2. cytotrophoblast
3. ectoderm
4. endoderm
5. endometrium
6. exocoelomic membrane
7. lacunae
8. primary yolk sac
9. trophoblast
10. uterine glands

B. A higher magnification of the embryo in **A** in a slightly more posterior transverse section. (×255)

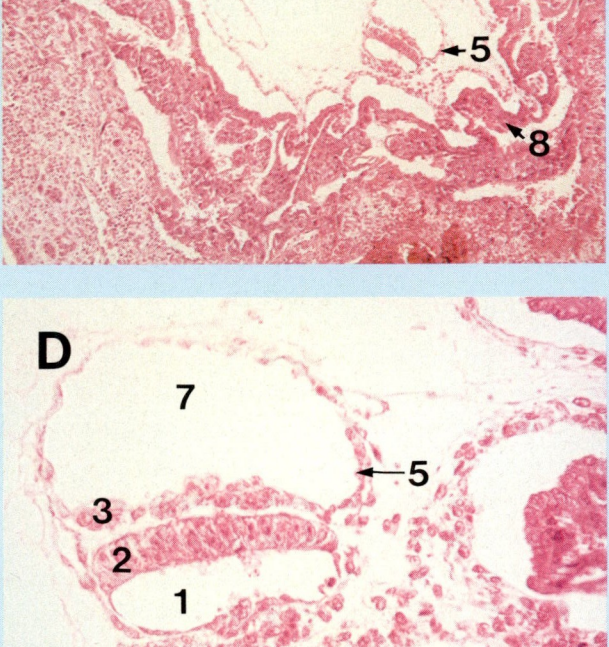

C. Horizon VI (Day 14). The bilaminar embryo sectioned transversely. (×48)

1. amniotic cavity
2. ectoderm
3. endoderm
4. endometrium
5. extra-embryonic endoderm
6. lacunae
7. secondary yolk sac
8. trophoblast

D. A higher magnification of the embryo in **C**. (×250)

A–D from C.C.H.M.S.

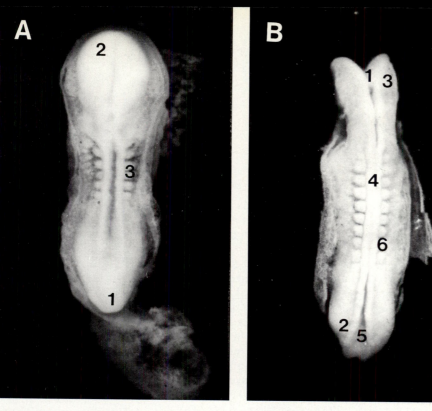

A

2
3
1

B

1 3
4
6
2 5

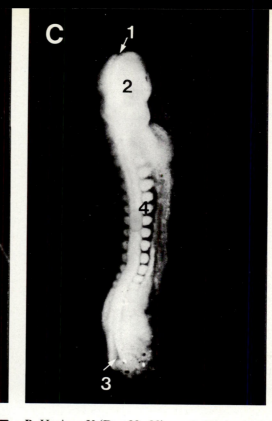

C

1
2
4
3

A. Horizon X (Day 22–23). The cephalic and caudal ends of the embryo can be distinguished at this stage, as well as right and left sides.

1. caudal
2. cephalic
3. somites

Figures **A–C** *from Professor H. Nishimura*

B. Horizon X (Day 22–23). The neural tube is fusing opposite the somites. The anterior and posterior neuropores remain widely opened.

1. anterior neuropore
2. caudal
3. cephalic
4. neural tube
5. posterior neuropore
6. somites

C. Horizon XI (Day 24–25). The anterior neuropore is closing while the posterior neuropore remains open.

1. anterior neuropore
2. brain
3. posterior neuropore
4. somites

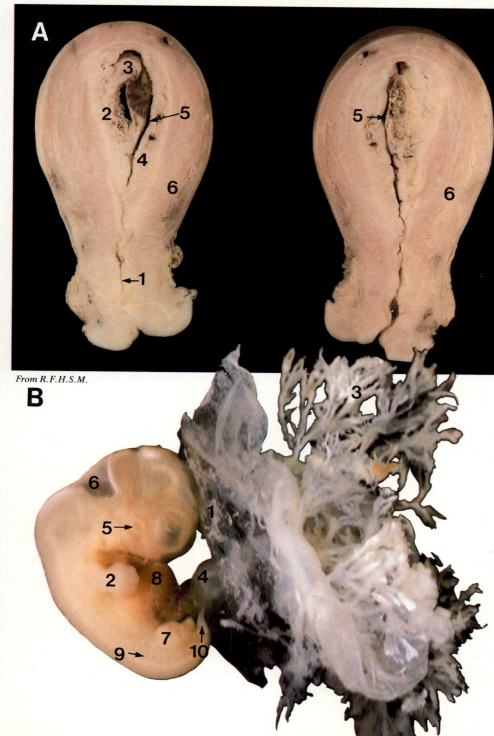

A

3
2 5
4
6
5
6
1

From R.F.H.S.M.

B

3
6
5→
1
2 8 4
9→ 7 →10

A. Horizon VI (Day 14). A sagittal section of a gravid uterus. (×1)

1. cervix
2. *decidua basalis*
3. *decidua capsularis*
4. *decidua parietalis*
5. uterine cavity
6. uterus

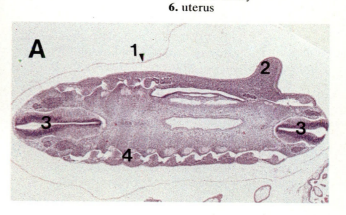

A

1
2
3
4
3

B. Horizon XVII (Day 35). Somites persist in the region of the tail as blocks of mesoderm. 12 mmCR (×5.7)

1. amnion
2. arm bud
3. chorionic villi
4. cord (umbilical)
5. eye
6. hindbrain
7. leg bud
8. liver
9. somites
10. tail

From L.H.S.M.

A. Horizon XV (Day 32). A transverse section through the lumbar region. 8 mmCR (×54)

1. amnion
2. leg bud
3. neural tube
4. somite

Coelom

Spaces appearing in the lateral plate and cardiogenic mesoderm of the primitive streak embryo coalesce to form the horseshoe-shaped coelom. The mesoderm is divided into two sheets; a somatic layer adjacent to the embryonic ectoderm and continuous with the mesoderm covering the amnion; and a splanchnic layer adjacent to the endoderm and continuous with the mesoderm covering the yolk sac.

The pericardial cavity will form in the curved portion of the horseshoe while the two straight portions become the pleural and peritoneal cavities. At the lateral edges of the embryo the cavities are continuous with the extra-embryonic coelom.

As the head, tail and lateral folds of the embryo form the future mouth (prochordal plate, oral membrane) and cloacal membrane are carried ventrally. The horseshoe-shaped coelom is also carried on to the ventral aspect. Then when the head fold forms, the future pericardial cavity is carried beneath the foregut, where it expands around the developing heart to form the pericardial cavity. Caudal to the pericardial cavity the coelom on each side narrows and each is called a pericardio–peritoneal canal. These two narrow canals connect the pericardial cavity with the two abdominal parts of the coelom.

The two peritoneal cavities become a single cavity except in the region of the caudal foregut. During Week 10 the peritoneal cavity is separated from the extra-embryonic coelom at the umbilicus as the intestines return to the abdomen (see Midgut rotation).

Divisions of the coelom

Four partitions form, one at each end of the two pericardio–peritoneal canals so separating the pericardial cavity from the pleural cavities and the pleural cavities from the peritoneal cavities.

The partition between the pericardial and pleural cavities is formed as the lung buds grow (see Lungs). They expand and press adjacent mesoderm into the pericardio–peritoneal canals. The mesoderm covering the lung buds forms visceral pleura, while the outer mesodermal wall of the coelom becomes parietal pleura.

The common cardinal veins further narrow the pericardo–peritoneal canals when they become invested with a ridge of mesoderm (pleuro-pericardial membrane).

As the lungs expand further, the pleural cavities extend around the heart ventrally and split the mesoderm into two layers; fibrous pericardium and body wall.

With the descent of the heart, growth of the common cardinal veins, and formation of the pleural cavities, the pleuro-pericardial membranes fuse in Week 7 with mesoderm ventral to the esophagus.

The pleuro-peritoneal membranes divide the pleural cavities and peritoneal cavity. These membranes form as the pleural cavities expand to extend around the heart. They grow medially and ventrally and in Week 6 their free edges fuse with the septum transversum and dorsal mesentery of the esophagus. With the extension of muscle into these membranes and the increase in liver size the pleuro-peritoneal openings are closed.

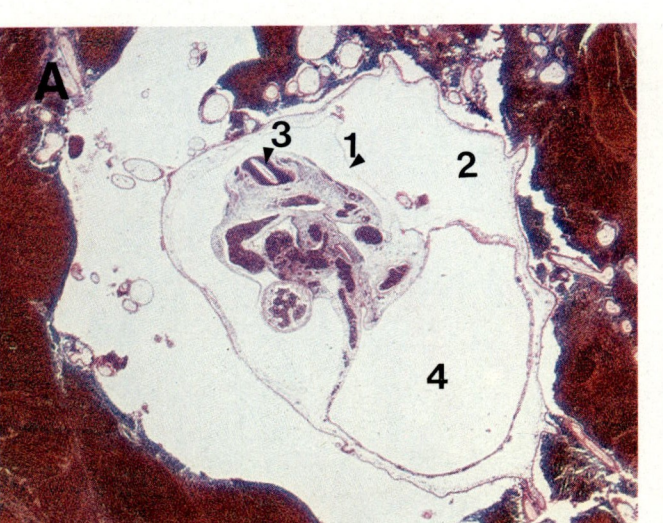

A. Approximately Horizon IX–X (Day 20–23). A transverse section of the embryo and embryonic membranes. (×12)

1. amnion
2. extra-embryonic coelom
3. neural tube
4. yolk sac cavity

Germ Layer Derivatives

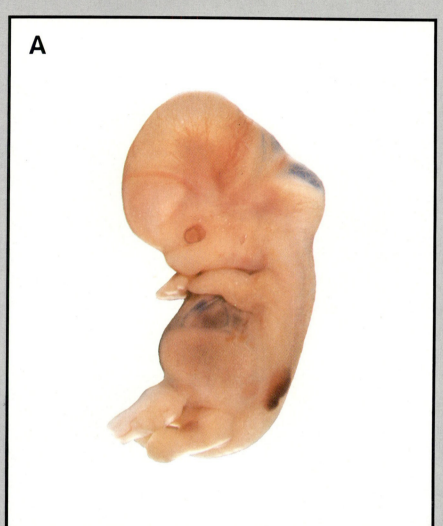

A

A. Horizon XX (Day 40–42). The arms curve over the heart bulge and the toe rays are present on the foot. 20mmCR (×5)

Ectoderm derivatives

Surface ectoderm
epidermis, hair, nails, sweat glands, sebaceous glands, mammary glands, lens of eye, inner ear, enamel of teeth and anterior pituitary

Neuroectoderm
Neural tube
   central nervous system, retina, pineal body and posterior pituitary
Neural crest
   cranial and spinal sensory nerves and ganglia, adrenal medulla, pigment cells, head mesoderm, branchial arch cartilages, sympathetic ganglia and nerves, Schwann cells

Endoderm derivatives

Epithelial parts of the tonsils, pharynx, thyroid, parathyroids, pharyngotympanic tube, tympanic cavity, trachea, bronchi and lungs
Epithelium of gastrointestinal tract, liver, pancreas, urachus and urinary bladder

Mesoderm derivatives

Head
skull, dentine, muscles and connective tissue

Paraxial
skeleton except skull, muscles of trunk, dermis of skin and connective tissue

Intermediate
urogenital system (gonads, ducts and accessory glands)

Lateral plate
cardiovascular system, blood cells, lymphatic system and cells of lymph, spleen, adrenal cortex, visceral and limb muscles, visceral connective tissue, serous membranes of pericardium, pleura and peritoneum

Fetal Membranes and Placenta

The embryonic (and fetal) membranes and the placenta protect the embryo (and fetus), providing for nutrition, respiration and excretion during development. These membranes are the amnion, chorion, allantois and yolk sac and they are formed by the zygote. The placenta forms from the fetal chorion and from the maternal endometrium. At birth the umbilical cord, placenta, amnion and chorion are expelled after the fetus as 'afterbirth'. (See Childbirth.)

As the blastocyst implants in the maternal endometrium (Day 7–10) a decidual reaction occurs. The stromal cells enlarge and increase in number. The glands and blood vessels also respond. Three regions develop in the decidua in relation to the implantation site; the area overlying the conceptus is the *decidua capsularis*; the area underlying the conceptus is the *decidua basalis*; the remainder of the maternal mucosa is the *decidua parietalis*.

Chorion

Between Day 13 and 14 the cytotrophoblast proliferates to form clumps that extend into the syncytiotrophoblast. These are the primary chorionic villi which soon branch. At about Day 15 the villi acquire connective tissue cores and are then called secondary villi. They cover the entire surface of the chorion. Capillaries develop in the villi (tertiary villi). All three types of villi may be present at the same time. Cytotrophoblast extensions from the villi penetrate the syncytiotrophoblast layer and join to form the cytotrophoblastic shell which anchors the chorionic sac to the maternal endometrium.

Up to Week 8 the chorionic sac is covered with villi. But as the sac grows the blood vessels in the *decidua capsularis* are compressed, and degenerate; and the chorion in this region becomes smooth *(chorion laeve)*. At the same time, the villi in the *decidua basalis* increase to form the *chorion frondosum (the fetal component of the placenta)*. The *decidua basalis* forms the maternal component (decidual plate). As the villi invade the *decidua basalis* they leave decidual tissue wedges called placental septa which divide the fetal part of the placenta into 10–38 cotyledons each of which contain two or more main stem villi.

As the fetus grows the *decidua capsularis* extends into the uterine cavity and eventually contacts and fuses with the *decidua parietalis*. By Week 22 the *decidua capsularis* degenerates owing to a reduced blood supply.

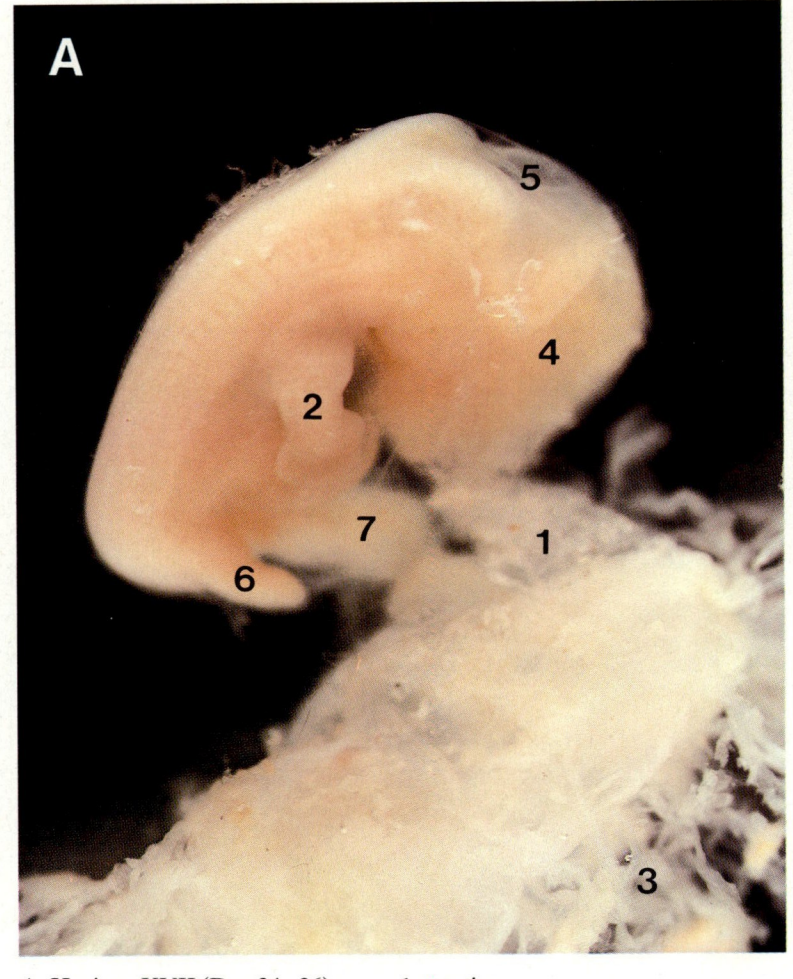

A. Horizon XVII (Day 34–36). The embryo connected to the amnion and chorion by the umbilical cord. 12 mm CR (×6.2)

1. amnion
2. arm bud
3. chorionic villi
4. head
5. hindbrain
6. leg bud
7. umbilical cord

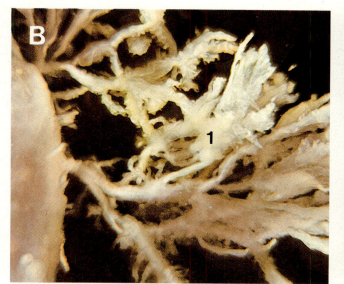

B. A higher magnification of the chorionic villi of the embryo in Figure **A**. (×9.3)

1. chorionic villi

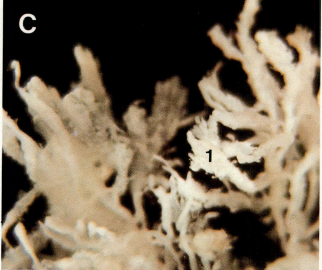

C. A higher magnification of the chorionic villi in Figure **A**. (×9.3)

A. Week 9. The fetus *in situ* in the chorionic sac. 46 mm CR ♂ (×2.1)

B. The fetus in Figure **A** with the chorionic sac opened. The amnion is present but is transparent. 46 mm CR ♂ (×2.1)

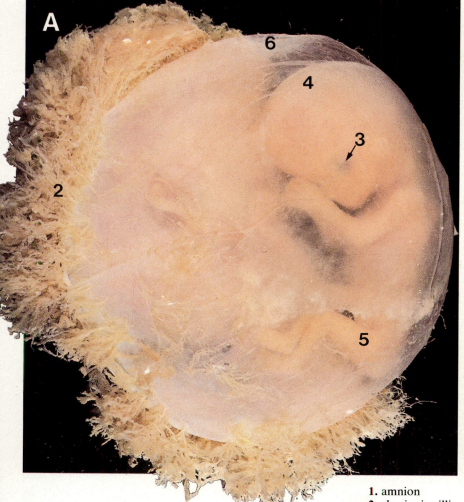

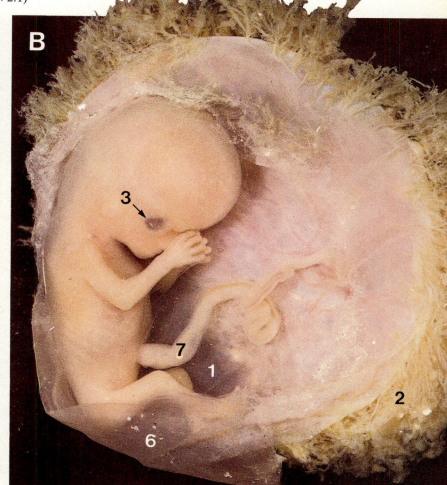

1. amnion
2. chorionic villi
3. eye
4. head

5. leg
6. smooth chorion
7. umbilical cord

Amnion

The amniotic cavity forms when spaces in the inner cell mass and trophoblast coalesce to form a cavity above the embryonic disc ectoderm. The epithelial roof forms from cytotrophoblast cells and its outer surface becomes covered with extra-embryonic mesoderm. As the extra-embryonic coelom extends, it separates the amniotic cavity from the chorion except in the region of the embryonic (connecting) stalk. When the embryo forms head and tail folds the amnion is carried around to the ventral side of the embryo.

The amniotic cavity enlarges at the expense of the extra-embryonic coelom which gradually disappears. The amnion lines the chorion which fuses first with the *decidua capsularis* and then with the *decidua parietalis* except in the region of the body stalk where it follows and lines the outer surface of the connecting stalk (later the umbilical cord).

The amniotic cavity initially contains fluid produced by its cellular walls, but the majority comes from maternal blood and in late pregnancy 500 ml of fetal urine is excreted daily into the cavity. The amniotic fluid physically cushions the embryo, maintains a constant temperature, prevents the amnion from adhering to the developing embryo and permits symmetrical growth and free movements of the fetus.

By Week 37 about 1000 ml of amniotic fluid is present; the fetus swallows and absorbs about 400 ml per day, and it produces 500 ml of urine daily back into the cavity. The water in the amniotic fluid is changed every 3 hours via the placental membranes and a small quantity exchanged through the amniochorionic membrane.

The amniotic fluid contains desquamated fetal epithelial cells, lanugo, *vernix caseosa*, proteins, fats, carbohydrates, hormones, enzymes, pigments, fetal urine and 98–99% water.

At term, a dilatation of amnion and chorion filled with amniotic fluid is present in the dilating cervix. (See Childbirth.)

- Amniocentesis: from about Week 14, amniotic fluid can be sampled by inserting a hollow needle through the maternal abdominal wall, the uterus, and into the amniotic cavity. Ultrasound can be used to guide the needle.

- Excessive quantities of amniotic fluid (polyhydramnios) and insufficient quantities (oligohydramnios) may be present in association with fetal abnormalities.

- Occasionally the amnion does not rupture at birth and the neonate is born enclosed in the amniotic sac or 'caul'.

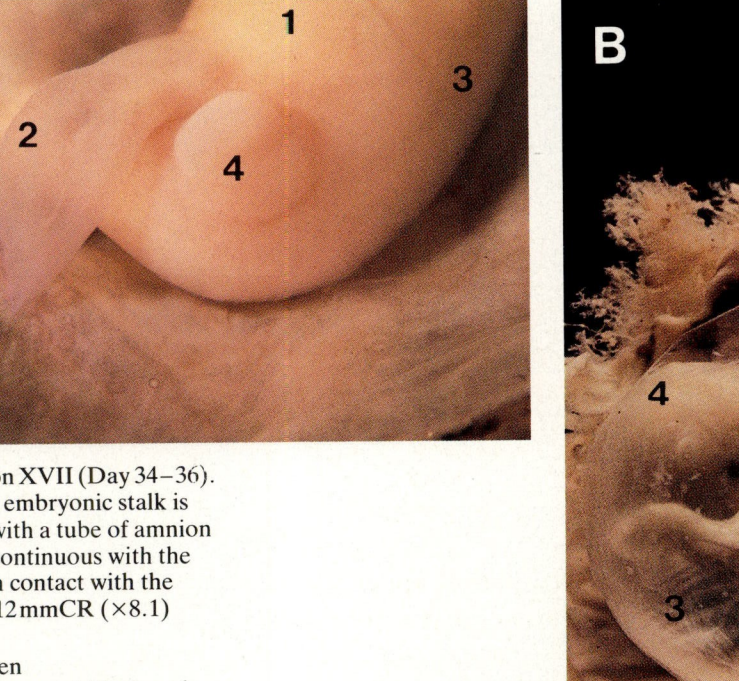

A. Horizon XVII (Day 34–36). The early embryonic stalk is covered with a tube of amnion which is continuous with the amnion in contact with the chorion. 12 mm CR (×8.1)

1. abdomen
2. amnion on umbilical cord
3. back
4. leg bud

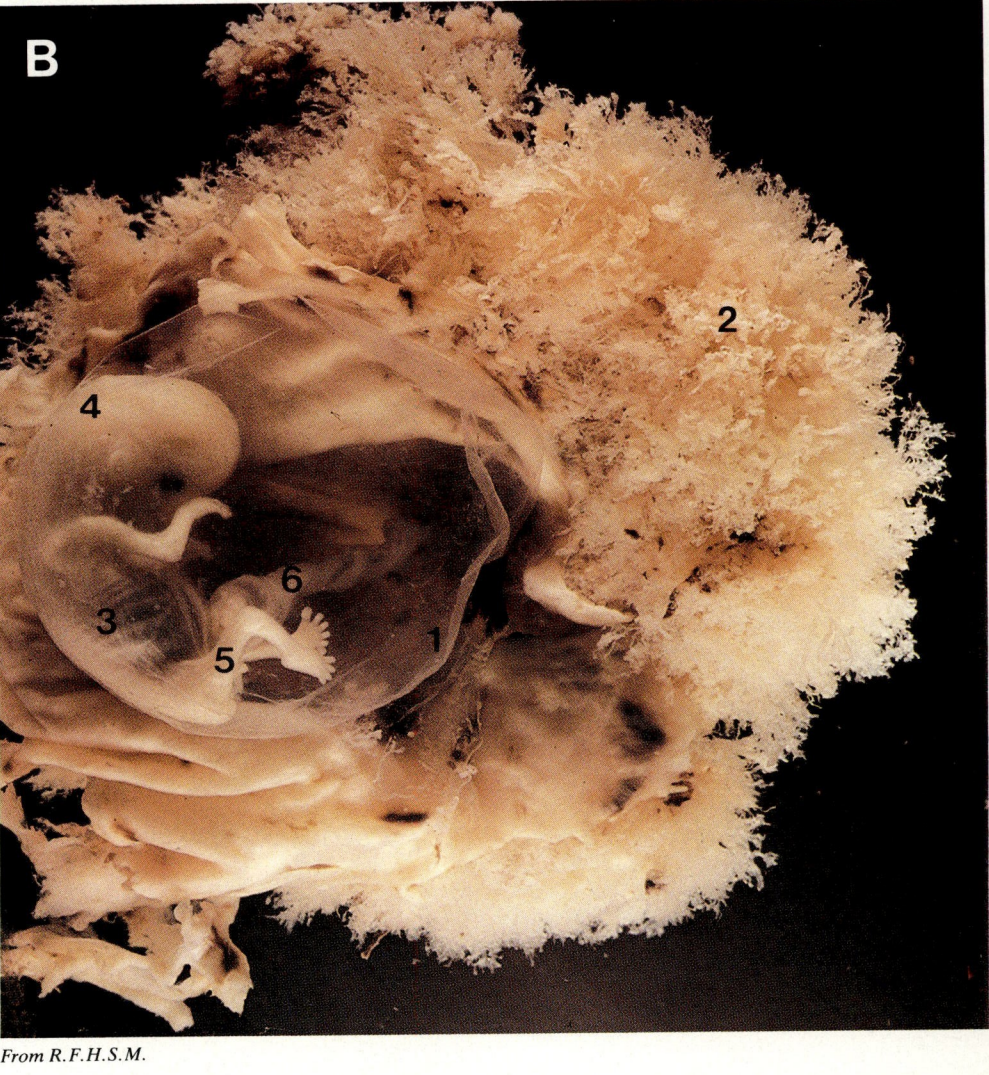

B. Week 7. The embryo suspended in the amniotic sac. 31 mm CR (×1.6)

1. amnion
2. chorionic villi
3. embryo
4. head
5. leg
6. umbilical cord

From R.F.H.S.M.

C. Week 12. The fetus
connected by the umbilical
cord to the fetal aspect of the
developing placenta.
85mmCR ♂ (×1.6)

1. amnion
2. chorionic villi
3. fetus
4. umbilical cord
5. umbilical vessels

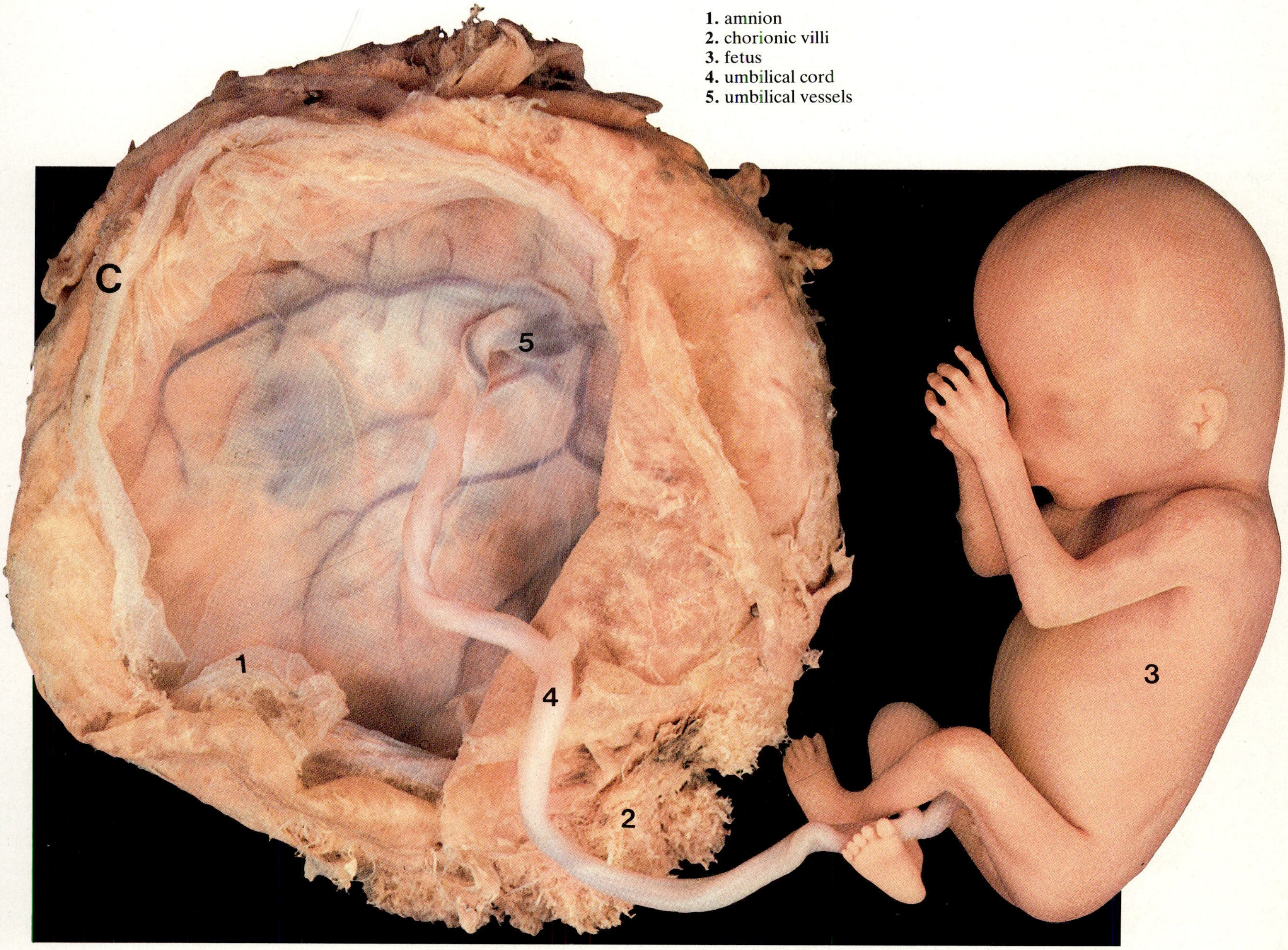

Yolk sac

The primary yolk sac is lined by a thin exocoelomic (Heuser's) membrane. As the extra-embryonic coelom forms the primary yolk sac degenerates and a smaller secondary yolk sac forms lined by endoderm. The first vascular blood forms from yolk sac mesoderm (Horizon VI, Day 13). This will provide embryonic blood until the liver starts to form blood (Week 5). It also provides nutrients during Week 2 and 3 while the chorioallantoic placenta develops. During Week 3 the primordial germ cells formed on the yolk sac migrate into the embryo. In Week 4 the body folds constrict the yolk sac and the portion incorporated into the embryo forms the epithelium of the gut tube. The extra-embryonic portion is the yolk sac remnant. The gut tube is divided into foregut, midgut and hindgut. The embryonic foregut includes the pharynx and its derivatives, the lower respiratory tract, esophagus, stomach, liver, pancreas, biliary apparatus and the duodenum to the entrance of the common bile duct. The celiac artery supplies all but the pharynx, respiratory tract and upper esophagus.

The embryonic midgut includes the small intestines from the entrance of the common bile duct, the cecum and the appendix, and the ascending and proximal part of the transverse colon. The superior mesenteric artery supplies the midgut.

The embryonic hindgut includes the distal part of the transverse colon, descending and sigmoid colon, rectum, upper anal canal and part of the urogenital system. The inferior mesenteric artery supplies the hindgut.

In Week 5–6 the yolk sac remnant (stalk) detaches from the gut (see Midgut rotation) and by Week 12 it is shrunken and hardened.

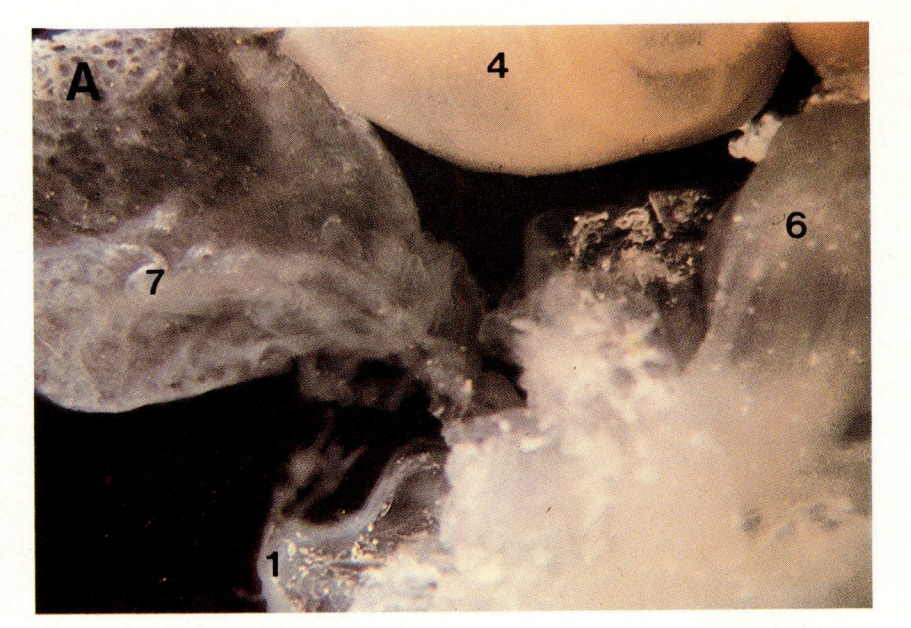

A. Horizon XVII (Day 34–36). The early yolk sac. 12 mmCR (×10.2)

1. amnion
2. chorionic villi
3. fetal surface of placenta
4. head of embryo
5. umbilical blood vessels
6. umbilical cord
7. yolk sac

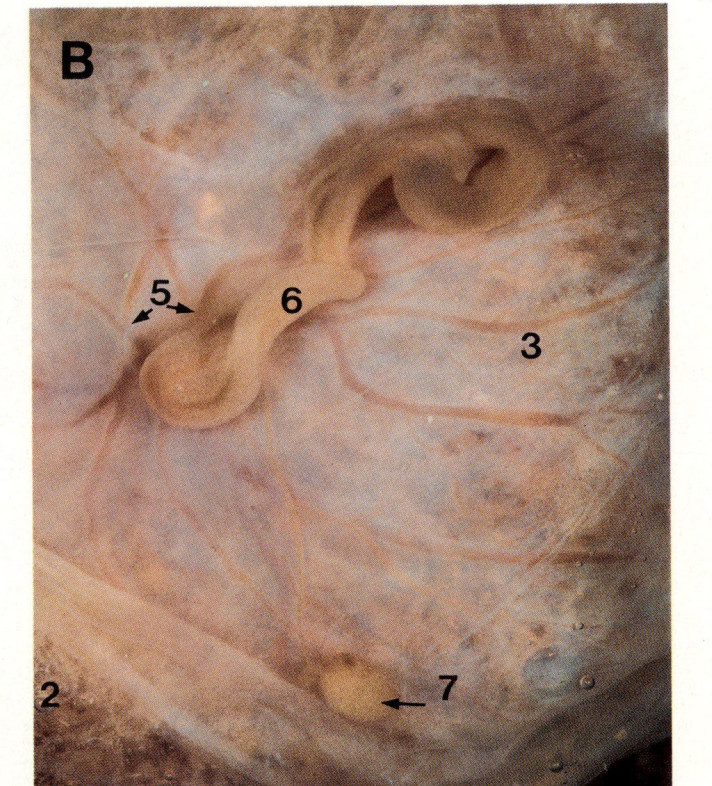

B. Week 9. The yolk sac is shrunken. 44 mmCR (×3.2)

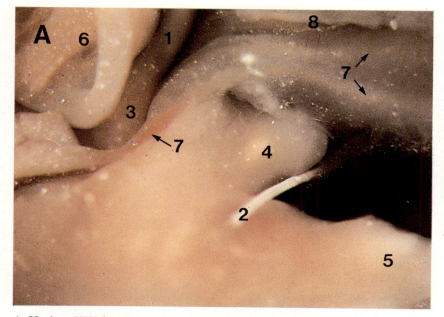

Allantois

The allantois appears on Day 16 as a diverticulum of the yolk sac. Between Week 3–5 blood forms in the walls of the allantois. The umbilical vein and arteries form from its blood vessels.

The intra-embryonic portion of the allantois extends from the umbilicus to the urinary bladder. As the bladder forms, the allantois becomes the urachus (see Bladder). During Week 5–8 the extra-embryonic portion degenerates.

● In the infant, the urachus becomes fibrous and forms the median umbilical ligament.

A. Horizon XIX (Day 38–40). The developing urinary bladder and allantois. The umbilical cord has been dissected open. 20 mmCR (×20.4)

1. allantois
2. cactus needle
3. developing urinary bladder (urogenital sinus)
4. genital tubercle
5. leg bud
6. midgut and hindgut
7. umbilical artery
8. umbilical cord dissected open

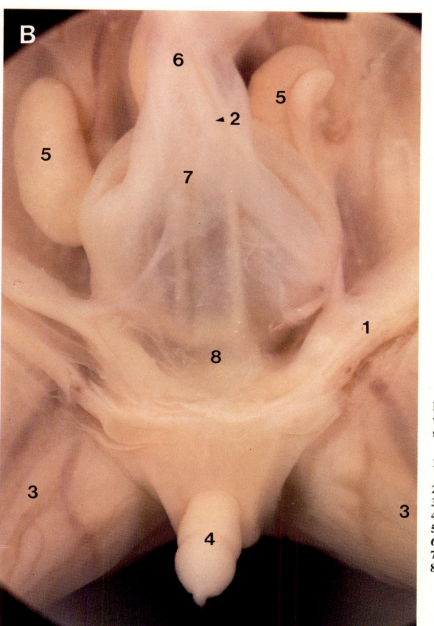

B. Week 11. The urachus viewed from the ventral surface. 65 mmCR ♂ (×11)

1. anterior abdominal wall (cut)
2. left umbilical artery
3. leg
4. penis
5. testis
6. umbilical cord
7. urachus
8. urinary bladder

Placenta

The placenta is interposed between fetal and maternal circulations and has several functions; these include metabolism and transfer of nutrients, wastes, antibodies, hormones and electrolytes. Drugs and infectious organisms may also cross the placenta. The placenta is a source of hormones.

The placental membrane is composed of syncytiotrophoblast, cytotrophoblast, a connective tissue core in each villus, and fetal capillary endothelium. Macrophage-like Hofbauer cells appear in the cores of villi in early pregnancy.

The villous tree grows by repeatedly branching and the fetal capillaries increase in number and size. In this way an initially terminal villus can become an intermediate villus. Eventually the capillaries come to lie close to the syncytiotrophoblast as the placental membrane becomes thinner in late pregnancy.

The mature placenta

The mature placenta is discoidal and flattened in shape and weighs approximately 500 g at birth. It is about 20 cm in diameter and 2.5 cm thick at the center. Implantation is usually in the upper part of the uterus on the dorsal aspect.

The fetal surface of the placenta is smooth with the umbilical cord attached near the centre. The cotyledonary vessels are visible through the amnion as they ramify in the chorionic mesoderm (chorionic plate).

The maternal oriented surface of the placenta is rough and raised into 10–38 cotyledons. Grooves between the cotyledons mark the site of the placental septa.

The amnion and chorion are continuous with the edges of the placenta. At parturition the umbilical cord, placenta, amnion and chorion follow the fetus as the 'afterbirth'.

- If implantation occurs in the lower uterus, the placenta may cover the internal os (placenta previa) and obstruct the fetus during parturition.

- Implantation may occur outside the uterus in an ectopic site (abdominal cavity, or uterine ((Fallopian)) tubes).

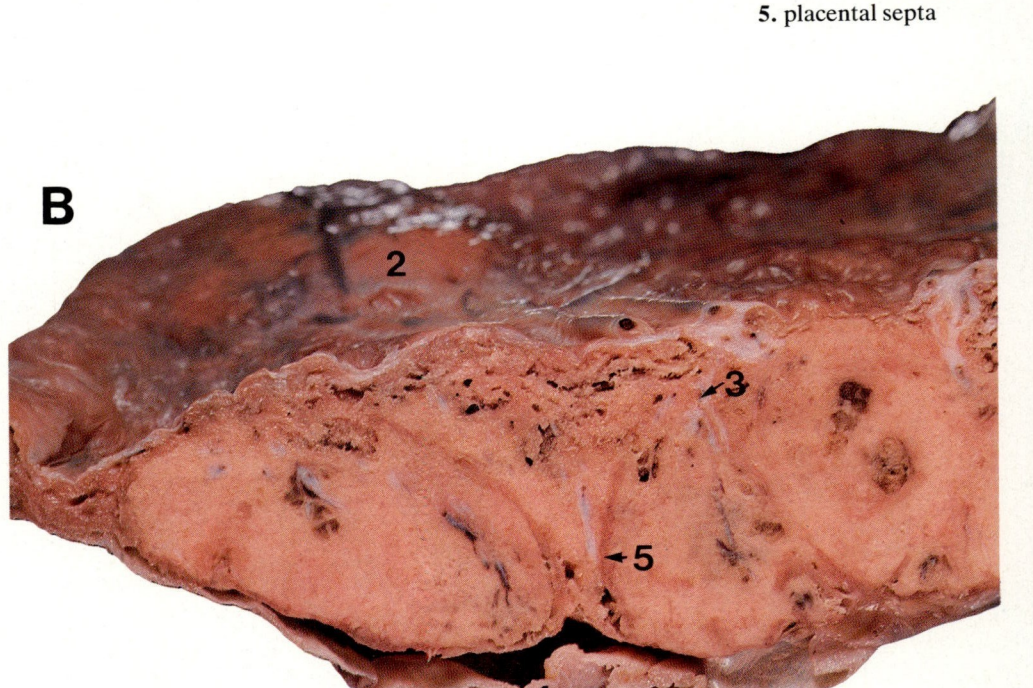

A. Week 23. Section of a placenta from a fetus. 220 mmCR ♂ (×0.98)

B. A higher magnification of the placenta in Figure **A**. (×2.1)

1. cotyledonary vessels
2. fetal surface
3. main stem villus
4. maternal surface
5. placental septa

A–D. Transverse sections of
developing umbilical cord.
A. Horizon XVIII (Day
36–38). 14 mmCR (×27)

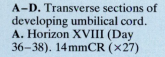

1. allantois
2. amniotic epithelium
3. coelom
4. umbilical vein (left)
5. umbilical artery
6. Wharton's jelly

B. Week 9. 48 mmCR ♀
(×15)

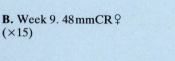

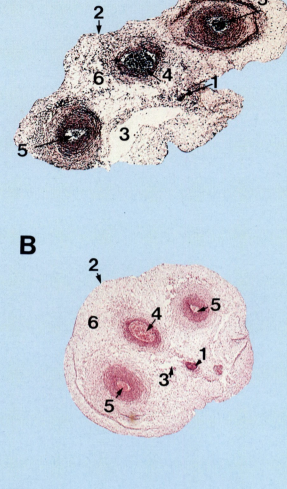

C. Week 13. 92 mmCR ♂
(×7.5)

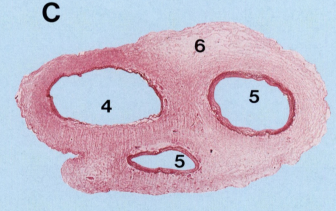

D. Week 23. 220 mmCR ♀
(×7)

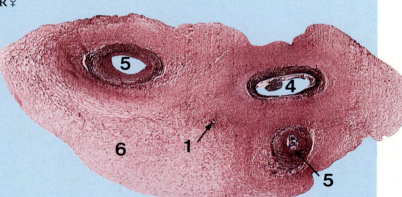

Umbilical cord

The early embryo has a very thick embryonic stalk
(body, connecting or umbilical stalk) containing two
umbilical arteries, one large umbilical vein, the allantois
and primary mesoderm cells. The arteries carry blood
from the embryo to the chorionic villi and the umbilical
vein returns blood to the embryo. The umbilical vein
and two arteries twist around one another.

In Week 5 the amnion expands to fill the entire extra-
embryonic coelom. This process forces the yolk stalk
against the embryonic stalk and covers the entire
contents with a tube of amniotic ectoderm so forming
the umbilical cord. The cord is narrower in diameter
than the embryonic stalk and it rapidly increases in
length. The connective tissue in the umbilical cord is
called Wharton's jelly and is derived from the primary
mesoderm cells. The early umbilical cord starts to twist
spirally on itself. It is not uncommon to find the cord
looped around the fetus. In Week 35–38 the attachment
of the umbilical cord becomes central in the abdomen.

● At birth the mature cord is about 50 cm in length and
  12 mm in diameter. There may be as many as 40 spiral
  twists present in the cord as well as false knots
  (irregular projections of blood vessels) and true
  knots (the fetus has moved through a loop of cord).

● When the blood flow is interrupted at birth the
  intra-embryonic parts of the umbilical arteries and vein
  gradually become fibrous cords.

● The course of the left umbilical vein is discernable in the
  adult as a fibrous cord from the umbilicus to the liver
  (*ligamentum teres*) contained within the falciform
  ligament.

● The umbilical arteries are retained proximally as the
  internal iliac arteries and give off the superior vesical
  arteries, and distally as the medial umbilical ligaments
  within the medial umbilical folds to the umbilicus.

● The umbilical cord remains stiff during development
  because of the blood flowing through it.

● The normal regression of the cord stump may be an
  important medico-legal factor in determining infant
  survival time.

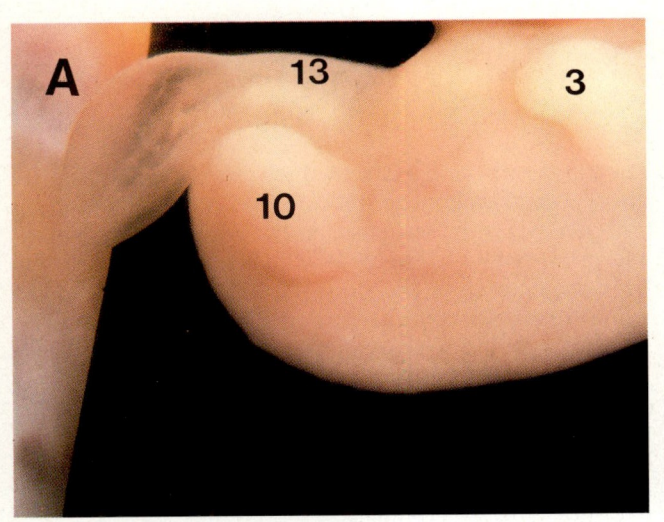

A. Horizon XVII (Day 34–36).
12 mmCR (×8.6)

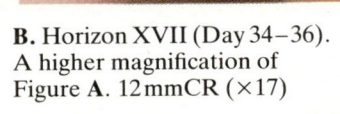

B. Horizon XVII (Day 34–36).
A higher magnification of
Figure A. 12 mmCR (×17)

A–I. Development of the
umbilical cord.

1. abdomen
2. amnion
3. arm bud
4. brain
5. branchial arch
6. buttock
7. external genitals
8. genital tubercle
9. leg
10. leg bud
11. spiral twist
12. tail
13. umbilical cord
14. umbilical vessels

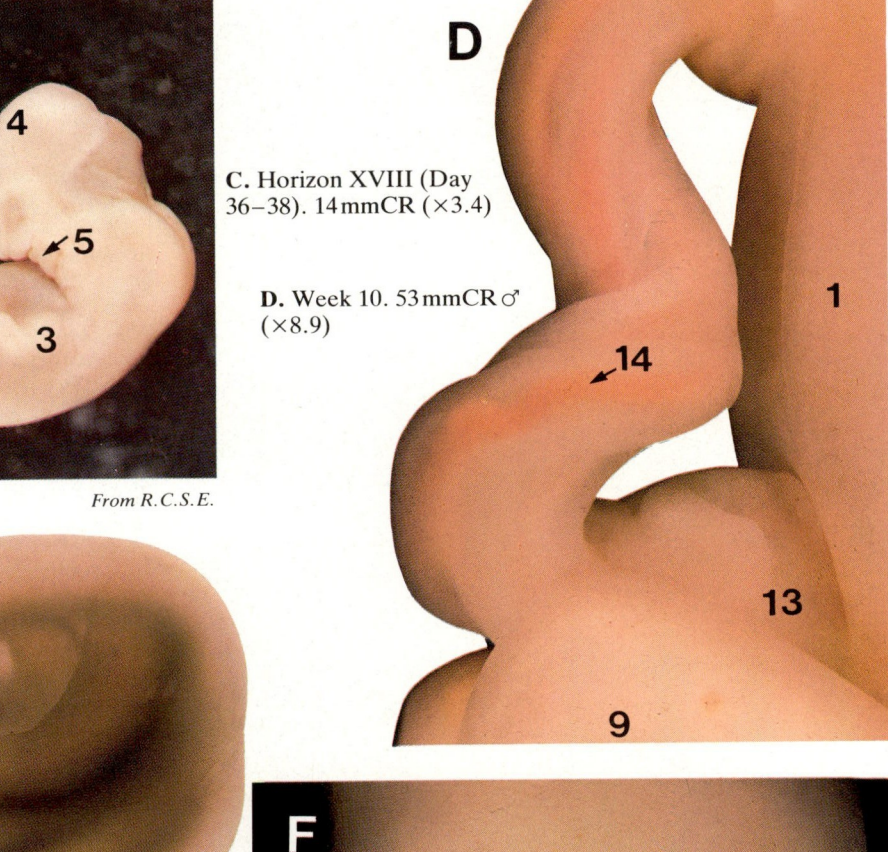

C. Horizon XVIII (Day
36–38). 14 mmCR (×3.4)

D. Week 10. 53 mmCR ♂
(×8.9)

From R.C.S.E.

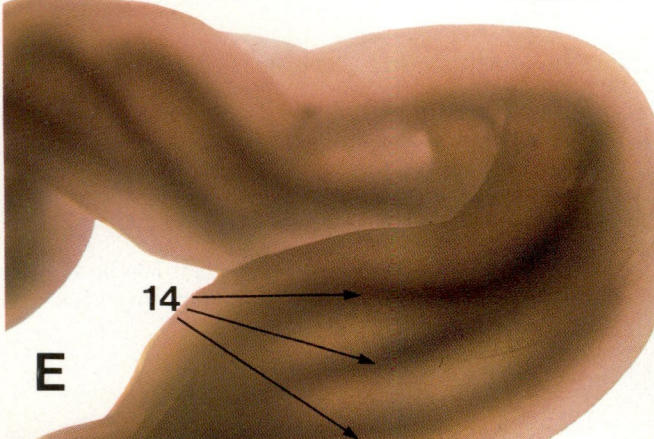

E. Week 10. 60 mmCR ♀
(×9)

F. Week 15. 130 mmCR ♀
(×0.9)

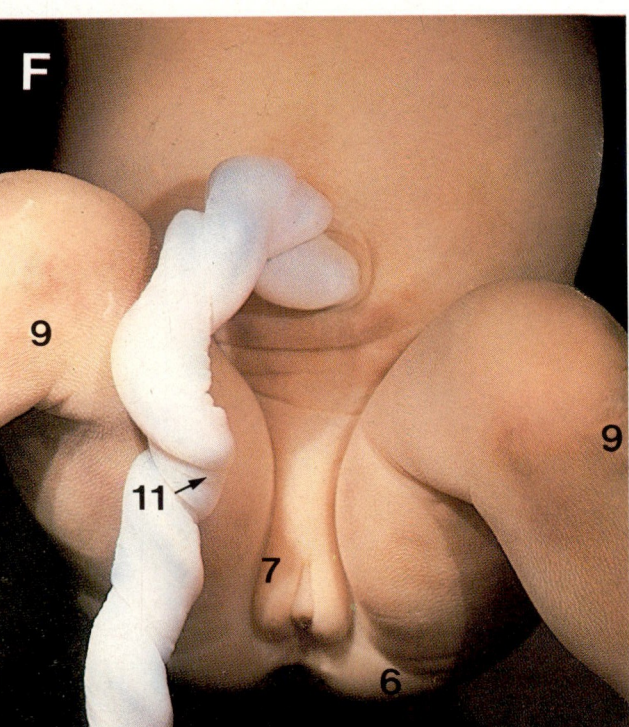

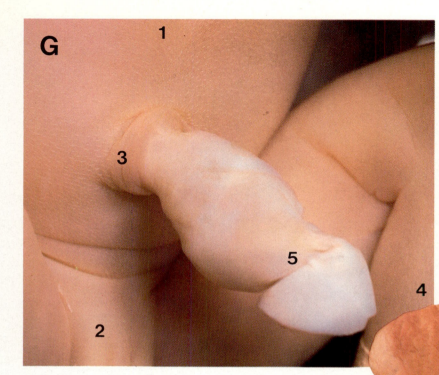

G. Week 15. Continuation of the amniotic cord epithelium and fetal epidermis. 130 mm CR ♀ (×3.3)

1. abdomen
2. external genitals
3. fetal epidermis
4. leg
5. umbilical cord covered with amnion

From C.C.H.M.S.

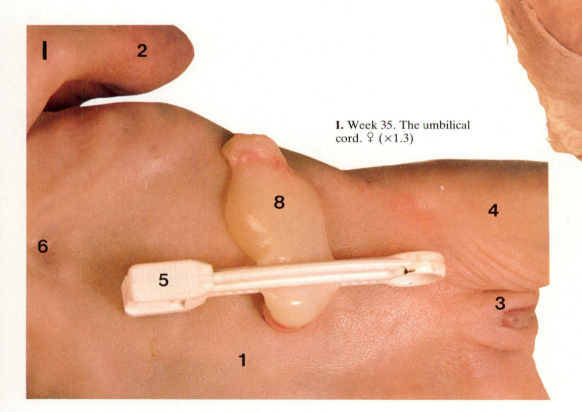

I. Week 35. The umbilical cord. ♀ (×1.3)

H

H. Week 28. The fetus *in situ* with a 'true' knot in the umbilical cord. (×0.5)

1. abdomen
2. arm
3. external genitals
4. leg
5. plastic clamp
6. thorax
7. true knot
8. umbilical cord
9. uterus

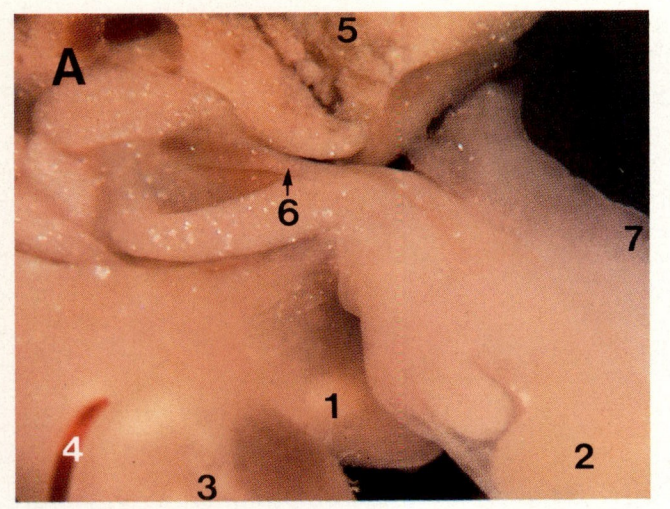

A. Horizon XIX (Day 38–40). The course of the umbilical artery to the umbilical cord. 20mmCR (×17)

1. genital tubercle
2. herniated midgut
3. leg bud
4. red cactus needle
5. right lobe of liver removed
6. umbilical artery
7. umbilical cord

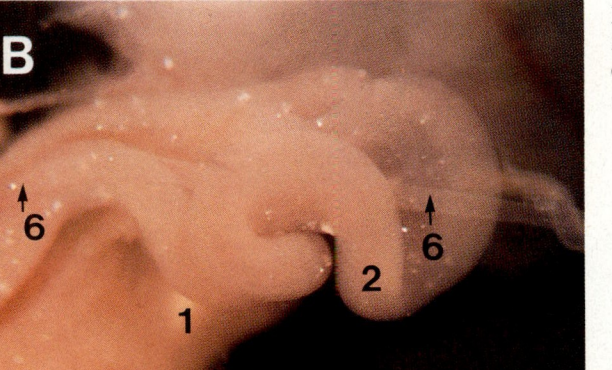

B. The same embryo as Figure **A** with the umbilical cord dissected away. 20mmCR (×17)

C. Week 10. The course of the umbilical vein from the umbilical cord viewed from the right. 56mmCR (×8.6)

1. intestine
2. left lobe of liver
3. right lobe of liver removed
4. umbilical cord
5. umbilical vein

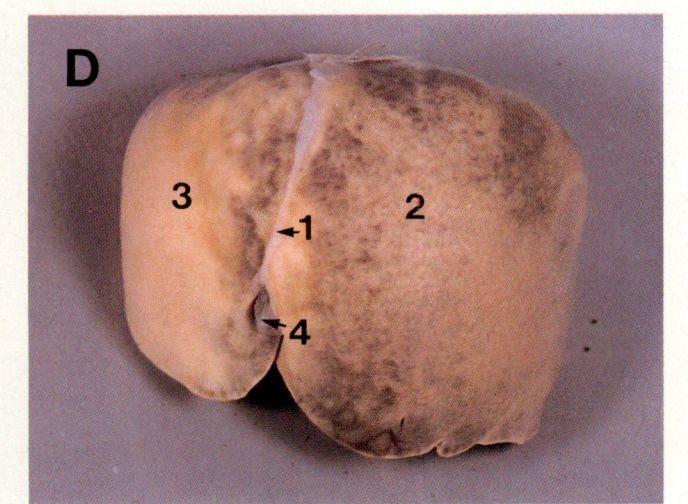

D. Week 13. Anterior view of the liver. 92mmCR ♀ (×2.3)

1. falciform ligament
2. left lobe
3. right lobe
4. umbilical vein

A. The anterior thoracic and abdominal wall in a full-term fetus. View from behind. Peritoneum and parts of muscles and the rectus sheaths have been removed. (×0.7)

1. diaphragm
2. external oblique muscle
3. falciform ligament
4. inferior epigastric vessels
5. internal oblique muscle
6. internal thoracic artery
7. left umbilical vein
8. ribs
9. transversus abdominus muscle
10. umbilical artery
11. urinary bladder

From R.C.S.E.

Head and Neck Development

Brain

The first rudiment of the nervous system is the mid-line ectoderm neural plate (Week 2). Neural folds form which rise and fuse to form a tube starting in the midbrain region. Fusion proceeds both cranially and caudally leaving both ends open; these are the anterior (rostral) and posterior (caudal) neuropores. The pores will eventually close. The *lamina terminalis* forms the cephalic end of the neural tube when the anterior neuropore closes. The main divisions of the central nervous system are established at this stage (Week 4): forebrain, midbrain, hindbrain and spinal cord. The optic cup is an outgrowth of the forebrain. In Week 5 the forebrain (prosencephalon) divides into three vesicles: a median diencephalon and two hemispheres (telencephalon). The midbrain (or mesencephalon) remains as before, but the hindbrain (or rhombencephalon) forms two regions: metencephalon and myelencephalon.

Cavities of the brain

A pair of cerebral hemispheres grows out from the telencephalon. The hollow space in each hemisphere is called the lateral ventricle which is continuous with the third ventricle (the original forebrain cavity) via the interventricular foramen. The third ventricle is continuous with the wide lumen of the midbrain, the cerebral aqueduct, which is continuous with the hindbrain lumen through a constriction, the isthmus. The diamond-shaped hindbrain's fourth ventricle merges into the central canal of the spinal cord without a distinct boundary.

Flexures

Three flexures appear in the brain due to unequal growth. The first, the midbrain flexure, appears during Week 4 when the forebrain bends in a ventral direction. The second flexure, the cervical or neck flexure, occurs during Week 5–7 between the hindbrain and spinal cord. This flexure diminishes and eventually disappears after the head extends during Week 8 (see Neck).

The third flexure, the pontine flexure, occurs in the region of the pons (Week 5). It does not noticeably alter the outline of the head as the first two flexures do. It does, however, cause the rhombencephalon's lateral walls to splay and thin so that the roof forms a diamond shape. The alar and basal laminae come to lie in the floor of the rhombencephalon with the *sulcus limitans* between the two.

Layers of the brain

Initially the brain and spinal cord have the same three layers; the ependymal, mantle and marginal layers. In the brain a fourth layer is added when cells from the mantle layer migrate through the marginal zone to the outside and form a layer of cortex. Therefore, grey matter (cortex) is on the outside of the brain and the axons from cell bodies pass centrally. This is unlike the spinal cord where the axons pass peripherally.

A and B. Flexures of the brain.

1. cervical flexure
2. eye
3. forebrain
4. heart
5. hindbrain
6. liver bulge
7. midbrain
8. midbrain flexure
9. pontine flexure
10. umbilical cord

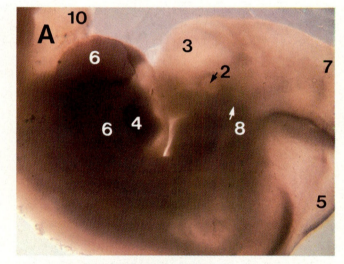

A. Horizon XVII (Day 34–36). 12mmCR (×8.4)

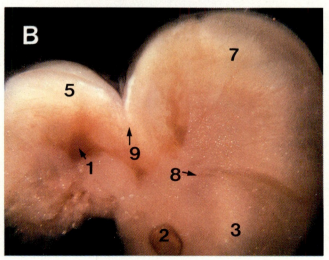

B. Horizon XIX (Day 38–40). The hindbrain roof has been removed. 20mmCR (×8.4)

Forebrain

The forebrain has two lateral expansions, the cerebral vesicles (telencephalon), connected by an intermediate region (diencephalon). The cavities of the cerebral vesicles are the lateral ventricles and these are continuous with the third ventricle of the diencephalon. The third ventricle is reduced by three swellings in its lateral walls; the epithalamus, thalamus and hypothalamus. The two thalami expand and usually fuse in the midline. Two mamillary bodies form on the ventral surface of the hypothalamus. The pineal gland is a midline diverticulum of the diencephalic roof.

Telencephalon: the cerebral vesicles are originally in wide communication with the third ventricle via the interventricular foramina though these openings are later reduced. The medial walls of the cerebral vesicles become very thin and are penetrated by vascular pia mater to form the choroid plexus at this site (choroid fissure). The cerebral hemispheres expand like two large balloons and cover the diencephalon, the midbrain and finally the hindbrain. As the hemispheres meet in the midline they flatten medially and trap mesoderm which forms the falx cerebri. The caudal end of the hemisphere turns ventrally, and then cranially to bury the insula, and form the temporal lobe adjacent to the lateral sulcus. Thus the cerebral hemisphere becomes 'C' shaped. The choroid fissure follows its line of growth.

In the floor of each hemisphere the corpus striatum develops and fibers passing to and from the cerebral cortex divide it into the caudate and lentiform nuclei (Week 6). This fiber pathway (internal capsule) becomes 'C' shaped.

As the cerebral hemispheres grow several groups of fibers (or commissures) connect the corresponding areas of the two hemispheres; these are the anterior commissure, the hippocampal (fornix) commissure, the corpus callosum and the optic chiasma.

The surface of the hemispheres is smooth until Week 25 and 26 when sulci and gyri develop and the brain volume is increased.

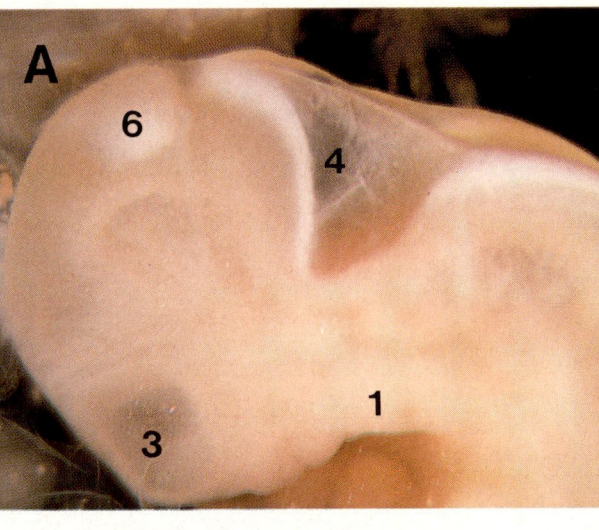

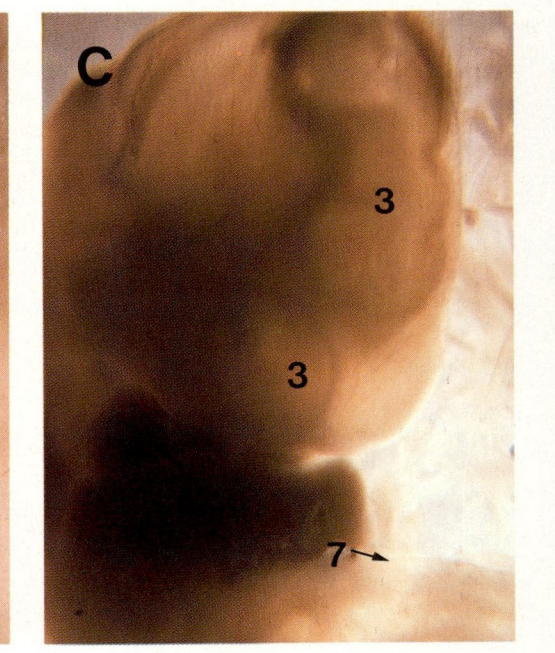

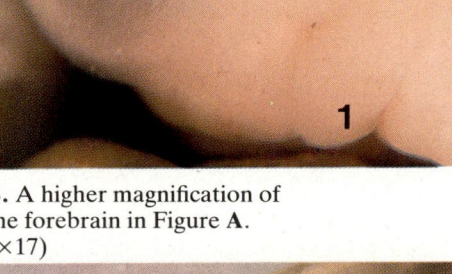

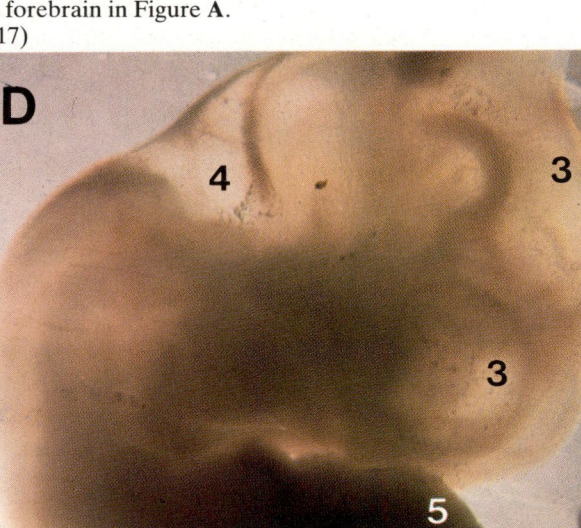

A–D. Horizon XVII (Day 34–36). Forebrain development. 12 mm CR

1. branchial arch
2. eye
3. forebrain
4. hindbrain
5. liver shadow
6. midbrain
7. umbilical cord

A. Note the diamond-shaped hindbrain and lateral vesicles of the forebrain. Viewed from the left. (×8.6)

B. A higher magnification of the forebrain in Figure **A**. (×17)

C. The same embryo as in Figure **A** seen by transmitted light. Viewed from the right and front. (×8.4)

D. Lateral view of the same embryo as in Figure **A**. Viewed from the right. (×8.4)

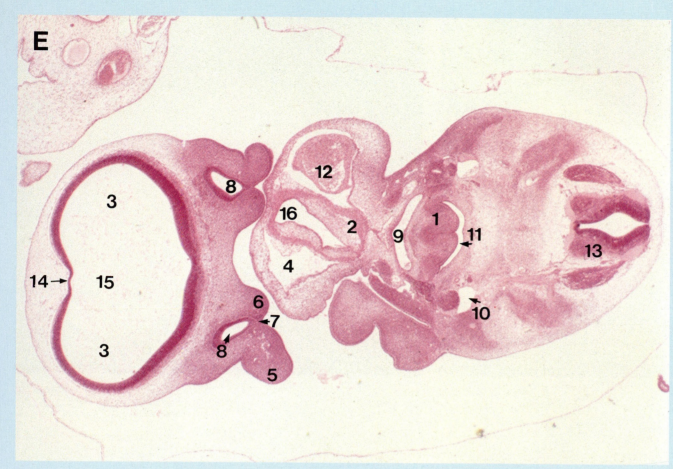

E. Horizon XVI (Day 32–34).
The telencephalon in
transverse paraffin wax
section. 10 mm CR (×28)

1. arytenoid swelling
2. heart (truncus)
3. lateral ventricle
4. left atrium
5. maxillary process
6. medial nasal prominence
7. nasal fin
8. nasal pit
9. primitive larynx
10. precardinal vein
11. pharynx
12. right atrium
13. spinal cord
14. telencephalon
15. third ventricle
16. truncus arteriosus

F. Horizon XVI (Day 32–34).
A transverse section of the
midbrain and fourth ventricle.
10 mm CR (×26)

1. fourth ventricle
2. mesencephalon
3. neural canal
4. neuromere
5. spinal ganglion
6. glosso pharyngeal ganglion
7. otocyst

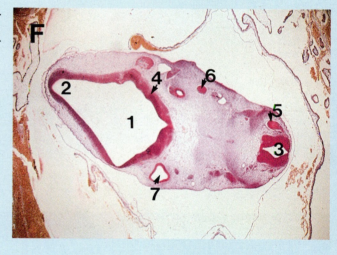

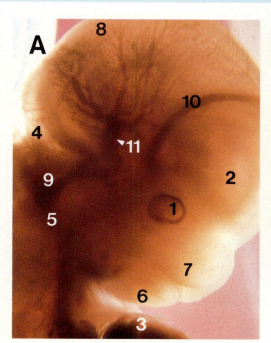

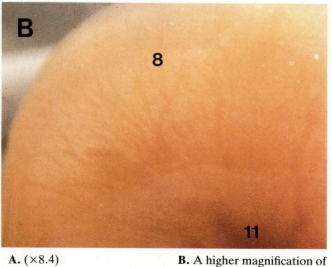

A and B. Horizon XIX (Day
38–40). Blood supply to the
developing brain. 20 mm CR

1. eye
2. forebrain
3. heart
4. hindbrain
5. internal jugular vein
6. mandible
7. maxilla
8. midbrain
9. sigmoid sinus
10. superior sagittal sinus
11. transverse sinus

A. (×8.4)

B. A higher magnification of
the midbrain in **A.** (×16.8)

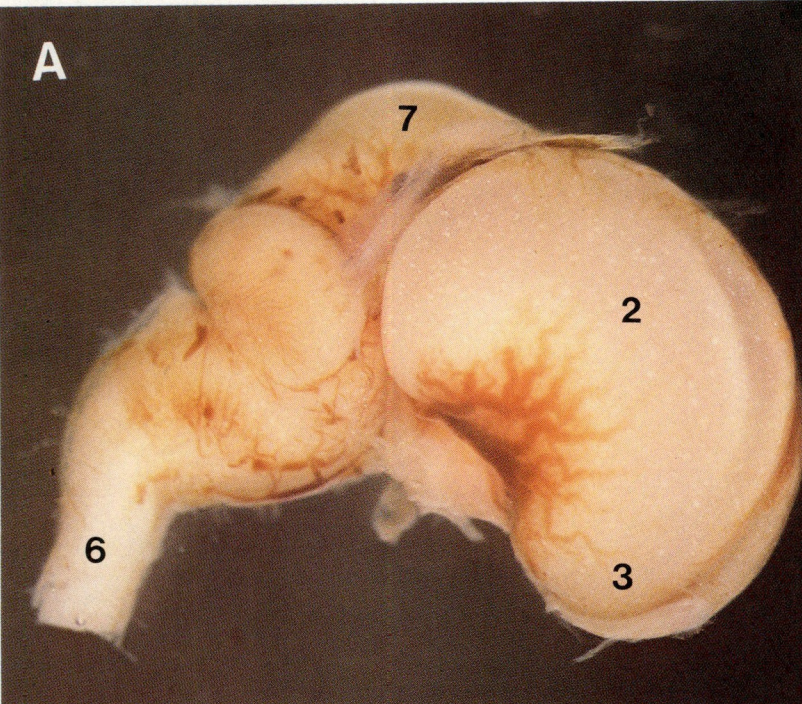

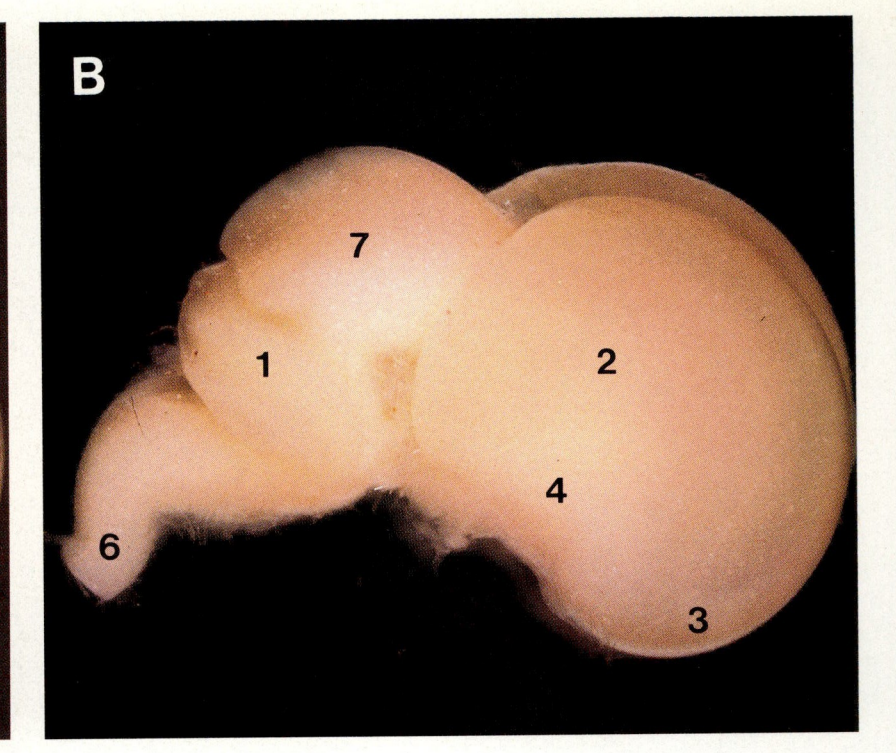

A. Week 8. 34 mm CR
(×5.8)

B. Week 8. 40 mm CR
(×5)

A–F. Development and rapid relative growth of the cerebral hemispheres, compared with midbrain, and the development of the gyri. Note the straight central sulcus.

1. cerebellum
2. cerebral hemispheres (telencephalon)
3. frontal lobe
4. insula
5. lateral sulcus
6. medulla
7. mesencephalon
8. occipital lobe
9. parietal lobe
10. temporal lobe

C. Week 10. 57 mm CR ♂
(×4)

D. Week 13. 101 mm CR ♀
(×2)

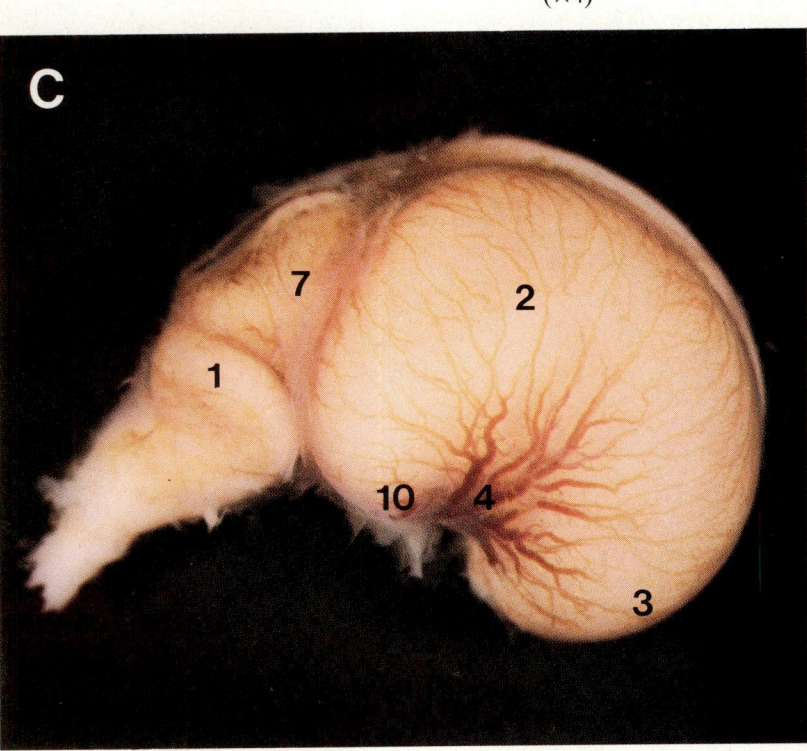

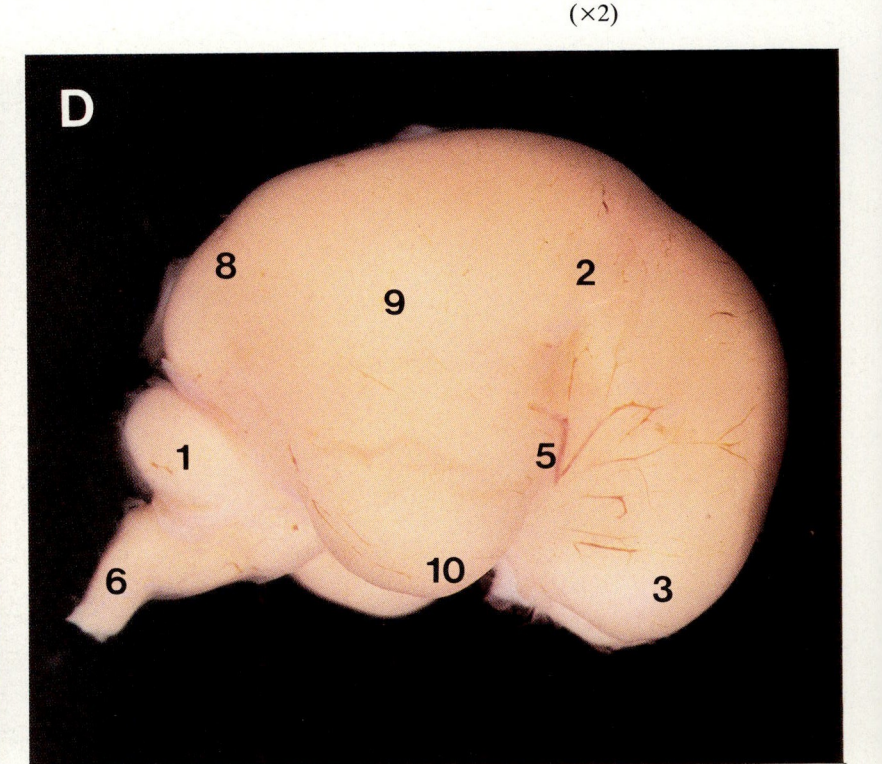

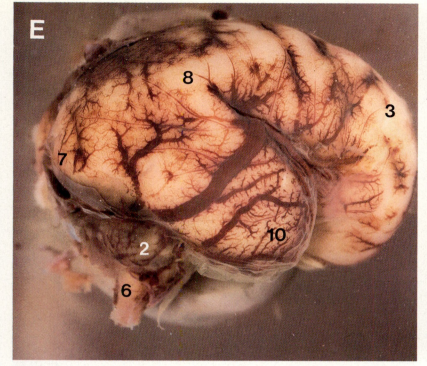

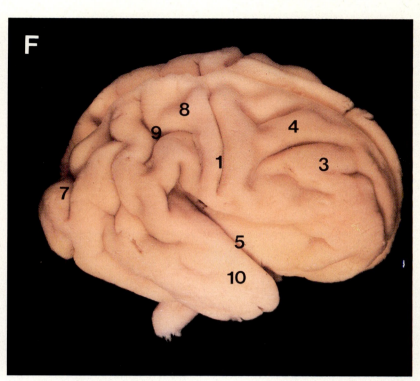

E. Week 18. 152 mmCR ♂
(×1.5)

F. Week 28. (×1.4)

From R.F.H.S.M.

1. central sulcus
2. cerebellum
3. cerebral hemispheres (telencephalon)
4. gyri
5. lateral fissure
6. medulla
7. occipital lobe
8. parietal lobe
9. sulci
10. temporal lobe

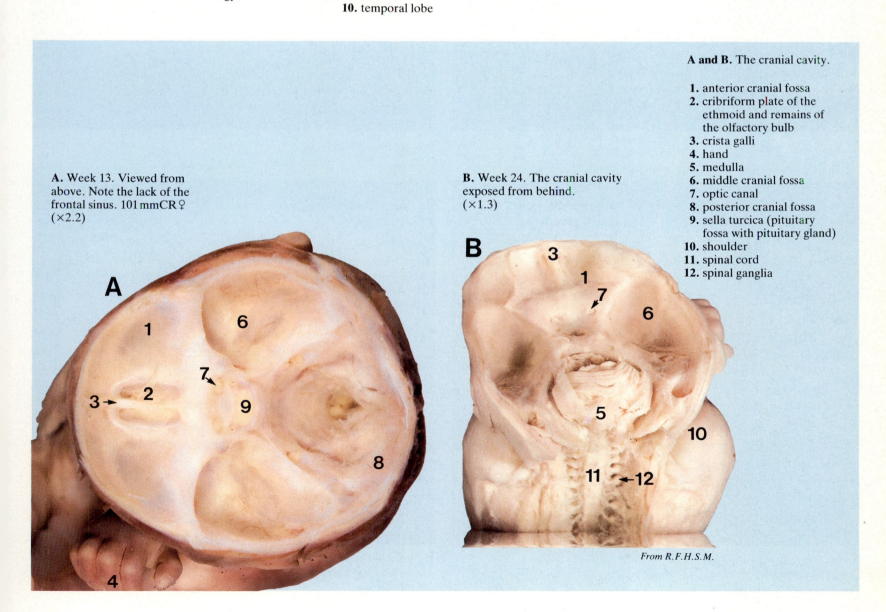

A. Week 13. Viewed from above. Note the lack of the frontal sinus. 101 mmCR ♀ (×2.2)

B. Week 24. The cranial cavity exposed from behind. (×1.3)

A and B. The cranial cavity.

1. anterior cranial fossa
2. cribriform plate of the ethmoid and remains of the olfactory bulb
3. crista galli
4. hand
5. medulla
6. middle cranial fossa
7. optic canal
8. posterior cranial fossa
9. sella turcica (pituitary fossa with pituitary gland)
10. shoulder
11. spinal cord
12. spinal ganglia

From R.F.H.S.M.

A–D. Cerebral hemispheres overgrowing the midbrain. Viewed from above (superior or cranial surface).

1. cerebellum
2. cerebral hemispheres
3. falx cerebri
4. hindbrain
5. mesencephalon
6. spinal cord

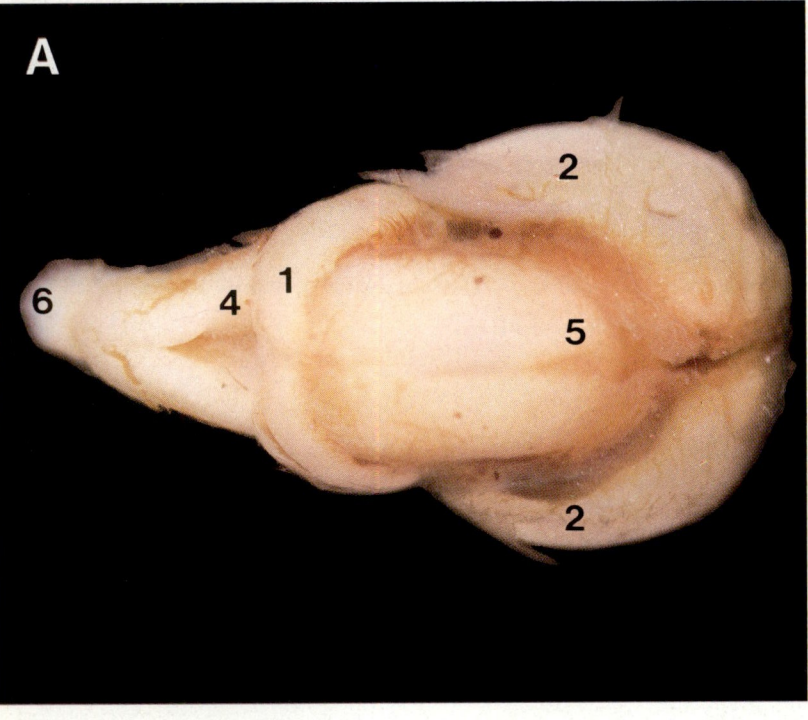

A. Week 8. 34 mm CR (×5.4)

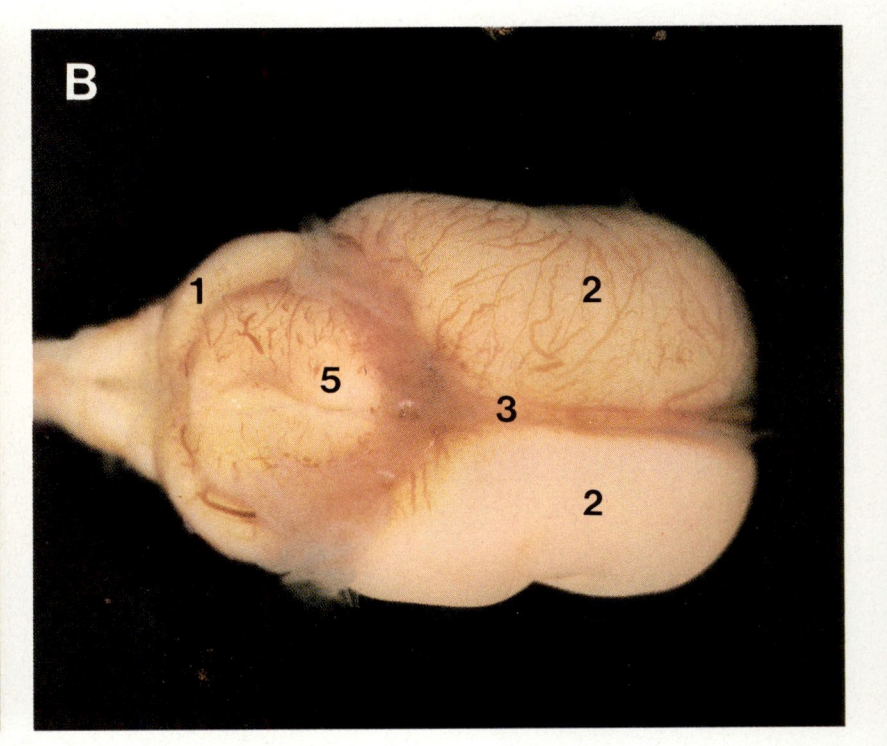

B. Week 10. 57 mm CR ♂ (×4)

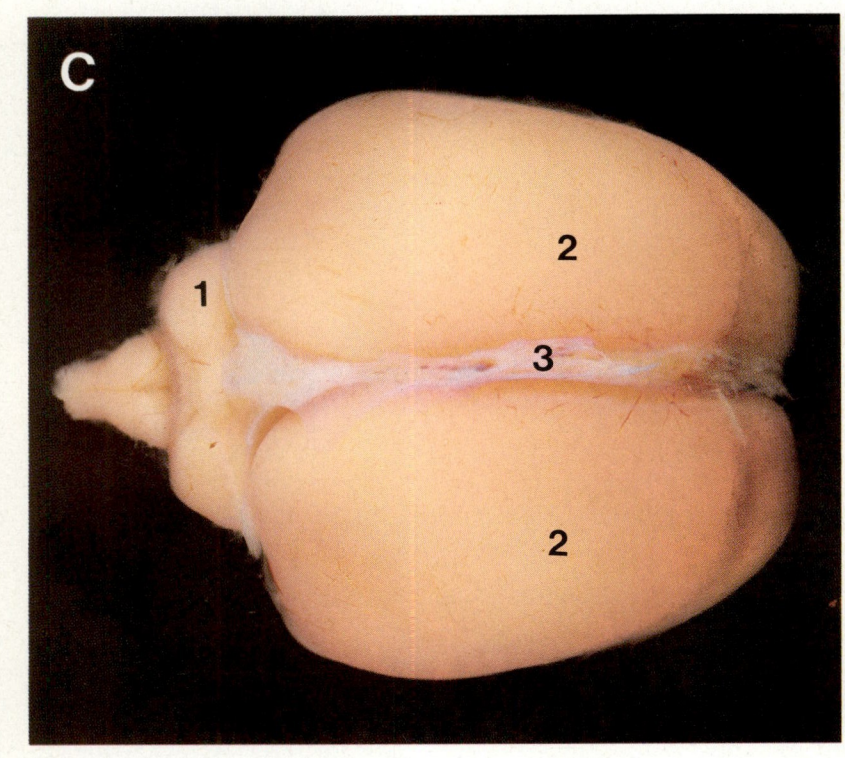

C. Week 13. Note the smooth surface of the cerebral hemispheres. 101 mm CR ♀ (×2)

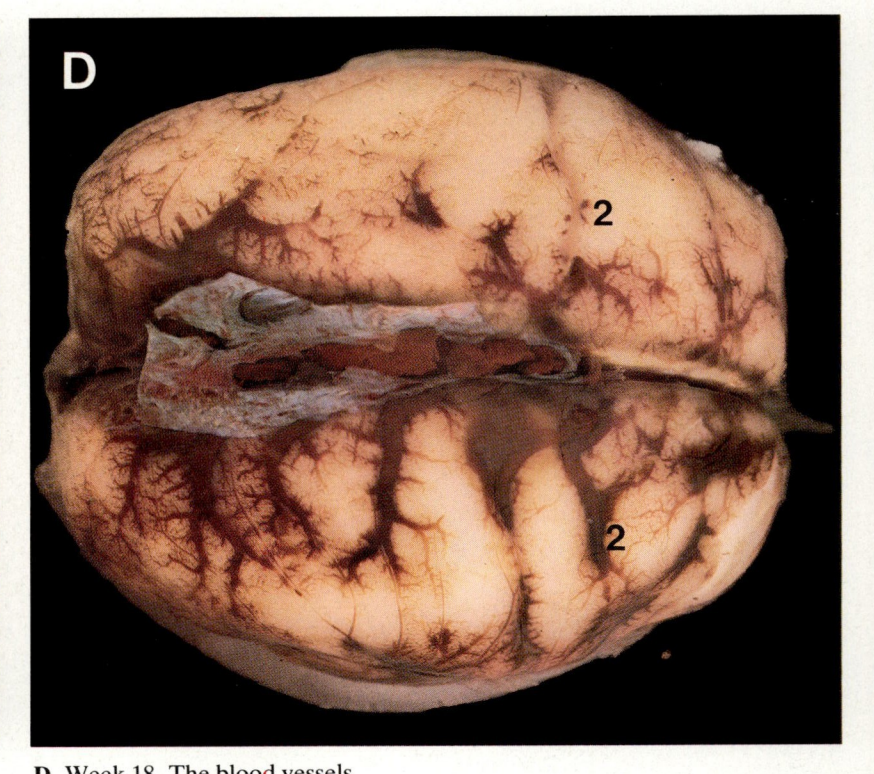

D. Week 18. The blood vessels are enlarged in this fetus. 152 mm CR ♂ (×1.5)

A–D. The fetal brain at various stages of development viewed from below.

1. anterior cerebral artery
2. basilar artery
3. cerebellum
4. frontal lobe
5. internal carotid artery
6. medulla
7. olfactory bulb
8. optic chiasma
9. pituitary stalk (cut)
10. pons
11. temporal lobe

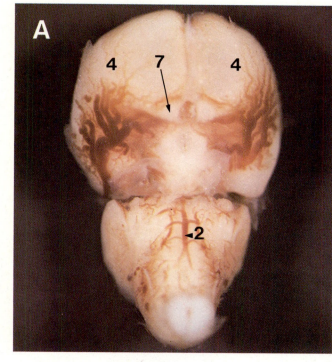

A. Week 8. 34 mm CR (×5.3)

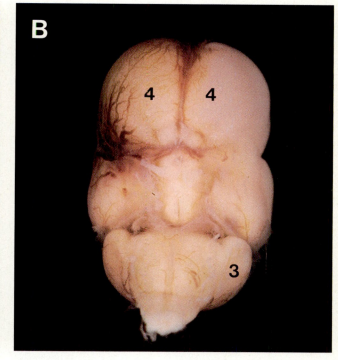

B. Week 10. 57 mm CR ♂ (×3.5)

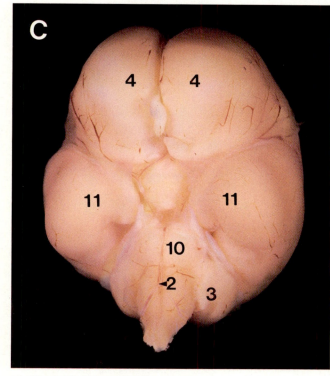

C. Week 13. 101 mm CR ♀ (×1.8)

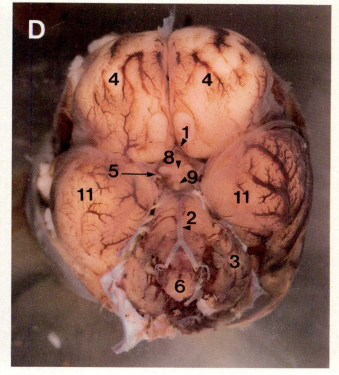

D. Week 18. 152 mm CR ♂ (×1.5)

Midbrain

The midbrain is most prominent at the midbrain flexure. Caudally it is constricted at the isthmus. Rostrally, its wide lumen is the mesocoele and its roof the smooth tectum. It joins the third and fourth ventricles. The lateral walls are divided into dorsal (or alar) and ventral (or basal) laminae.

The wide lumen is reduced to a narrow channel, the cerebral aqueduct when four colliculi form in the tectum from neuroblasts in the alar laminae. The walls are thickened laterally and ventrally by the formation of the red nucleus, the nuclei of cranial nerves III and IV and reticular nuclei. The cerebral peduncles and substantia nigra also reduce the lumen of the aqueduct.

A. Viewed from the left. (×17)

B. A higher magnification of the midbrain in Figure A. (×34)

A and B. Horizon XVII (Day 34–36). The midbrain in the 12mmCR embryo.

1. back
2. branchial arches
3. forebrain
4. heart
5. hindbrain roof
6. midbrain

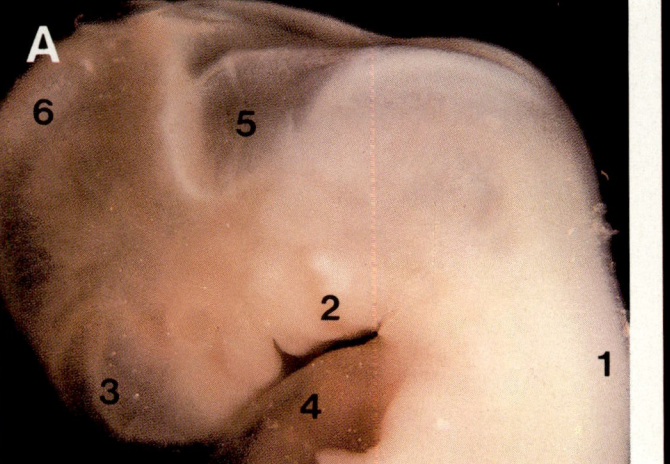

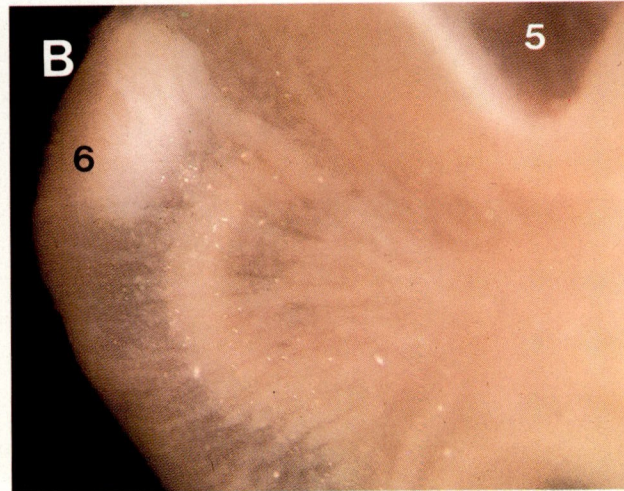

A. Horizon XIX (Day 38–40) The midbrain in a 20mmCR embryo. The ectoderm and roof plate have been removed from the region of the hindbrain. (×17)

1. eye
2. forebrain
3. hindbrain
4. midbrain

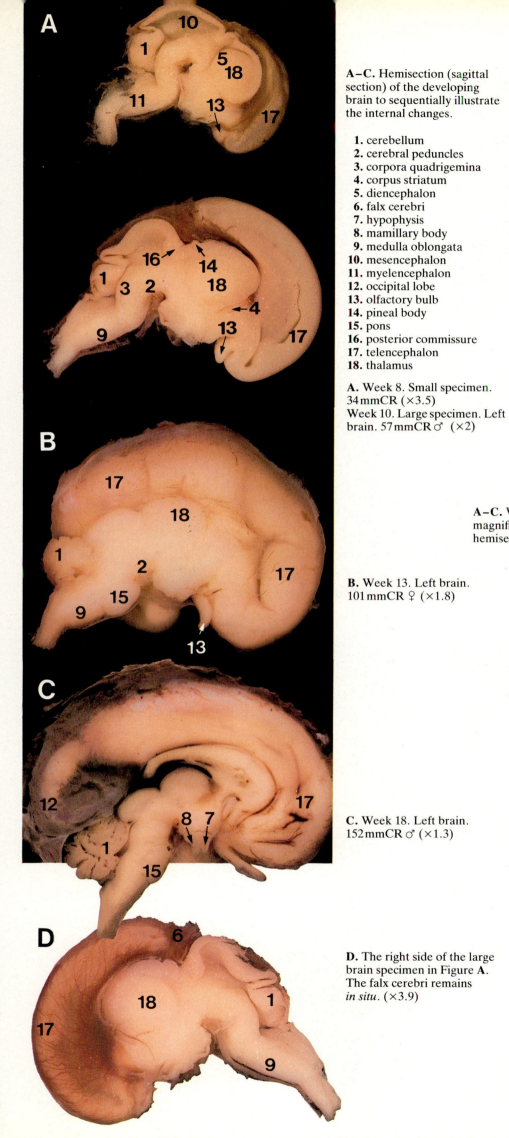

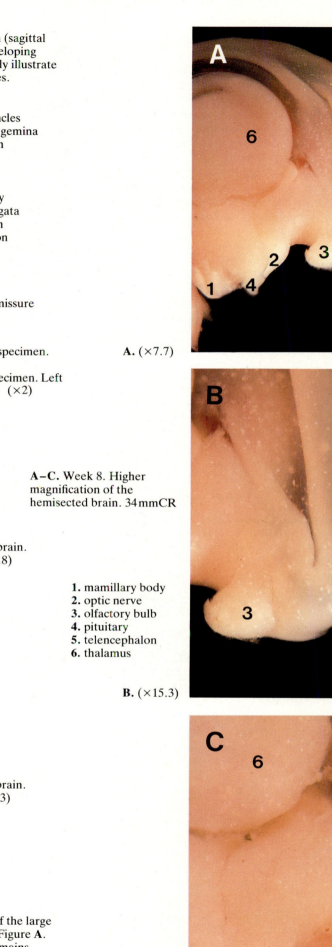

A–C. Hemisection (sagittal section) of the developing brain to sequentially illustrate the internal changes.

1. cerebellum
2. cerebral peduncles
3. corpora quadrigemina
4. corpus striatum
5. diencephalon
6. falx cerebri
7. hypophysis
8. mamillary body
9. medulla oblongata
10. mesencephalon
11. myelencephalon
12. occipital lobe
13. olfactory bulb
14. pineal body
15. pons
16. posterior commissure
17. telencephalon
18. thalamus

A. Week 8. Small specimen. 34 mmCR (×3.5)
Week 10. Large specimen. Left brain. 57 mmCR ♂ (×2)

A. (×7.7)

A–C. Week 8. Higher magnification of the hemisected brain. 34 mmCR

B. Week 13. Left brain. 101 mmCR ♀ (×1.8)

1. mamillary body
2. optic nerve
3. olfactory bulb
4. pituitary
5. telencephalon
6. thalamus

B. (×15.3)

C. Week 18. Left brain. 152 mmCR ♂ (×1.3)

D. The right side of the large brain specimen in Figure **A**. The falx cerebri remains *in situ*. (×3.9)

C. (×16.5)

Hindbrain

The diamond-shaped hindbrain (rhombencephalon) is continuous with the spinal cord. The pontine flexure divides the hindbrain into two parts; metencephalon (cephalically) and myelencephalon (caudally). The roof is very thin and the floor is thrown into a series of waves (neuromeres) which later disappear. The cavity is the fourth ventricle and the central canal of the lower medulla. The otocyst lies caudal to the widest part of the diamond-shape of the hindbrain. The isthmus (from the midbrain) forms the anterior medullary velum, the superior cerebellar peduncles and the cranial part of the fourth ventricle.

The metencephalon roof thickens to form the cerebellum and the floor becomes the pons. The middle part of the fourth ventricle is of metencephalic origin.

The floor of the myelencephalon contributes to the medulla oblongata and in Week 14–17 the pyramids are formed by the downgrowing corticospinal fibers from the telencephalon. Its lumen is the caudal part of the fourth ventricle. The alar and basal laminae separated by the sulcus limitans are clearly distinguishable.

The choroid plexus invaginates into the roof. As cerebrospinal fluid (CSF) is formed by the choroid plexus, pressure increases in the fourth ventricle and three foramina form in the thin roof; the median foramen of Magendie, and the two paired lateral foramina of Luschka. These allow the CSF to escape into the subarachnoid space.

● If the aqueducts or foramina of Magendie or Luschka are blocked by scar tissue from intrauterine infection the CSF cannot escape and congenital hydrocephalus results.

Cranial nerves. The olfactory (I) and optic (II) nerves are atypical in origin as they are outgrowths of the brain. The remaining cranial nerves can be divided into those with ganglia, i.e. having some sensory and/or autonomic components (V, VII, IX, and X) and those without ganglia. Sensory and autonomic cranial nerve ganglia form from neural crest similar to the spinal dorsal root or sympathetic ganglia.

The remaining cranial nerves are without ganglia and have no sensory or autonomic fibers.

The cranial nerves are therefore either purely sensory, purely motor or mixed, while all spinal nerves are mixed.

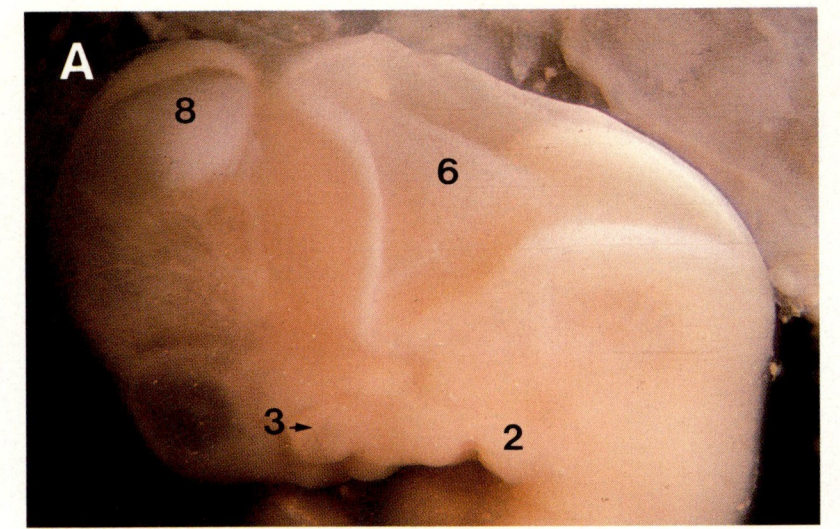

A. Viewed from above left. (×8.6)

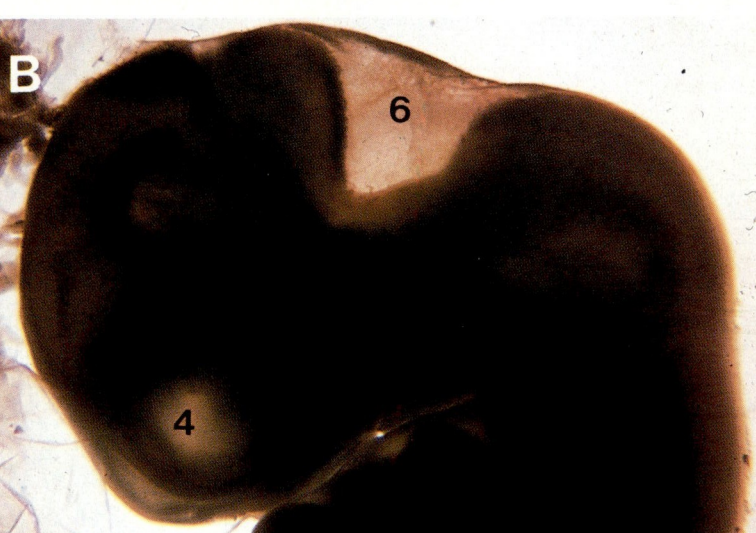

B. The same embryo as in Figure **A** viewed with transmitted light. (×8.6)

A–C. Horizon XVII (Day 34–36). The hindbrain. 12mmCR.

1. arm bud
2. branchial arch
3. eye (left)
4. forebrain
5. heart
6. hindbrain roof
7. liver
8. mesencephalon
9. umbilical cord

C. Another view of the embryo in Figure **A** viewed with transmitted light. (×11)

A and B. Horizon XVIII (Day 36–38). The hindbrain viewed in sagittal section. 14 mmCR

1. neuromeres
2. pontine flexure
3. roof plate

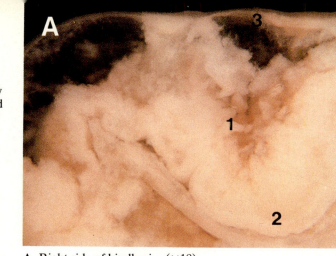

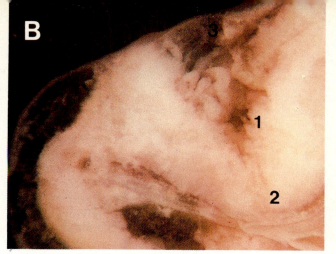

A. Right side of hindbrain. (×18)

B. Left side of hindbrain in Figure **A**. (×18)

A–C. Horizon XIX (Day 38–40). The midbrain and hindbrain viewed from the right. 20 mmCR

1. blood supply
2. choroid plexus
3. ear
4. eye (right)
5. hindbrain
6. midbrain

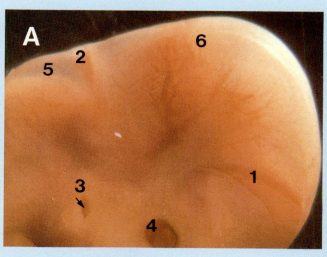

A. (×6.2)

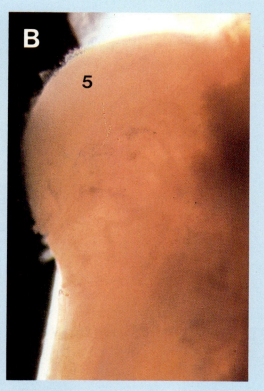

B. A higher magnification of the hindbrain (medulla) in Figure **A**. (×17.4)

C. A higher magnification of the hindbrain (cerebellum) in Figure **A**. View from the left. (×17)

A and B. Horizon XIX (Day 38–40). The hindbrain viewed from above. The ectoderm and roof plate have been removed. 20 mmCR

1. cerebellum
2. entrance to aqueduct of mesencephalon
3. fourth ventricle
4. medulla

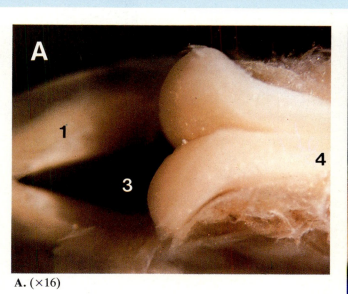

A. (×16)

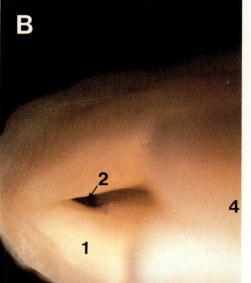

B. (×17)

Cerebellum. The cerebellum develops as swellings formed from cells in the rhombic lip and dorsal part of the alar lamina of the metencephalon. Initially (Horizon XVII, Day 34–36) the swellings bulge into the fourth ventricle, fuse in the midline, enlarge externally at the expense of the interventricular portion, and overgrow the rostral half of the fourth ventricle so overlapping the pons and medulla by Week 12. Transverse grooves appear on the dorsal aspect (Week 13) and the flocculonodular lobe is demarcated from the rest of the cerebellum.

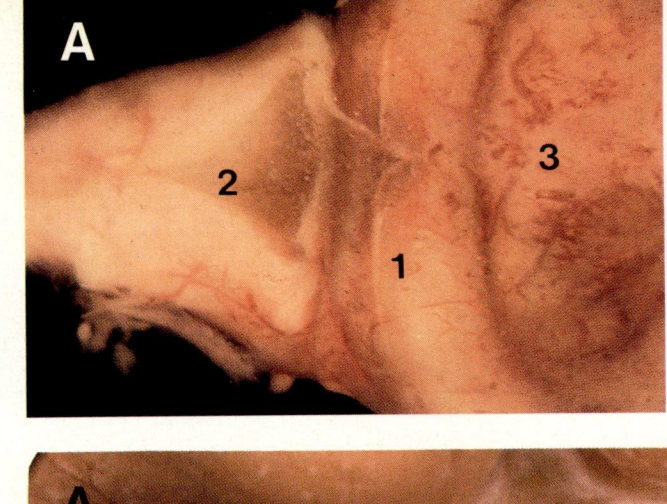

A. Week 10. The hindbrain and developing cerebellum. 57 mmCR ♂ (×7.8)

1. cerebellum
2. fourth ventricle with roof removed
3. mesencephalon

A. Week 15. The cerebellum. 123 mmCR ♀ (×5.6)

1. cerebellar hemisphere
2. colliculus facialis
3. culmen
4. flocculus
5. lobules of vermis
6. medulla oblongata
7. mesencephalon

A. Top: Week 16. (×0.9)
Bottom: Week 18.

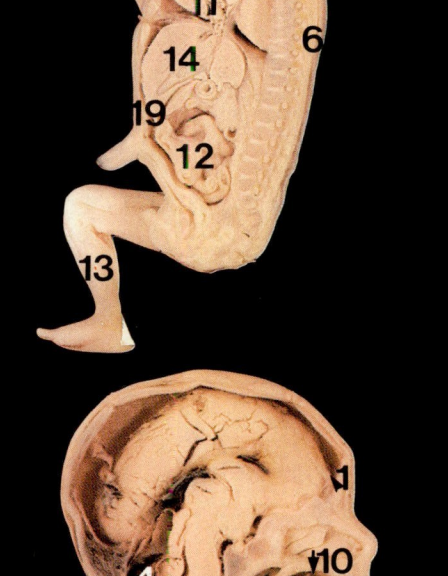

A–E. The development of the brain as seen in sagittal section.

1. anterior cranial fossa
2. arm
3. body of mandible
4. cerebellar fossa
5. confluence of sinuses
6. dorsal
7. dorsum of tongue
8. esophagus
9. falx cerebri
10. hard palate
11. heart
12. intestines
13. leg
14. liver
15. nose
16. pituitary gland
17. sella turcica
18. soft palate
19. ventral
20. vertebrae

A–E *from R.C.S.E.*

B. Week 19. The two halves of the same head. (×0.8)

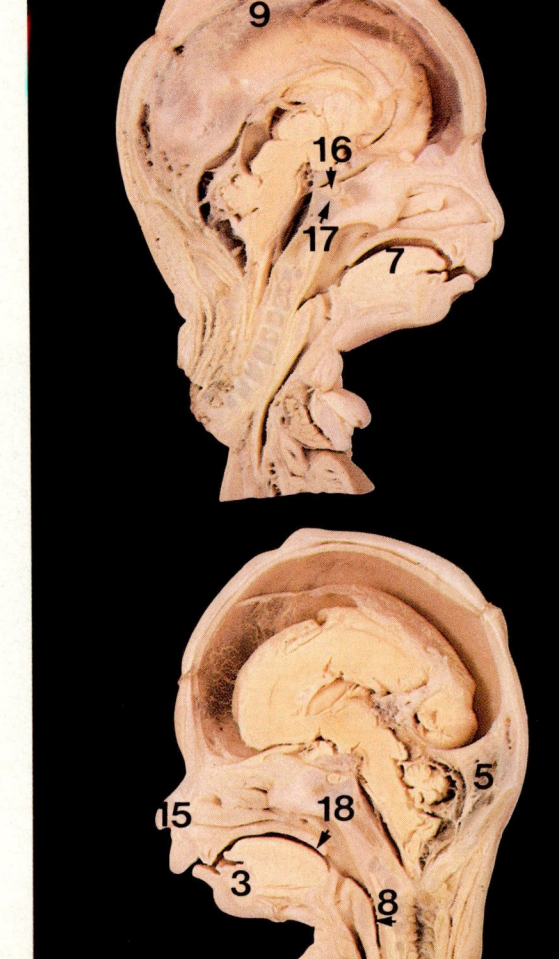

C. Week 19. (×0.7)

D. Week 19. A higher magnification of Figure **B**. (×1.2)

E. The same head as in Figure **B**. (×1)

1. anterior cranial fossa
2. arm
3. body of mandible
4. cerebellar fossa
5. confluence of sinuses
6. dorsal
7. dorsum of tongue
8. epiglottis
9. esophagus
10. falx cerebri
11. genioglossus muscle
12. geniohyoid muscle
13. hard palate
14. heart
15. intestines
16. leg
17. lip
18. liver
19. middle cranial fossa
20. mylohyoid muscle
21. nasal septum
22. nose
23. pituitary gland
24. posterior nasal aperture (choana)
25. sella turcica
26. soft palate
27. tentorium cerebelli
28. tongue
29. tracheal rings
30. ventral
31. vertebrae
32. vestibular fold
33. vocal fold

A. The cranial cavity of the neonate. The skull has been flattened slightly in handling. (×1.4)

From R.F.H.S.M.

Meninges

The meninges are formed when the mesoderm surrounding the neural tube condenses to form the primitive meninx. Dura mater forms from the outer layer of primitive meninx, the inner layer (pia-arachnoid) which may have neural crest contributions remains thin. Fluid filled spaces appearing within this layer coalesce and so form the subarachnoid space.

Choroid plexus

Pia mater and blood vessels invaginate the thin inner wall of the hemispheres and the thin thalamic and hindbrain grooves to form the choroid plexus of the lateral, third, and fourth ventricles (Horizon XIX, Day 38–40). These plexuses form CSF.

A–F. Development of the choroid plexus from Day 34 to Week 9.

1. arm bud
2. branchial arch
3. choroid plexus
4. eye
5. forebrain
6. hindbrain
7. leg bud
8. liver bulge
9. midbrain

A. Horizon XVII (Day 34–36). The hindbrain region. 12 mm CR (×8.1)

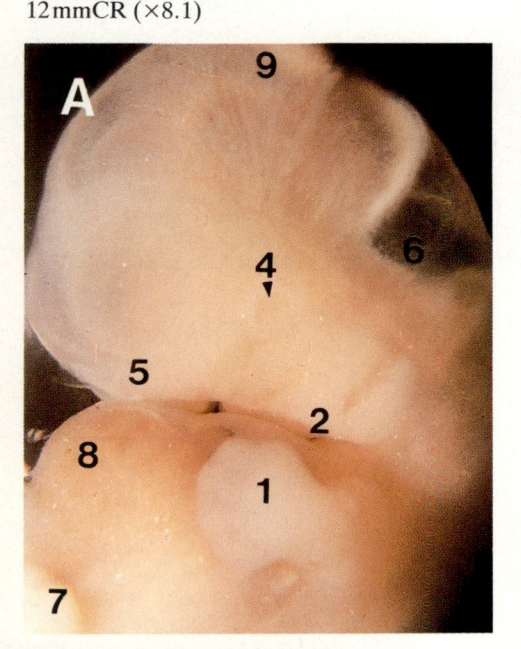

B. Horizon XIX (Day 38–40). The hindbrain region and the developing choroid plexus of the fourth ventricle. 20 mm CR (×5)

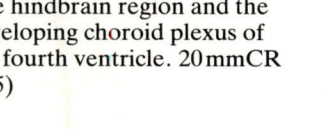

C. A higher magnification of Figure **B**. The hindbrain roof has been removed. (×15)

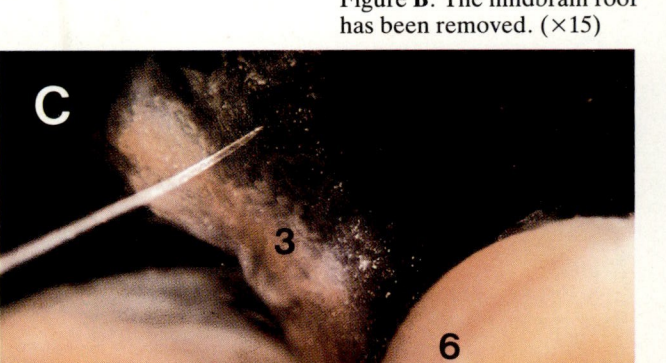

D. The developing choroid plexus of the cerebral vesicles. (×2.6)
Week 8. Small specimen. 34 mm CR
Week 10. Larger specimen. 57 mm CR ♂

1. choroid plexus
2. corpus striatum
3. forebrain
4. hindbrain
5. lateral lobe of cerebellum
6. midbrain
7. spinal cord

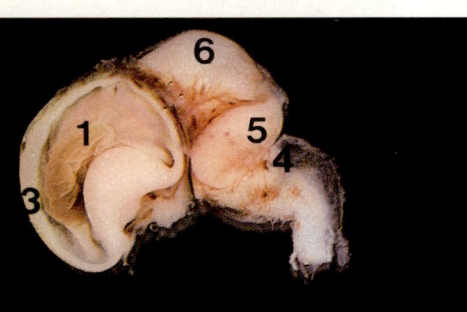

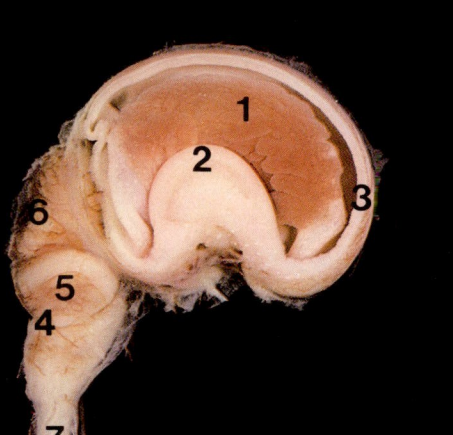

E. Week 9. Further development of the choroid plexus of the cerebral vesicles. 48 mm CR ♂ (×4.3)

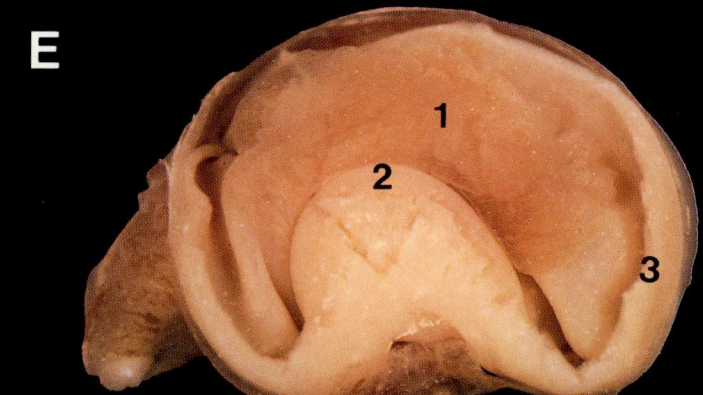

F. Week 9. Choroid plexus removed from specimen in Figure **E**. (×4.5)

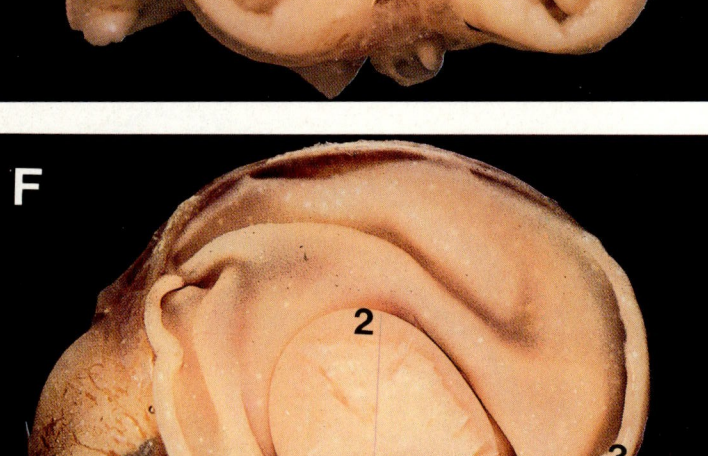

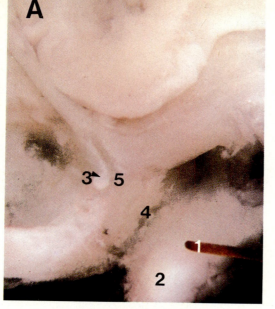

A. Horizon XVIII (Day 36–38). Neurohypophysis in sagittal section. 14mmCR (×17.7)

1. cactus needle
2. mandibular prominence
3. neurohypophysis
4. pharynx
5. Rathke's pouch

Pituitary gland (hypophysis)

The pituitary gland has dual origins: one part, the adenohypophysis, is an outpouching of the stomodeum (Rathke's pouch) and the other part is a diverticulum of the diencephalon called the neurohypophysis. At Horizon XI (Day 24) the pouch tissue enlarges and its connection with the mouth eventually atrophies (Week 9). Rathke's pouch forms the *pars distalis, pars tuberalis* and *pars intermedia*. The neurohypophysis and its cavity form the *pars nervosa*, the infundibular stem and median eminence.

During Week 9–17 the pituitary assumes its characteristic shape and histology.

At Week 9, gonadotrophins are produced by the fetal pituitary and at Week 10 the neurohypophysis produces small quantities of growth and lactogenic hormones. Between Week 8 and 9 adrenocorticotrophic hormone is released and thyrotrophic hormone is released by Week 19.

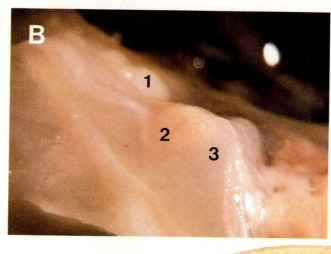

B. Week 13. The pituitary gland in the sella turcica. 95mmCR ♂ (×7.9)

1. middle cranial fossa
2. pituitary gland
3. sella turcica

C. The neonatal pituitary gland. (×1.1)

1. anterior cranial fossa
2. cerebellar fossa
3. epiglottis
4. hard palate
5. laryngopharynx
6. mandible
7. maxilla
8. middle cranial fossa
9. nasal conchae
10. nasopharynx
11. nose
12. oropharynx
13. pituitary gland
14. soft palate
15. tongue
16. vertebral column

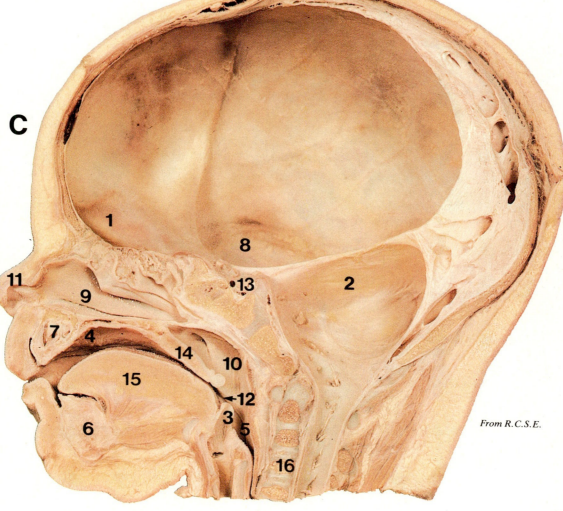

From R.C.S.E.

Eye

Facial development

One eye forms on each side of the head. They then move medially (Week 5–8) on to the front of the face so allowing for binocular vision in later life.

Eye formation

The optic vesicles are two lateral outgrowths of the forebrain (prosencephalic) with lumina at first continuous with the forebrain lumen. The proximal part constricts to form the optic stalk, while the distal portions (optic vesicle) form the retina, part of the iris and ciliary body. The optic bulb induces a lens placode in the head ectoderm and indents to form the optic cup. This indentation continues on to the inferior aspect of the optic stalk (fetal or choroidal fissure). The two layers of the optic cup appose and together form the retina. As these changes occur the lens placode sinks beneath the ectoderm, detaches and forms a hollow vesicle.

Vascular mesoderm enters the choroidal fissure and blood vessels grow from the proximal to the distal parts of the optic cup. In Week 7 the fetal fissure fuses and the blood vessels are incorporated into the optic stalk. These vessels form the hyaloid artery and vein which pass from the fissure to the lens. Distally they degenerate and disappear after Week 31, proximally they persist as the central artery and vein of the retina.

Lens

The lens begins as a hollow vesicle in which the posterior wall cells hypertrophy and eventually obliterate the cavity. The anterior wall cells persist as a cuboidal anterior lens epithelium. The hypertrophied cells form lens fibers. New lens fibers are added to the mature lens by the equatorial cells. The lens capsule is produced by the underlying epithelial cells.

Retina

The retina forms from the two apposed layers of the optic cup. The outer layer forms the pigmented layer of the retina (Horizon XVI, Day 32–34); the inner layer forms the other layers of the retina. Differentiation is confined to the cells in the caudal part of the cup (pars optica) which form three zones: ependymal, mantle and marginal.

The ependymal zone gives rise to the mantle neuroblasts which form two layers: an outer which forms the bipolar cell layer and possibly the rods and cones, and an inner which forms the ganglion cells which give rise to the optic nerve. The optic nerve cell axons converge on to the future optic disc region, then change direction to grow centripetally in the marginal zone of the optic stalk. Eventually the stalk lumen disappears. Spongioblasts of the cup give rise to the retinal neuroglia (Muller's fibers).

The inner margin of the optic cup does not differentiate in this manner. The inner layer remains single and together with the single cell layer of the outer cup forms first the pars caeca retinae, and later the adult pars iridica retinae, and the pars ciliaris retinae, the posterior epithelial components of the iris and ciliary body.

Choroid, sclera and cornea

Mesoderm surrounding the optic cup gives rise to the choroid and dura mater of the optic nerve, the sclera, and the substantia propria corneae. The stratified squamous corneal epithelium forms from surface ectoderm.

Iris

Mesoderm immediately anterior to the developing lens gives rise to the pupillary membrane, whose peripheral part together with the pars iridica retinae form the iris. The dilator and sphincter pupillae muscles differentiate in situ. The centre of the pupillary membrane degenerates to form the pupil.

The anterior chamber forms in the mesoderm between the lens and substantia propria of the cornea. The posterior chamber is an extension of the anterior chamber.

Lacrimal glands

Ectodermal buds from the conjunctival sac branch, canalize, and form the ducts and alveoli during Week 8.

Nasolacrimal duct

The nasolacrimal duct forms from an ectodermal cord along a line where the frontonasal and maxillary processes meet. The cord later canalizes.

Eyelids

The eyelids are mesodermal folds covered with ectoderm which first appear above and below the lens placode and grow toward each other. They fuse at Week 9 to 10 and remain fused until Week 25 to 26. The mesodermal fold gives rise to the tarsal plate and musculature; the ectodermal covering gives rise to the tarsal glands and eyelashes.

● Myelination of the optic nerve occurs mainly in the first three weeks after birth.

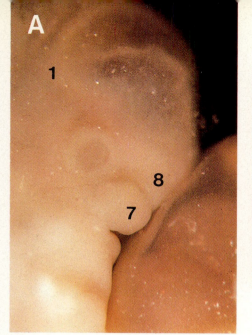

A

1

8

7

A. Horizon XVII (Day 34–36). Viewed from the side. 12 mmCR (×34)

B. Horizon XVIII (Day 36–38). Viewed from the side. 14 mmCR (×16.2)

C. Horizon XIX (Day 38–40). Viewed from the side. 20 mmCR (×16.2)

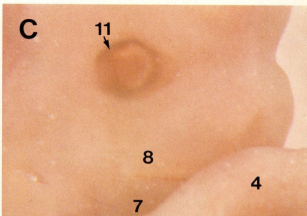

B

11

6

8

7

C

11

8

7

4

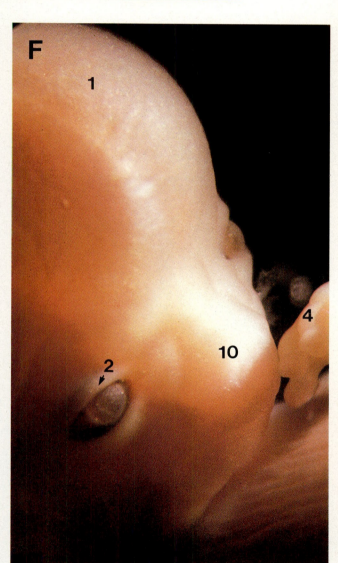

F

1

4

10

2

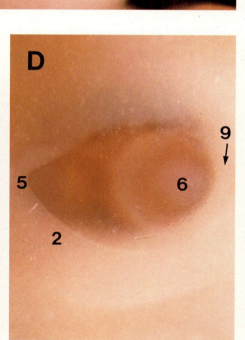

D

9

5

6

2

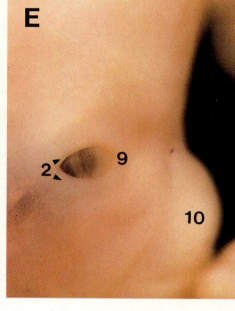

E

2

9

10

D. Horizon XXII (Day 44–46). Viewed from the side. 25 mmCR (×34)

E. Horizon XXII (Day 44–46). Viewed from the side. 27 mmCR (×16)

H. Week 9. Viewed from the front. 48 mmCR (×8)

F. Horizon XXII (Day 44–46). Viewed from the side. 27 mmCR (×12)

A–I. Development of the eyelids from Day 34 to Week 15.

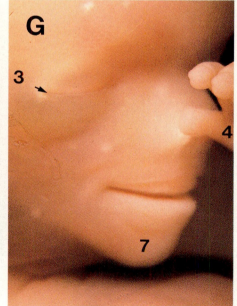

G

3

4

7

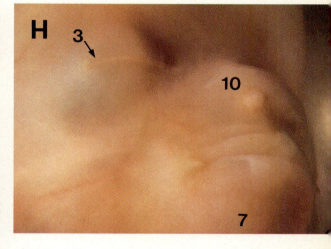

H

3

10

7

G. Week 9. Viewed from the front. 46 mmCR (×8)

I. Week 15. Viewed from the front. 130 mmCR ♀ (×4.1)

I

3

5

9

1. brain
2. eyelid
3. fused eyelids
4. hand
5. lateral angle (outer canthus)
6. lens
7. mandible
8. maxilla
9. medial angle (inner canthus)
10. nose
11. pigment

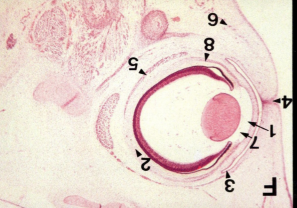

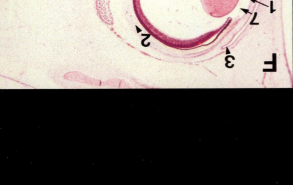

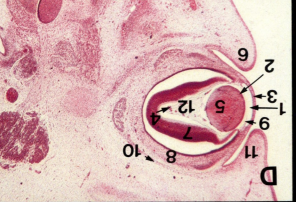

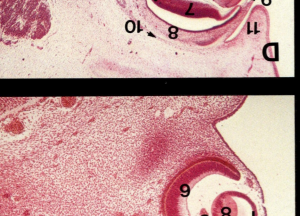

A–F. Coronal sections of the developing eye from Horizon XVI (Day 32–34) to Week 8.

A. Horizon XVI (Day 32–34). 10 mm CR (×60)
1. anterior lens cells
2. fetal fissure
3. hyaloid artery
4. optic cup
5. posterior lens cells

B. Horizon XVII (Day 34–36). 12 mm CR (×60)
1. anterior lens cells
2. corneal ectoderm
3. corneal mesoderm
4. fetal fissure
5. hyaloid artery
6. optic cup: inner layer
7. optic cup: outer layer
8. posterior lens cells

C. Horizon XVII (Day 34–36). The other eye as in Figure B. 12 mm CR (×60)

D. Horizon XXII (Day 44–46). 25 mm CR (×17.5)
1. anterior chamber
2. anterior lens epithelium
3. cornea
4. hyaloid artery
5. lens
6. lower eyelid
7. optic cup: inner layer
8. optic cup: outer layer
9. pupillary membrane
10. sclera
11. upper eyelid
12. vitreous

E. Horizon XXIII (Day 46–48). The width of the intraretinal space is exaggerated. 30 mm CR (×17.5)
1. anterior chamber
2. conjunctival sac
3. intraretinal space
4. lens
5. vitreous

F. Week 8. The eyelids have fused. 40 mm CR (×15)
1. anterior chamber
2. choroid
3. conjunctival sac
4. fused eyelids
5. inferior rectus muscle
6. orbicularis oculi muscle
7. pupillary membrane
8. sclera

A–F from C.H.M.S.

Spinal cord

The walls of the neural tube are composed of neuroepithelium which forms three regions; an inner ependymal zone, a mantle zone and an outer marginal zone. The ependymal layer gives rise to all the spinal cord neurons and macroglial cells. These pass into the mantle layer and differentiate into neuroblasts and supporting cells so forming the gray matter. The mantle layer sends axons into the outer marginal zone which forms the white matter of the cord which contains no cell bodies, only afferent and efferent nerve fibers.

The neuroepithelial cells initially produce neuroblasts, then glioblasts, and finally differentiate into ependymal cells.

As the neuroepithelial cells proliferate and differentiate the lateral walls of the neural tube thicken until the spinal cord has thin roof and floor plates and a small central canal. Each lateral wall is divided by the *sulcus limitans* into two halves, the dorsal alar and ventral basal lamina. The alar lamina with the neural crest will form the sensory apparatus (dorsal or posterior horn) and its associated structures, while the basal lamina will form the motor apparatus (ventral or anterior horn). The two sides of the cord are separated by the dorsal septum and the ventral median fissure and septum.

Microglial cells form from mesoderm surrounding the neural tube.

Spinal nerves: dorsal root

Dorsal root ganglia, containing the primary sensory neurons, form from segmental aggregations of neural crest cells. The dorsal root itself consists of processes from these cells extending peripherally (towards sensory receptors) and centrally into the dorsal horn.

Spinal nerves: ventral root

Cell axons grow out from the ventral (anterior) horn of gray matter to each somite.

Tracts

The marginal layer becomes thickened by the development of longitudinally running bundles of nerve fibers (tracts). The first to form are short intersegmental tracts (fasciculi proprii) later followed by the major ascending and descending pathways connecting the spinal cord with the brain.

Spinal cord levels

In the embryo the spinal cord and its associated nerves are present throughout the length of the embryo at Week 8. As the spinal cord grows more slowly than the dura mater and vertebral column, the caudal end of the cord comes to lie at higher vertebral levels. By Week 24 the tip of the cord lies at S1, while in the neonate it is at L3. As these levels are reached, the spinal nerves run obliquely towards the intervertebral foramina to leave the vertebral column. The dura mater extends the – length of the vertebral column, while the pia mater forms the *filum terminale* as the cord retreats.

Myelination begins at about Week 17–20 and continues until age of 1 year.

● In the adult the spinal cord ends at the lower border of L1. The changes in level should be considered when performing a lumbar puncture on a child.

A. Week 13. Sagittal (longitudinal) section of the thoracic spinal cord. 95 mmCR ♂ (×6.8)

1. dorsal body wall
2. lamina of vertebra
3. spinal cord
4. vertebral body

B. Week 11. Transverse section of developing lower sacral spinal cord. 65 mmCR (×19)

1. central canal
2. centrum
3. dorsal horn
4. dorsal nerve root
5. dorsal root ganglion
6. dorsal septum
7. ependymal layer
8. marginal zone
9. neural arch
10. ventral horn
11. ventral median fissure

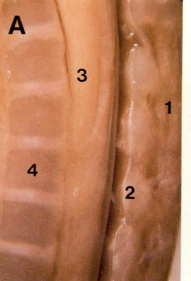

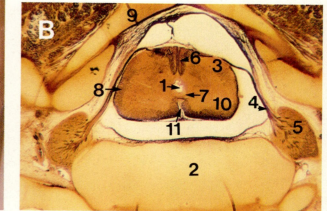

From C.C.H.M.S.

C. Week 24. The spinal cord no longer occupies the total length of the canal. Exposed from behind. (×1.3)

1. cervical enlargement
2. head
3. lumbar enlargement
4. ribs
5. spinal cord
6. spinal nerve

From R.F.H.S.M.

Peripheral nervous system

During Week 5 peripheral nerves grow into the upper and lower limb buds and into the trunk. Dermatomes, or areas of skin supplied by a single spinal nerve and its dorsal root ganglion, are distributed in segmental bands to supply both dorsal and ventral limb surfaces. These patterns are altered as the limbs grow and rotate, but remain relatively unaltered in the trunk.

Autonomic ganglion cells arise from the neural crest. In the case of the sympathetic system the ganglion cells pass through an intermediate stage in the spinal ganglia then migrate ventrally. Some come to lie alongside the aorta forming the ganglia of the sympathetic trunk. Initially this exists only in the thoracic and upper lumbar regions but later extends cranially and caudally. Some neural crest cells migrate more extensively and form collateral ganglia such as the celiac and superior mesenteric and the chromaffin cells of the adrenal medulla.

The parasympathetic (craniosacral) ganglia are derived from neural crest in the appropriate regions, along with sensory cranial nerve ganglia such as the trigeminal and facial ganglia.

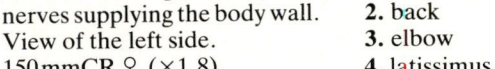

A. Week 18. Segmental spinal nerves supplying the body wall. View of the left side. 150 mm CR ♀ (×1.8)

1. abdomen
2. back
3. elbow
4. latissimus dorsi muscle (position)
5. leg (left)
6. segmental spinal nerves
7. serratus anterior muscle (position)

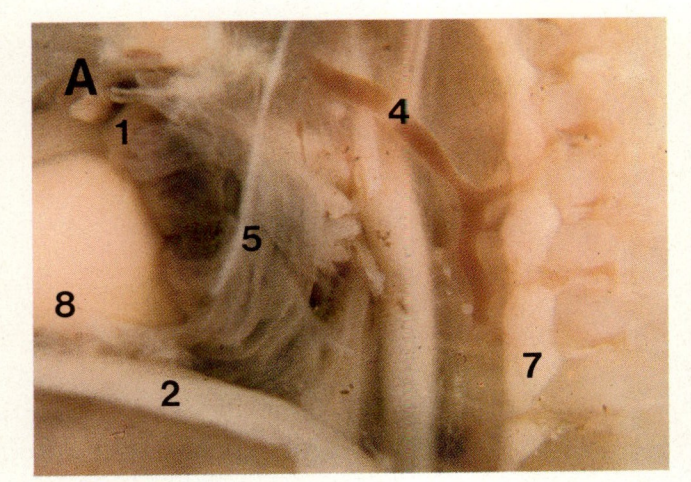

A. 56 mm CR (×7.8)

B. 56 mm CR (×16.8)

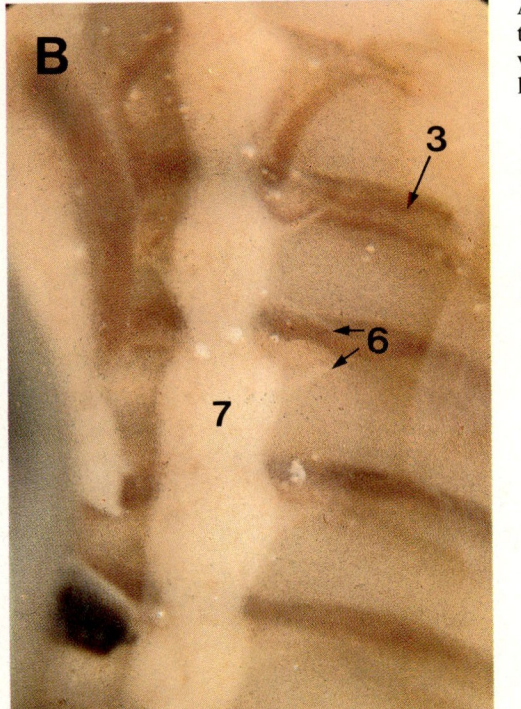

A and B. Week 10. The thoracic sympathetic trunk viewed from the left side. The left lung has been removed.

1. auricle of heart
2. diaphragm
3. intercostal vessels
4. left superior intercostal vein
5. pericardium (reflected)
6. rami communicantes
7. sympathetic trunk
8. ventricle of heart

Face development

The face develops over a period of time. Initially the eyes are on the sides of the head, the nostrils are widely separated, the nose flattened, and the ears on the side of the neck.

The face forms as a result of changes in relative position and proportion. The eyes move medially on the face, the nostrils move medially and the ears rise on to the head (see Face profile).

A–L. Development of the face from Day 36 to Week 18.

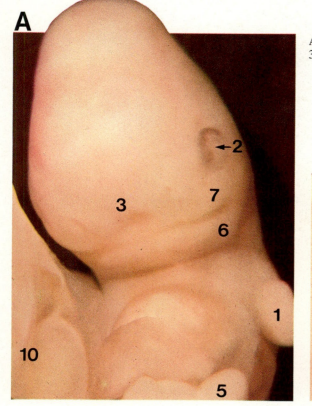

A. Horizon XVIII (Day 36–38). 14 mmCR (×8)

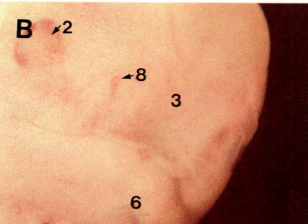

B. Horizon XVIII (Day 36–38). 14 mmCR (×15.6)

1. arm
2. eye
3. frontonasal process
4. hand
5. leg
6. mandibular prominence
7. maxillary prominence
8. nasal pit
9. nostril
10. umbilical cord

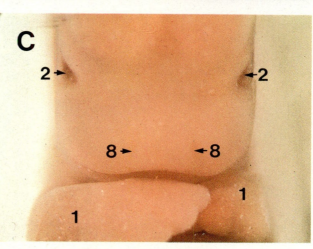

C. Horizon XIX (Day 38–40). 20 mmCR (×15.6)

D. Horizon XIX (Day 38–40). 20 mmCR (×15.6)

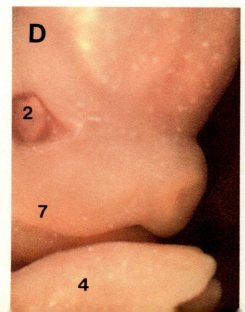

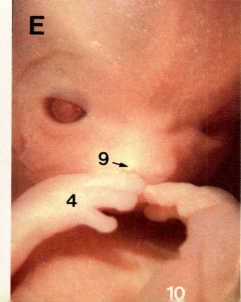

E. Horizon XXII (Day 44–46). 27 mmCR (×7.8)

71

10

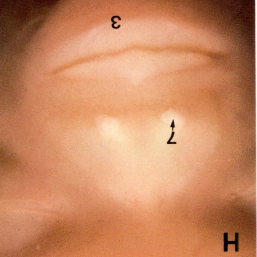
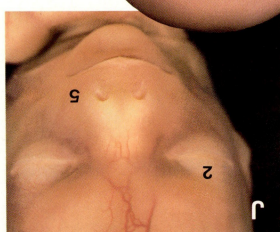
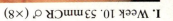
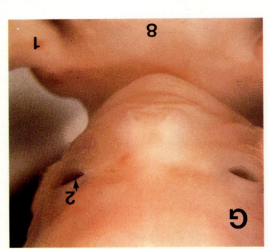
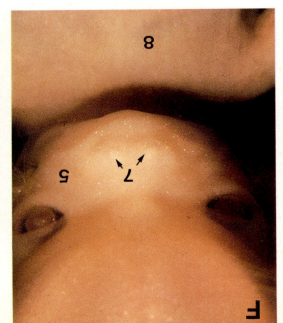

L. Week 18. 160mmCR♀ (×1.2)

K. Week 18. 152mmCR♂ (×1.6)

J. Week 12. 85mmCR♂ (×2.6)

I. Week 10. 53mmCR♂ (×8)

1. arm
2. eye
3. lips
4. mandible
5. maxilla
6. nose
7. nostril
8. thorax

H. Week 9. 48mmCR♀ (×9)

G. Week 8. 32mmCR (×4.8)

F. A further view of the face in Figure E. (×9)

Nose

At Week 5 the embryo's eyes are on either side of the head. The nasal placodes are well separated on the front of the face and sinking into the underlying mesoderm to form the nasal pits. The pits are partly on the face and partly in the stomodeum.

The pits or nostrils are blind sacs directed caudally. The extent of the pit is reflected on the surface by the position of the nasal fin.

During Week 6 the nostrils move toward one another on the face and the medial nasal prominences fuse with the maxillary prominences to form the intermaxillary segment which gives rise to the philtrum of the lip, middle portion of the upper jaw and primary palate. The frontonasal process forms the forehead, bridge and apex of the adult nose and the lateral nasal prominences the alae of the adult nose. Ectoderm in the floor of the nasolacrimal groove between the lateral nasal prominence and maxillary prominences forms the nasolacrimal duct.

The nasal fin on the face breaks down and the mesoderm cells of the maxillary prominences and medial nasal prominence fuse. The nerve supplies grow across the fusion.

The caudal part of the fin remains attached to the roof of the stomodeum and, as the blind end of the nostril grows rapidly inward on either side of the mid-line, the nasal fin becomes short and stretched. The stretched membrane called the oronasal membrane breaks down and connects the blind tubes of the nostrils (the nasal cavity) with the stomodeum. The opening is called the primitive choana (naris). The sheet of mesoderm left hanging between the two posterior primitive choanae is called the nasal septum and it is in contact with the dorsum of the tongue.

Projections of the lateral walls form the inferior, middle and superior conchae. The ectodermal roof of each nasal cavity forms the olfactory region some of whose cells form olfactory cells whose nerve fibers grow into the olfactory bulb through the cribriform plate of the ethmoid bone.

● If fusion is incomplete (hare lip) the maxillary division of the trigeminal nerve is unable to spread to the philtrum of the lip. Instead the ophthalmic division enters the philtrum from above.

● The neonate breathes primarily through the nose and will only breathe through the mouth when nasal obstruction produces stress.

A–N. Development of the nose from a nasal pit to nostril.

1. eye
2. forehead
3. frontonasal process
4. lateral nasal prominence (alar process)
5. mandibular prominence
6. maxillary prominence
7. medial nasal prominence
8. nasal fin
9. racket-shaped nasal pit
10. stomodeum
11. thorax

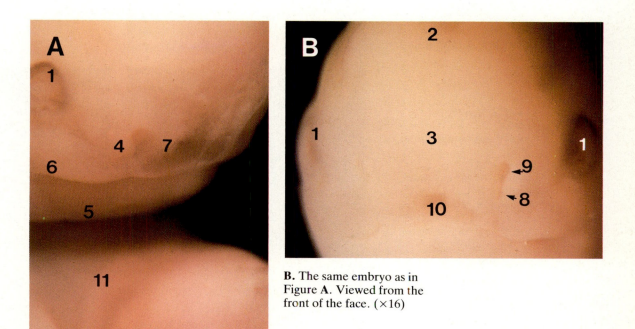

A. Horizon XVIII (Day 36–38). The nasal pits are widely separated on the developing face. Viewed from the right side and front. 14mmCR (×16)

B. The same embryo as in Figure **A**. Viewed from the front of the face. (×16)

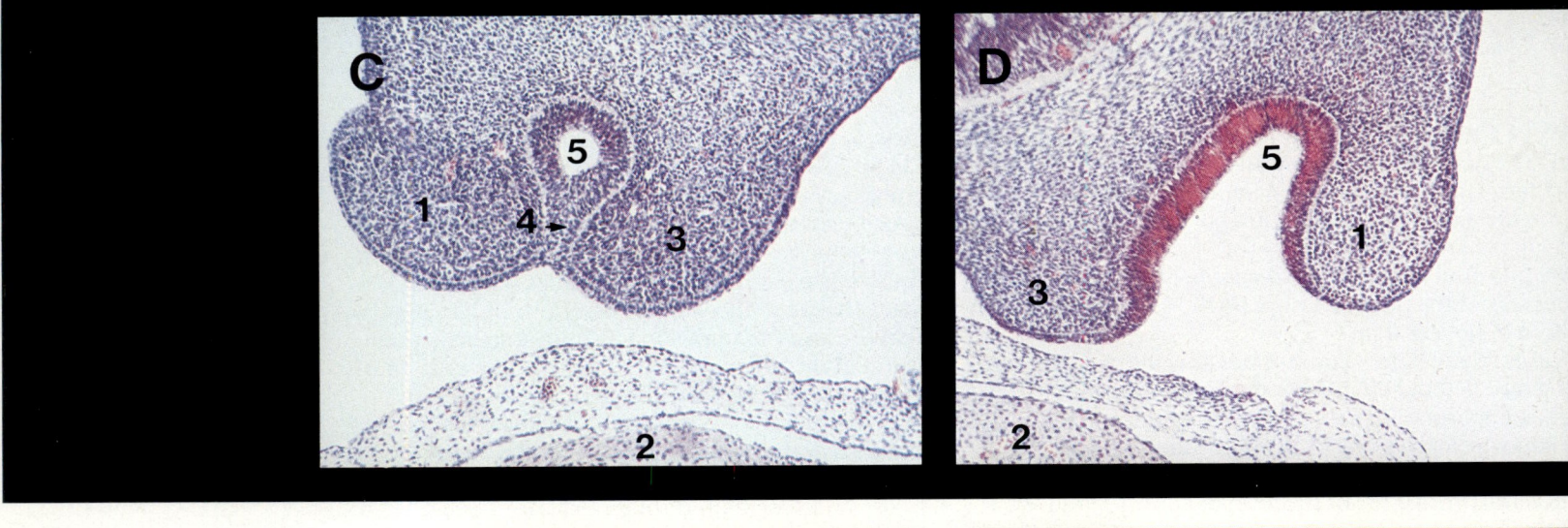

C. Horizon XVI (Day 32–34). Transverse paraffin wax section through the developing nasal pit which ends as a blind sac. 10mmCR (×167)

D. Section posterior to that shown in Figure C. (×167)

1. lateral nasal prominence (alar process)
2. heart
3. medial nasal prominence
4. nostril
5. nasal pit

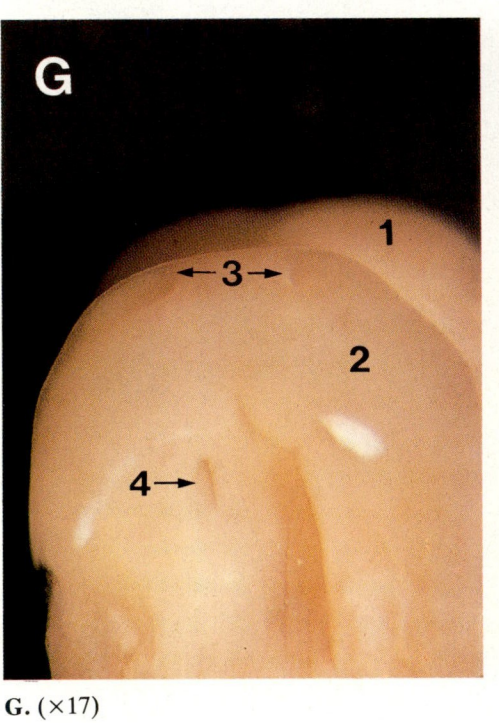

E. Horizon XIX (Day 38–40). Embryo viewed from the front of the face. The eyes and nostrils are still widely separated, but have moved toward the front and mid-line of the face. 20mmCR (×17)

1. eye
2. forebrain
3. hand paddle
4. maxillary prominence
5. nostril

F. Higher magnification of the embryo in Figure E. (×34)

G and H. The roof of the stomodeum (oral cavity) of the embryo shown in Figure E.

1. forehead
2. maxillary prominence
3. nostril
4. posterior choana (naris)

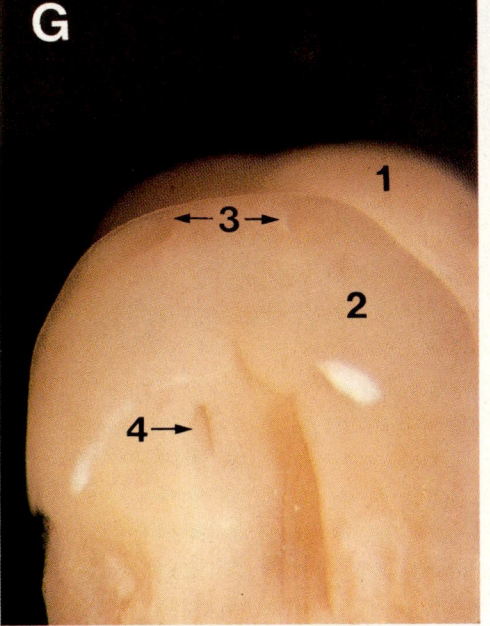

G. (×17)

H. (×34)

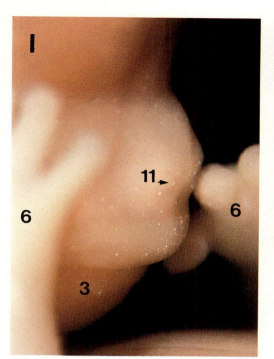

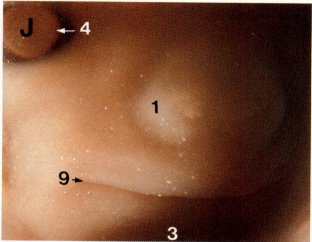

I. Horizon XXII (Day 44–46). The developing nostril in profile. Note the plugged nostril. 27 mmCR (×17)

J. Same embryo as in Figure **I**. Viewed from the front and right side. (×17)

1. alae
2. bridge of the nose
3. chin
4. eye
5. forehead
6. hand
7. lanugo hair
8. lip
9. mouth
10. nose
11. nostril
12. palate
13. philtrum of the lip
14. plug in the nostril

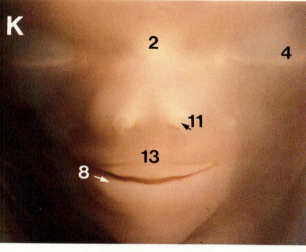

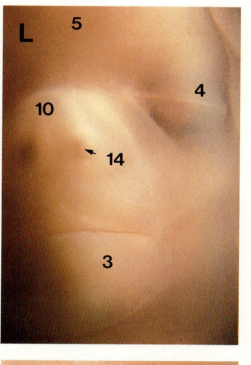

K. Week 9. Viewed from the front. The nostrils are widely separated and directed forward. 46 mmCR (×8)

L. Week 10. Viewed from the front. 53 mmCR ♂ (×8)

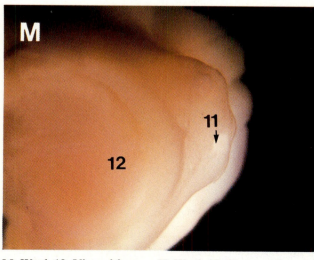

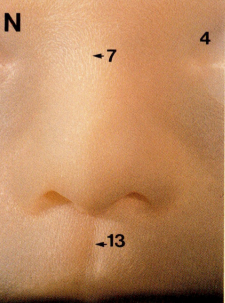

M. Week 10. Viewed from below. 60 mmCR ♀ (×8)

N. Week 15. The nostrils are pointed downward. 130 mmCR ♀ (×4.1)

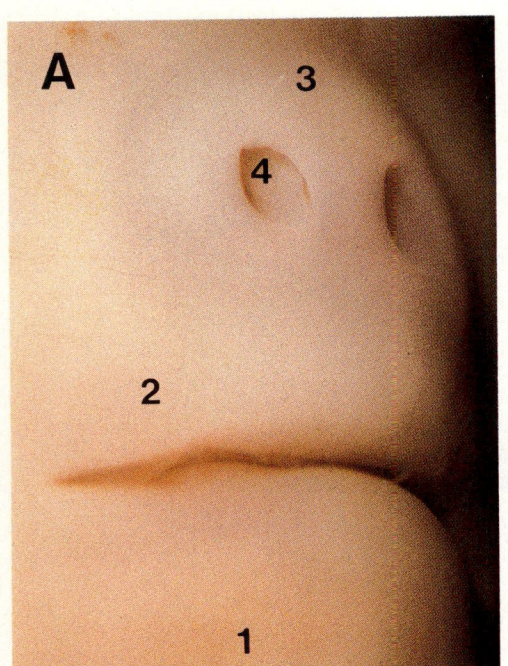

A. Week 9. Fetus with the plugs washed from the developing nostril. 41 mm CR (×17)

1. mandible
2. maxilla
3. nose
4. nostril

A. Week 18. A hemisection (sagittal) of the head. The black thread through the nostril marks the extent of the nasopharynx. (×1.3)

1. cranial fossa (middle)
2. diaphragm
3. heart
4. mandible
5. nose
6. nasopharynx
7. spinal cord
8. sternum
9. thymus
10. tongue
11. vertebrae

From R.C.S.E.

A. Week 13. The normal sensory distribution of the trigeminal nerve on the face. 92 mm CR ♀ (×3.2)

1. maxillary division
2. mandibular division
3. ophthalmic division

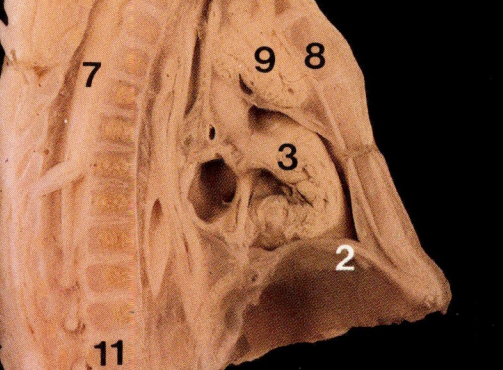

A. Horizon XVII (Day 34–36). 12 mm CR (×7.5)

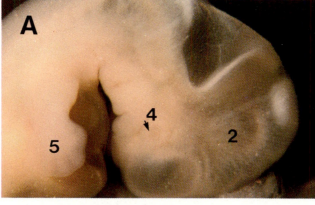

B. Horizon XVIII (Day 36–38). 14 mm CR (×7.2)

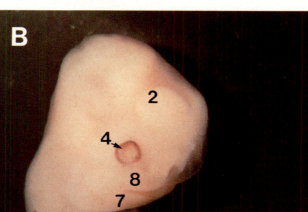

C. Horizon XIX (Day 38–40). 20 mm CR (×7.2)

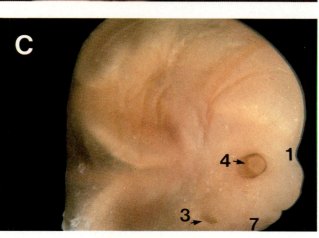

Face profile

The profile changes dramatically; originally the forehead dominates the face (Horizon XVI, Day 32–34) and the mandible is more advanced in development than the maxilla. The nose and maxilla then grow rapidly (Horizon XIX, Day 38–40) and the mandible lags behind so the embryo lacks a well developed chin and its face has a simian appearance.

During Week 8–12 the mandible grows rapidly, and the deep indentation between the nose and forehead is lost as the bridge of the nose is elevated. The nostrils which were widely separated and directed forward are then pointed downward.

A–K. The developing profile of the face.

1. bridge of the nose
2. brain
3. ear
4. eye
5. hand
6. lips
7. mandible
8. maxilla
9. nose
10. nostril

D. Week 8. 34 mm CR (×9.3)

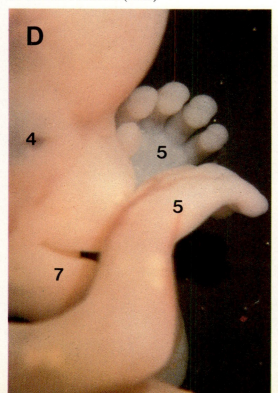

E. Week 9. 43 mm CR (×9.3)

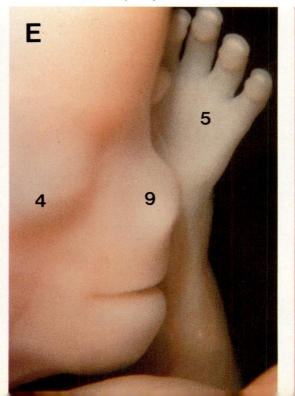

F. Week 9. 48 mm CR ♀ (×9.3)

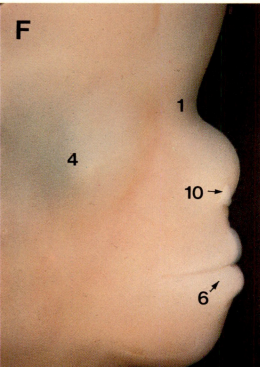

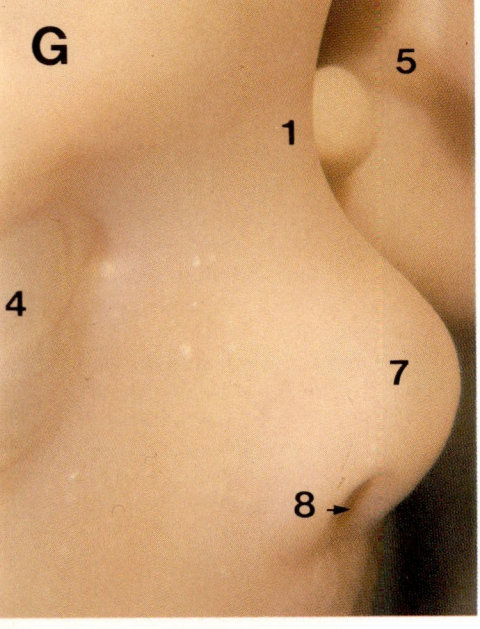

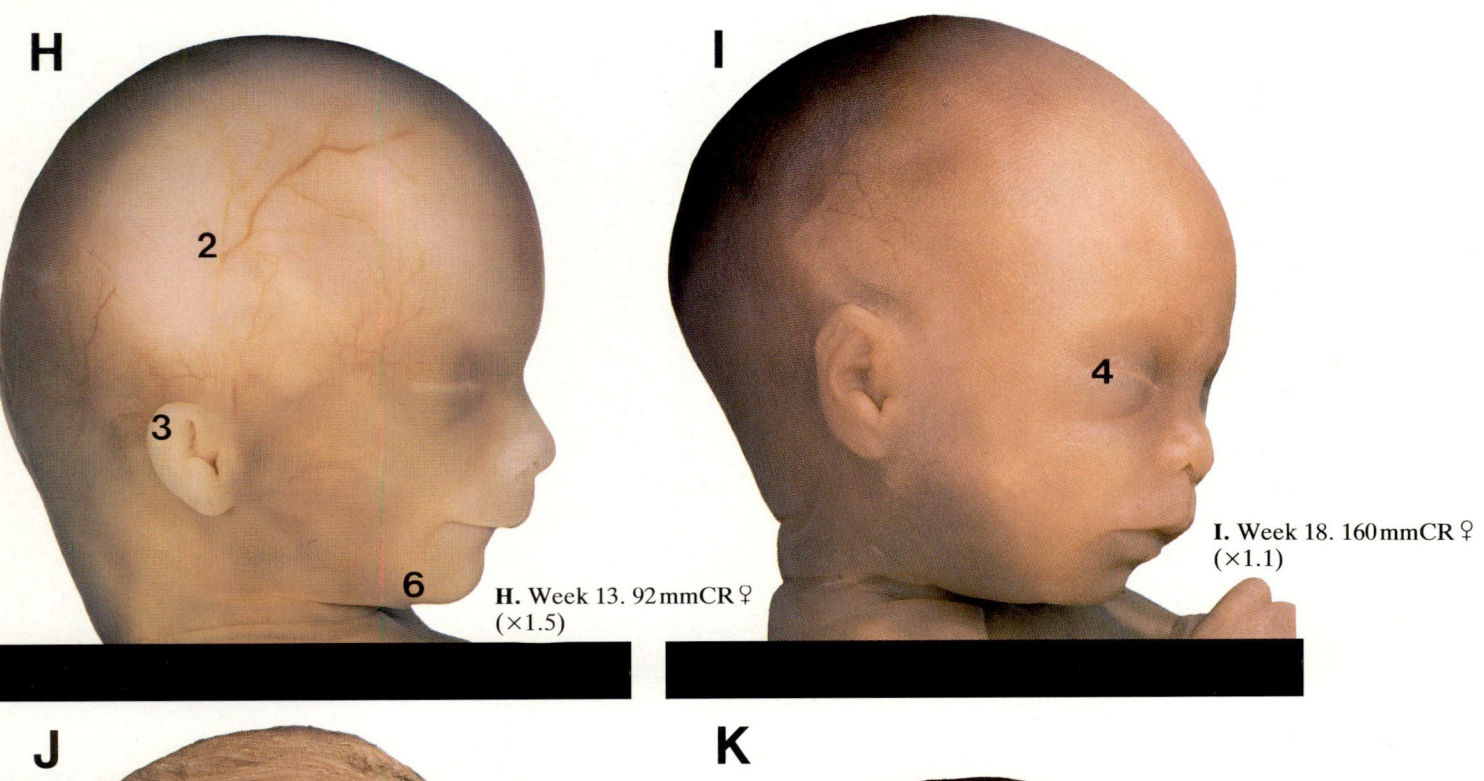

G. Week 12. 85 mmCR ♂
(×8.3)

1. bridge of nose
2. brain
3. ear
4. eye
5. hand
6. mandible
7. nose
8. nostril

H. Week 13. 92 mmCR ♀
(×1.5)

I. Week 18. 160 mmCR ♀
(×1.1)

J. Week 24. 228 mmCR
♂ (×0.8)

K. The profile of the neonate.
(×0.7)

From R.C.S.E.

Mandible and maxilla

The first branchial arch on each side of the head divides into two processes; maxillary and mandibular prominences which grow toward the mid-line. The two mandibular prominences (processes) fuse first (Week 4) and the maxillary processes fuse with the frontonasal process in Week 6 and 7. The outer corners of the mouth are defined by Week 5 and this broad mouth opening is later reduced during Week 6 to 6½ by the lips fusing laterally at the corners. The cheeks then form. The labial and buccal muscles form from the second branchial arch mesoderm.

Meckel's cartilage forms by Day 28 from the first arch and serves as 'scaffolding' for the membrane bone of the mandible. Neural crest cells in the arches form skeletal and connective tissue of the lower face and anterior neck.

The primitive mouth is an ectoderm-lined depression (stomodeum) separated from the foregut by the oral (buccopharyngeal) membrane. In Week 4 the oral membrane ruptures and the foregut communicates with the amniotic cavity.

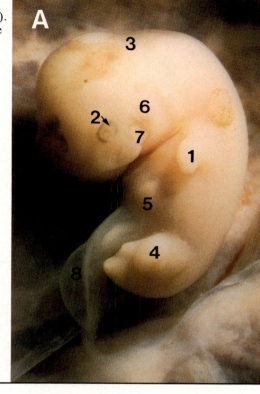

A. Horizon XVII (Day 34–36). The mandible and maxilla are represented by two arch prominences from the first branchial arch. 12 mmCR (×5.9)

1. arm bud (left)
2. eye
3. hindbrain
4. leg bud
5. liver bulge
6. mandibular prominence (process)
7. maxillary prominence (process)
8. umbilical cord

A–G. Development of the mandible and maxilla.

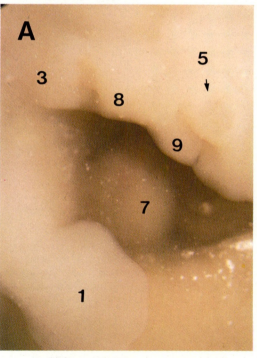

A. Horizon XVII (Day 34–36). View from the right side. 12 mmCR (×17)

1. arm bud (right)
2. brain
3. branchial arch
4. buccopharyngeal membrane
5. eye
6. frontonasal process
7. heart
8. mandibular process
9. maxillary prominence (process)

B. Horizon XVIII (Day 36–38). View from the front. 14 mmCR (×17)

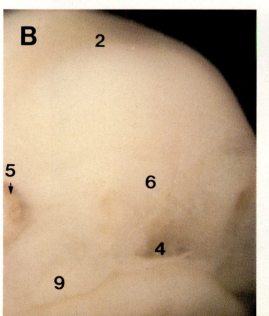

C. Horizon XVIII (Day 36–38). A hemisection of the head. View from the medial surface. 14 mmCR (×9)

1. buccopharyngeal membrane
2. forebrain
3. hindbrain
4. mandibular prominence (process)
5. pharynx

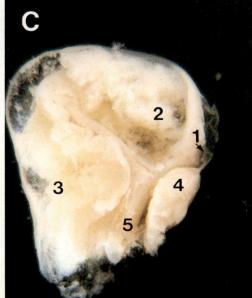

D. Horizon XIX (Day 38–40). View from the front. The maxillary prominences (processes) and frontonasal process have fused to form the maxilla. Note the wide mouth and the eyes still placed on either side of the head. 20 mm CR (×18)

1. angle of mouth
2. eye
3. mandibular prominence
4. maxillary prominence
5. thorax

E. Horizon XXII (Day 44–46). View from the right side. Note the angles of the mouth are fusing to form a less broad mouth. 27 mm CR (×9)

1. angle of mouth
2. arm
3. eye (right)
4. hand
5. mandible
6. maxilla
7. ribs

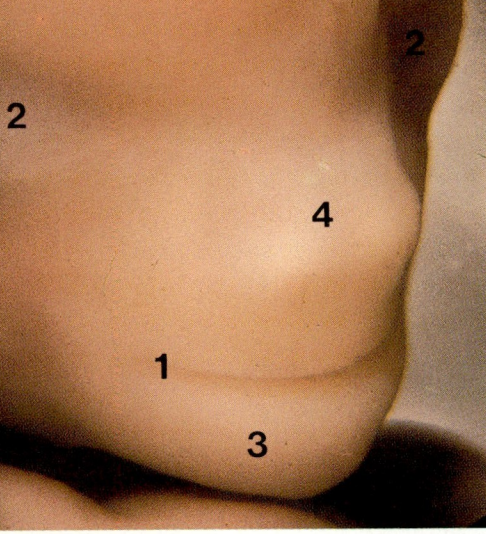

F. Week 9. View from the right and front of the fetus. Note the eyes and nose are not yet in their final positions on the face. 43 mm CR (×9)

1. angle of mouth
2. eye
3. mandible
4. nose

G. Week 8. The skin has been removed from the mandible to illustrate the developing bone. Viewed from the right side. 40 mm CR (×18)

1. chin
2. lip
3. mandible

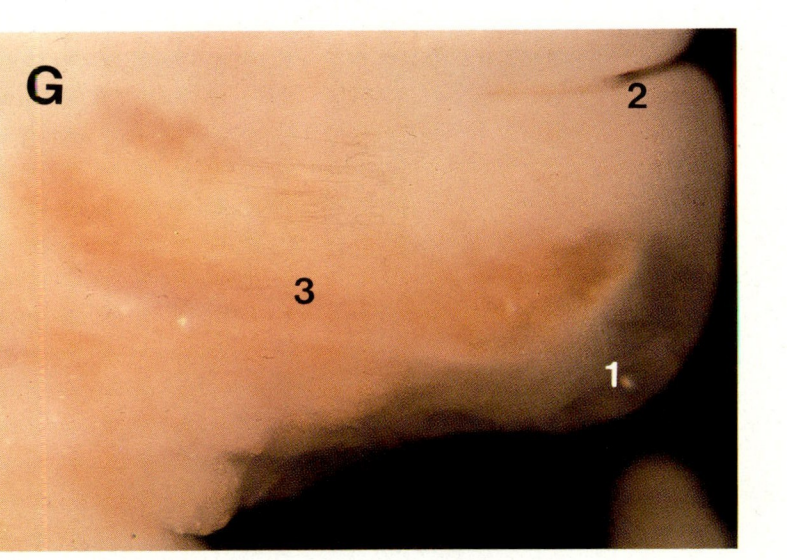

Lips and teeth

The early mouth is bounded by the fused mandibular processes and the fused maxillary and medial nasal processes. These boundaries divide (Week 6–10) into the lips (labia) and gums (gingiva). In Week 6 an ectodermal thickening, the dental lamina, grows into the underlying mesoderm. A second ectodermal thickening, the labio-gingival lamina grows into the mesoderm between the dental lamina and the future lip. As the teeth develop the labio-gingival lamina degenerates and leaves a groove which deepens and separates the lips, cheeks and gums. One small area does not completely degenerate and forms the mid-line frenulum attaching the upper lip to the gingiva.

The dental laminae in each jaw form ten oval buds which will form the enamel organ primordia of the deciduous teeth (milk teeth). These are followed at Week 10 by the first permanent teeth buds which form lingual to the deciduous teeth. The laminae then disappear.

Based on their appearance the tooth buds progress through a cap stage and finally a bell stage.

Early in Week 7 the gum mesoderm deep to the enamel organ condenses to form a dental papilla (cap stage). The dental papilla will give rise to the dentine and pulp.

In the bell stage, the dental papilla mesoderm differentiates into dentine forming odontoblasts. The earliest dentine formed is the outermost layer until the papilla is reduced and the remaining mesoderm cells form the pulp. Odontoblast processes remaining in the dentine are called Tomes' dentinal fibers. Mesoderm surrounding the enamel organ and dental papilla condenses and will form cementum and the peridontal ligament. By Week 14 cells of the inner part of the enamel organ differentiate into ameloblasts and form enamel, the deepest layer being the first to be laid down. Enamel is laid down at the cusp first and progresses toward the root as does dentine formation. The root is formed as the enamel epithelium (epithelial root sheath) grows into adjacent mesoderm. Odontoblasts within the sheath form dentine continuous with the crown.

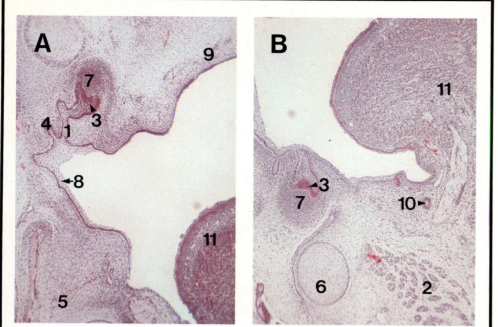

A. (×80)

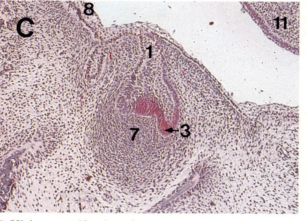

B. (×80)

C. Higher magnification of Figure **B**. (×155)

A–C. Week 8. Coronal sections of cap stages of tooth development. 32 mmCR

1. dental ledge
2. developing muscles
3. enamel organ of milk teeth (deciduous teeth)
4. labiogingival lamina
5. mandible
6. Meckel's cartilage
7. mesodermal pulp primordium (dental papilla)
8. oral epithelium
9. palate
10. submandibular duct
11. tongue

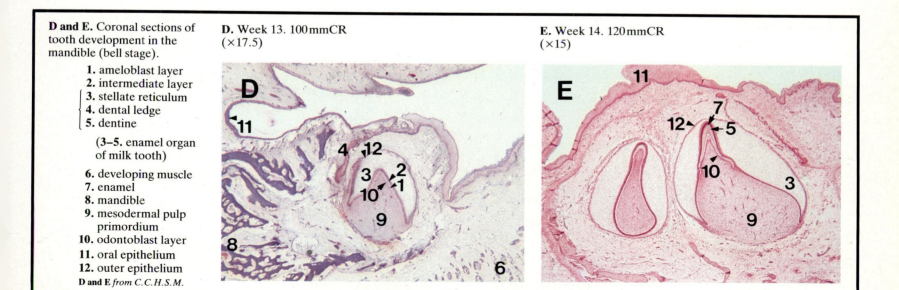

D and E. Coronal sections of tooth development in the mandible (bell stage).

1. ameloblast layer
2. intermediate layer
3. stellate reticulum
4. dental ledge
5. dentine

   (3–5. enamel organ of milk tooth)

6. developing muscle
7. enamel
8. mandible
9. mesodermal pulp primordium
10. odontoblast layer
11. oral epithelium
12. outer epithelium

D and E *from C.C.H.S.M.*

D. Week 13. 100 mmCR (×17.5)

E. Week 14. 120 mmCR (×15)

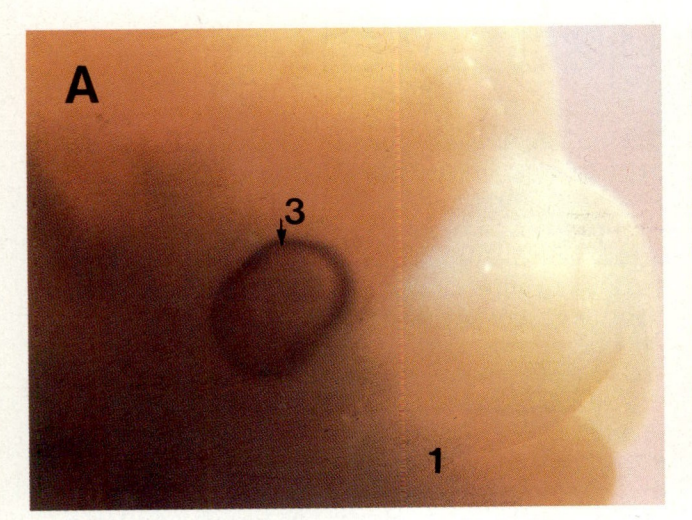

A. Horizon XIX (Day 38–40). View from the right side. 20 mmCR (×18)

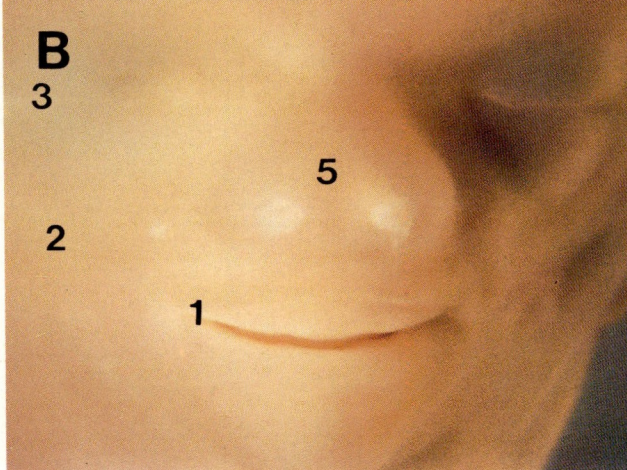

B. Week 9. View from the front. 46 mmCR (×8.4)

A–C. Development of the lips.

1. angle of the mouth
2. cheek
3. eye
4. lip
5. nose
6. nostril with plug

- Permanent molars with no deciduous predecessors develop as buds from the dental laminae.

- The teeth do not all develop at the same time.

- The root of the tooth forms shortly before eruption.

- The neonatal jaw contains the completed crowns of the 20 deciduous teeth and the primordia of all the 32 permanent teeth except the second and third molars.

C. Week 9. View from the right side. 48 mmCR ♀ (×12)

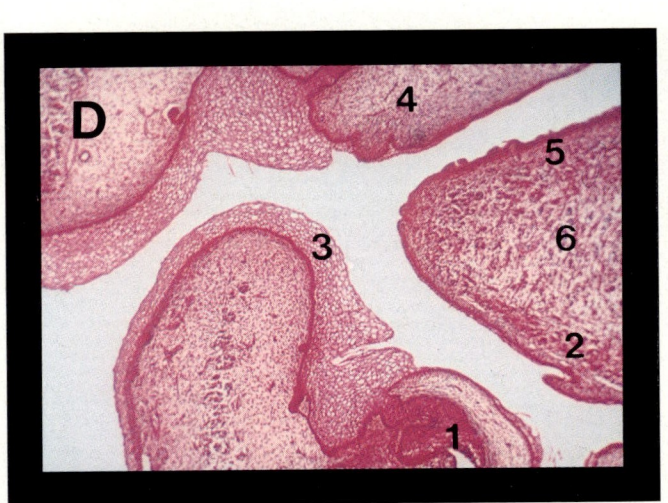

D. Week 8. Sagittal section through the lips, palate and tongue. 35 mmCR (×60)

1. dental ledge
2. inferior longitudinal muscle
3. oral epithelium
4. palate
5. superior longitudinal muscle
6. tongue

From Mr G. Bottomley

A and B. Horizon XIX (Day 38–40). The palate. Two views of the same embryo. 20mmCR (×35)

1. developing gum
2. developing lip
3. eye
4. forehead
5. lateral palatine process
6. maxillary process
7. nasal septum
8. nostril

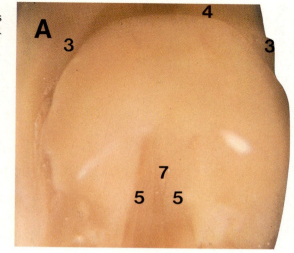

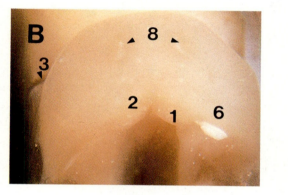

Palate

Three palatal processes develop which will separate the nasal cavity and the mouth: the primary palate (or median palatine process) and the secondary palate (two lateral palatine processes). The primary and secondary palate form between Week 5–12. The primary palate forms in Week 5 from the fusion of the two medial nasal prominences (see Nose). The secondary palate forms when the dorsum of the tongue which is pressed against the nasal septum (Week 7) withdraws. The two lateral palatine processes which originally projected vertically downwards on either side of the tongue meet in the midline and fuse. They also fuse with the primary palate and nasal septum and together form a horizontal shelf. Fusion occurs between Week 7–12.

Membrane bone in the primary palate forms the premaxilla; while bone from the maxilla and palatine bone extends into the lateral palatine processes to form the hard palate. The soft palate and uvula extend beyond the nasal septum and do not become ossified.

● If the processes fail to fuse the nasal cavity and mouth remain in continuity. This condition known as cleft palate interferes with feeding and speech.

● The neonatal hard palate is short and broad, while the adult palate is deeply arched.

C. The mandible and tongue of the embryo in Figure **A.** The tongue is positioned in a groove on the mandibular process. (×35)

1. chin
2. dorsum of the tongue
3. mandible
4. tip of the tongue

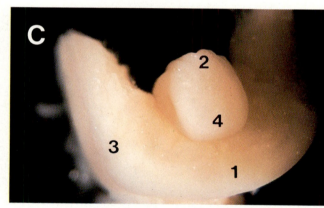

A. Week 8. The two lateral palatine processes and median palatine process have fused in the mid-line. The uvula remains unfused. 35mmCR (×17)

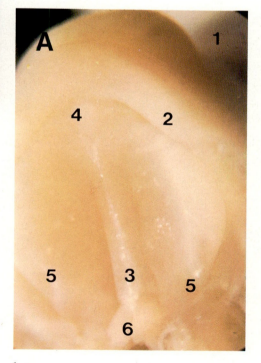

1. eye
2. maxilla
3. palatine raphe
4. primary palate
5. secondary palate
6. uvula

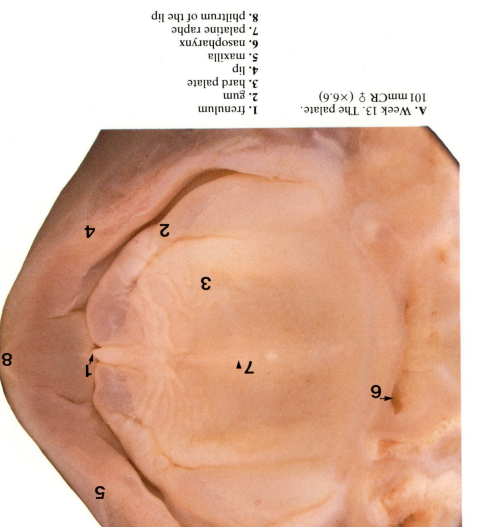

A. Week 13. The palate.
101 mmCR ♀ (×6.6)

1. frenulum
2. gum
3. hard palate
4. lip
5. maxilla
6. nasopharynx
7. palatine raphe
8. philtrum of the lip

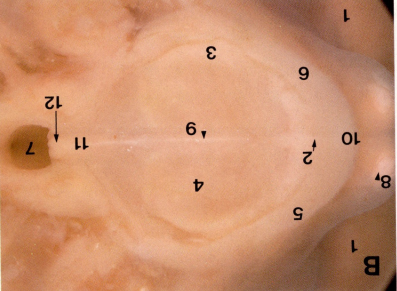

B. Week 11. The uvula has fused in the mid-line.
65 mmCR ♂ (×8.1)

1. eye
2. frenulum
3. gum
4. hard palate
5. lip
6. maxilla
7. nasopharynx
8. nostril
9. palatine raphe
10. philtrum of the lip
11. soft palate
12. uvula

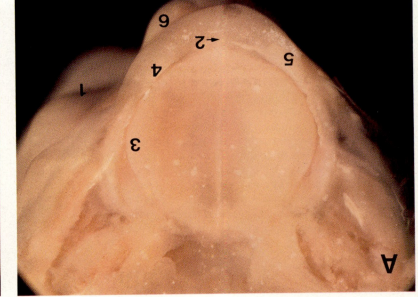

A. Week 9. The frenulum and gums of the maxilla are beginning to be distinguishable. The mandible has been removed. 48 mmCR ♂ (×9.6)

1. eye
2. frenulum
3. gum
4. lip
5. maxilla
6. nose

A and B. The unfused and fused palate in transverse paraffin wax sections.

1. arytenoid swelling
2. cartilagenous otic capsule
3. Eustachian tube
4. fused lateral palatine processes
5. hindbrain (medulla)
6. hyoid cartilage
7. lateral palatine processes
8. maxilla
9. Meckel's cartilage
10. nasal cavity
11. nasal septum
12. oral cavity
13. semicircular canals
14. submandibular gland
15. thyroid cartilage
16. tongue
17. tooth

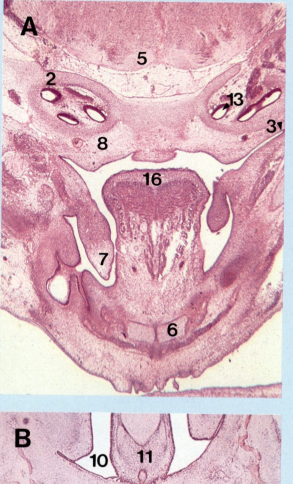

A. Horizon XXI (Day 42–44). 24 mmCR (×20)

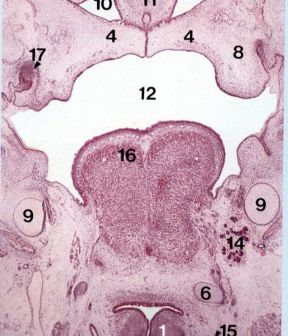

B. Week 8. 32 mmCR (×40)

A and **B** *from C.C.H.M.S.*

A. Week 17. The fused palate in a sagittal (longitudinal) section. 150 mmCR (×1.6)

1. aorta
2. atrium of heart
3. cerebellum
4. diaphragm
5. ductus venosus
6. esophagus
7. feet
8. fingers
9. hard palate
10. intestines
11. lip
12. liver
13. lung
14. nasal cavity
15. nose
16. phallus
17. pituitary
18. soft palate
19. sternum
20. urinary bladder
21. ventricle of heart
22. vertebrae

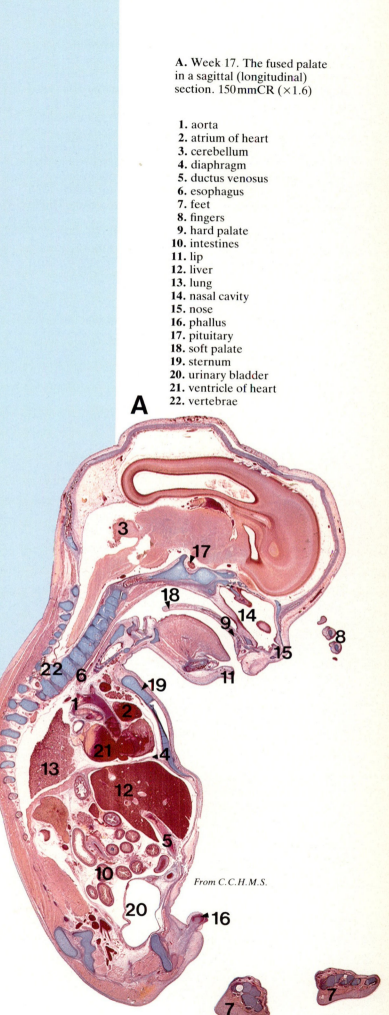

From C.C.H.M.S.

Tongue

The anterior two-thirds of the tongue (body) forms during Week 4 from the fusion of a medial swelling *(tuberculum impar)* in the floor of the pharynx between the first pair of branchial arches and the two lateral lingual swellings derived from each first arch. The two lateral swellings overgrow and bury the *tuberculum impar* as they grow medially. The median sulcus marks are the fusion of the two lateral lingual swellings.

The posterior third of the tongue (root) forms from the fusion of the ventromedial ends of the second arches to form the copula. A large hypobranchial eminence develops caudal to the copula from third and fourth arch mesoderm. This eminence overgrows the copula which disappears.

The boundary between the two areas is the sulcus terminalis with the thyroid rudiment the *foramen cecum* in the mid-line. The papillae develop at Week 7–9. Most of the muscles develop from occipital myotomes.

- The neonatal tongue is within the oral cavity. The posterior third will descend into the neck after birth (1–5 years) to form part of the anterior pharyngeal wall.

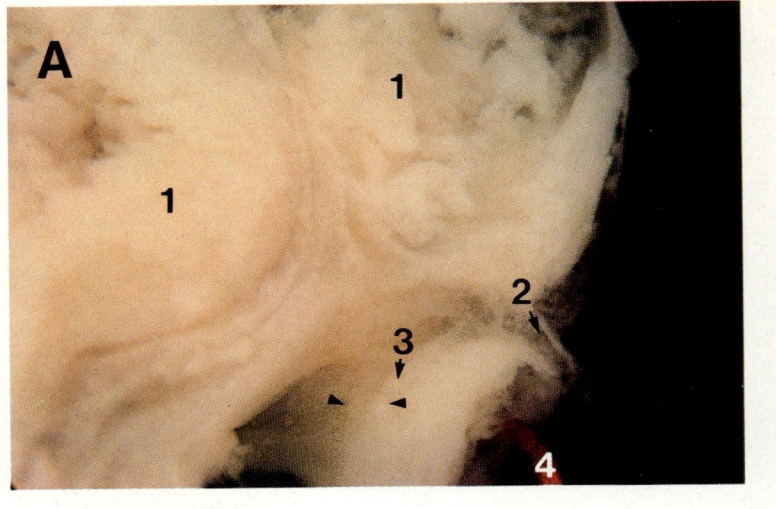

A. Horizon XVIII (Day 36–38). Sagittal section through the left side of the developing pharynx and brain. 14 mm CR (×17)

1. brain
2. buccopharyngeal membrane
3. floor of pharynx (one *tuberculum impar* and two mandibular swellings)
4. red cactus needle

Larynx

The proximal end of the respiratory diverticulum, the larynx, develops from the endodermal lining of the respiratory diverticulum and surrounding mesoderm (fourth and sixth branchial arches). In Week 5 and 6 three swellings appear, one called the epiglottal swelling (from third and fourth branchial arches), and two arytenoid swellings. Together the three swellings make the opening to the trachea 'Y' or 'T' shaped. Later the corniculate and arytenoid cartilages form from the arytenoid swellings.

In Week 7–10 the laryngeal epithelium fuses and the entrance ends blindly. In Week 10 the larynx recanalizes and two lateral recesses, the laryngeal ventricles, are formed as well as the vestibular and vocal folds and the laryngeal aditus slowly enlarges.

The laryngeal muscles are fourth and sixth branchial arch derivatives and the cartilages are from the fourth and fifth arches.

- Before the posterior third of the tongue descends into the neck (first to fifth years of postnatal development) the opening of the larynx is directly below the oral cavity.

- Owing to its high position in the neck, the neonatal epiglottis can make direct contact with the soft palate which assists in directing fluid and breathing freely during suckling.

A–E. Development of the tongue.

1. arytenoid swellings
2. developing tongue
3. dorsum of tongue
4. epiglottis
5. mandibular prominence
6. mandible
7. vallate papillae

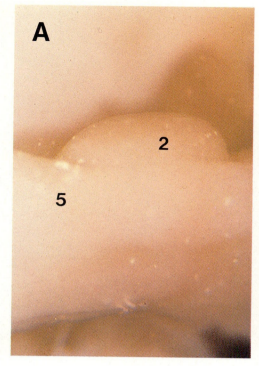

A

A. Horizon XVIII (Day 36–38). Viewed from the front of the face. 16 mm CR (×65)

B. Horizon XIX (Day 38–40). Dorsum of the tongue. 20 mm CR (×16.5)

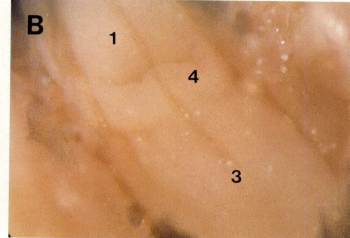

B

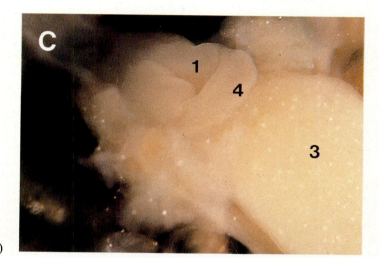

C

C. Week 8. 40 mm CR (×16.5)

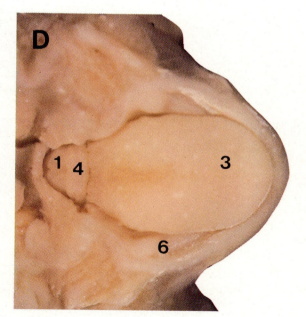

D

D. Week 9. 48 mm CR ♂ (×8.5)

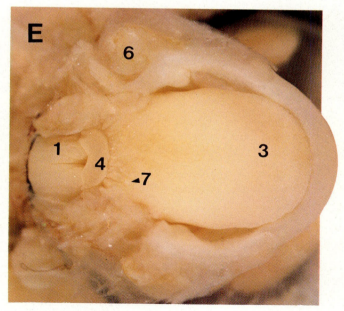

E

E. Week 11. 65 mm CR ♂ (×7.6)

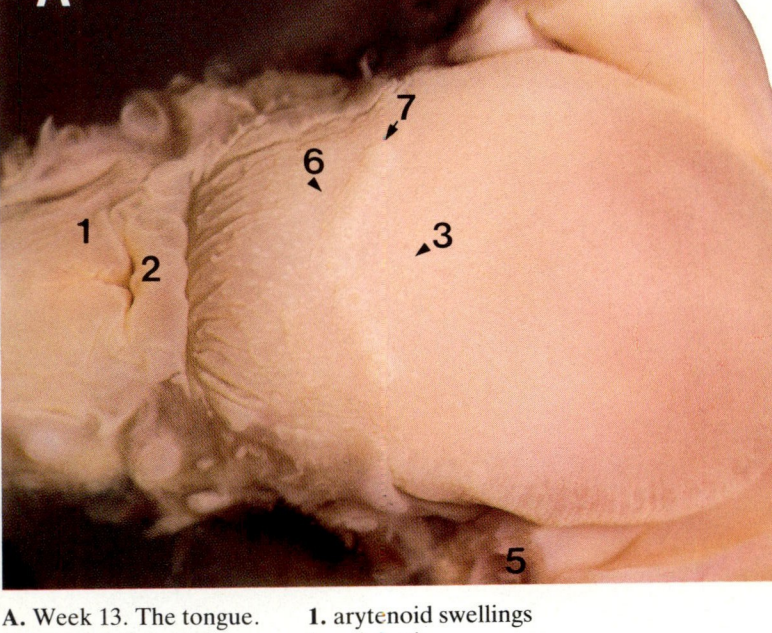

A

A. Week 13. The tongue. 101 mmCR ♀ (×5.6)

1. arytenoid swellings
2. epiglottis
3. fungiform papillae
4. lip
5. mandible
6. sulcus terminalis
7. vallate papillae

A

A. Sagittal section of a neonatal head to illustrate the position of the developed tongue and larynx. (×0.7)

From R.C.S.E.

1. cerebellar fossa
2. confluence of sinuses
3. epiglottis
4. genioglossus muscle
5. hard palate
6. lips
7. mandible
8. mylohyoid muscle
9. nasal cavity
10. note the absence of a developed frontal sinus
11. pharynx
12. soft palate
13. tentorium cerebelli

A. Week 8. Transverse section of the developing tongue. 32 mmCR (×25)

1. dental ledge
2. mandible
3. maxilla
4. Meckel's cartilage
5. tongue

A

A

From Mr G. Bottomley

A. Week 8. Longitudinal section of the developing tongue. 35 mmCR (×27)

1. dental ledge
2. genioglossus muscle
3. geniohyoid muscle
4. hard palate
5. lip
6. mandible
7. maxilla
8. nasal cavity
9. inferior longitudinal muscle
10. superior longitudinal muscle
11. vertical muscle and transverse muscle

(9–11 intrinsic muscles of the tongue)

A. Development of the epiglottis and arytenoid swellings. Views of the dorsum of the tongue. (×3.2)
Large: Week 13. 101 mmCR ♀
Small: Week 13. 92 mmCR ♀

1. arytenoid swellings
2. dorsum of the tongue
3. epiglottis
4. lip
5. mandible
6. sulcus terminalis

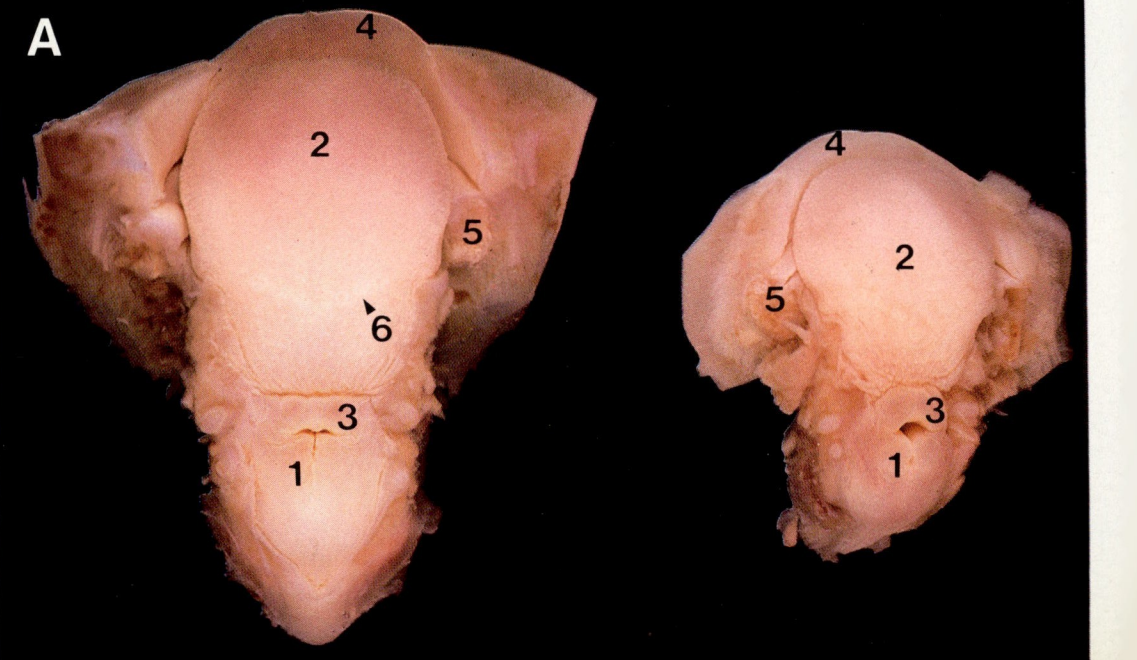

A

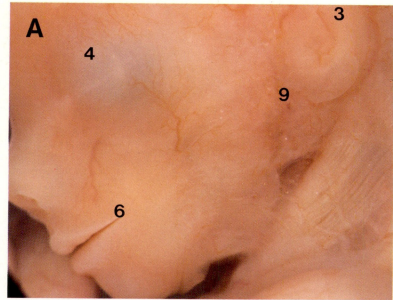

A. Week 11. 65 mm CR ♂ (×6.3)

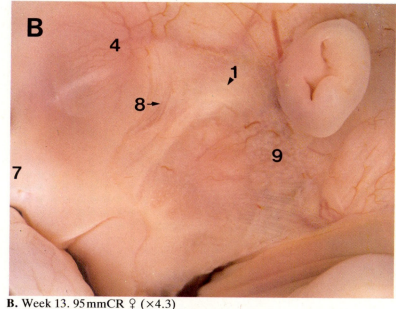

B. Week 13. 95 mm CR ♀ (×4.3)

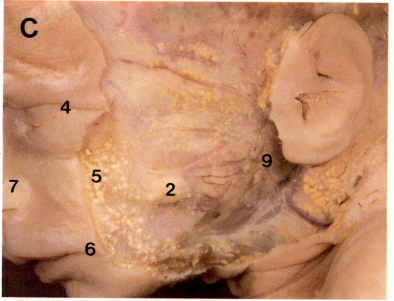

C. Week 18. 152 mm CR ♂ (×2.3)

Salivary glands

The first pair of salivary glands to develop are the parotid glands (Week 6 and 7). The submandibular glands develop late in Week 6 and the sublingual glands at Week 8.

All three pairs of glands develop from solid epithelial outgrowths which penetrate into the surrounding mesoderm. The tips of the outgrowths form branches and terminal acini. By Week 24 the solid outgrowths, branches and acini develop lumens. The main outgrowths form the main ducts of the salivary glands while the mesoderm forms the remainder of the glands apart from the epithelium lining the acini and ducts.

The parotid gland outgrowth develops from the ectodermal lining of the mouth; while the submandibular and sublingual glands develop from endodermal outgrowths.

● In the 2 years following birth, all three pairs of salivary glands develop the typical adult histological appearance.

● In the neonate the sublingual gland is continuous with the deep portion of the submandibular gland.

● The parotid gland is round at birth and gradually grows over the surface of the parotid duct in early childhood.

A–C. Lateral view of the left parotid gland.

1. branches of the facial nerve
2. buccal fat pad
3. ear
4. eye
5. fat
6. mouth
7. nose
8. orbicularis oculi
9. parotid gland

D. Week 8. Transverse paraffin wax section through the nasal septum and tongue. 32 mm CR ♂ (×31)

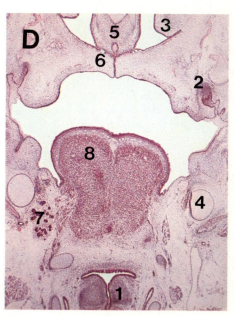

1. arytenoid swelling
2. developing tooth
3. inferior concha
4. Meckel's cartilage
5. nasal septum
6. palate
7. submandibular gland
8. tongue

Ear: external

Auricle

At Day 24–27 a series of six tubercles appears around the first branchial groove, three on each of the first (mandibular) and second (hyoid) arches.

The tubercles on each arch fuse together to form the auricle (pinna) of the ear, only the most ventral on the first arch is recognizable as the tragus. Mesoderm of the hyoid arch proliferates to complete the auricle. The auricles initially form in the neck region but move up on to the head by Week 10.

External auditory meatus

The external auditory meatus develops at the dorsal end of the first branchial groove as a funnel-shaped tube (primary meatus). Ectoderm cells at the inner end of the primary meatus proliferate to form a meatal plug. Later this degenerates forming a cavity, the inner part of the external auditory meatus.

The early tympanic membrane (or eardrum) is the branchial membrane. Later mesoderm enters and the tympanic membrane is formed from meatal plug ectoderm, mesoderm from the first and second branchial arches, and tubotympanic recess endoderm.

- The shape of the fully formed auricles varies greatly from individual to individual.

- The tympanic membrane completes its growth by birth.

- The lumen of the neonatal external auditory meatus is filled with a sebaceous secretion, the *vernix caseosa*, and desquamated epithelial cells.

- At birth amniotic fluid and fluid secreted by the respiratory tract are often found in the cavity of the middle ear.

- At birth the stylomastoid foramen and the emerging facial nerve lies unprotected near the surface as the mastoid process is not developed until 2 years of age.

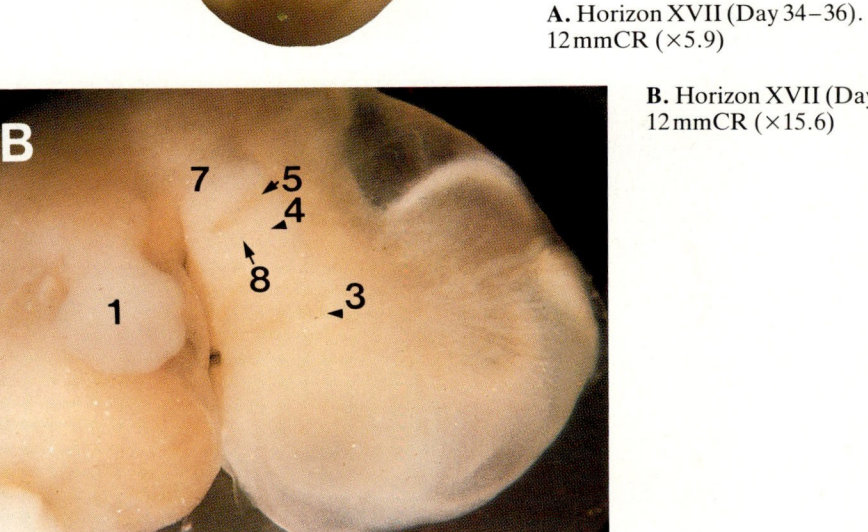

A–J. Development of the auricle and external auditory meatus.

1. arm bud
2. external auditory meatus
3. eye
4. first arch (mandibular)
5. first branchial groove
6. mandible
7. second arch (hyoid)
8. tubercles (hillocks)

A. Horizon XVII (Day 34–36). 12 mmCR (×5.9)

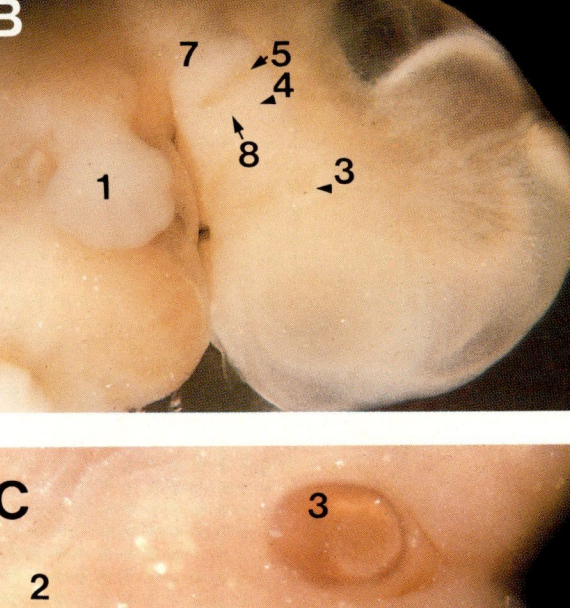

B. Horizon XVII (Day 34–36). 12 mmCR (×15.6)

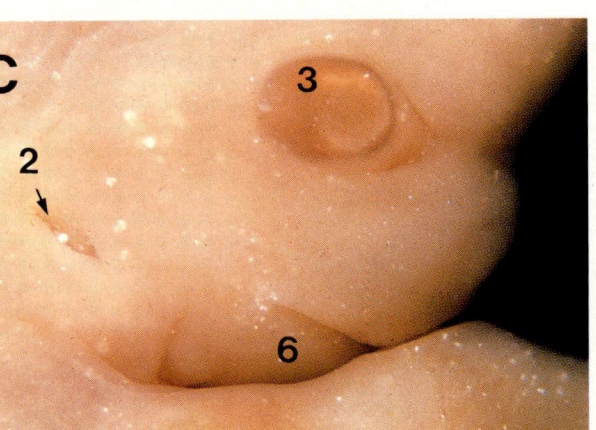

C. Horizon XIX (Day 38–40). 20 mmCR (×15.6)

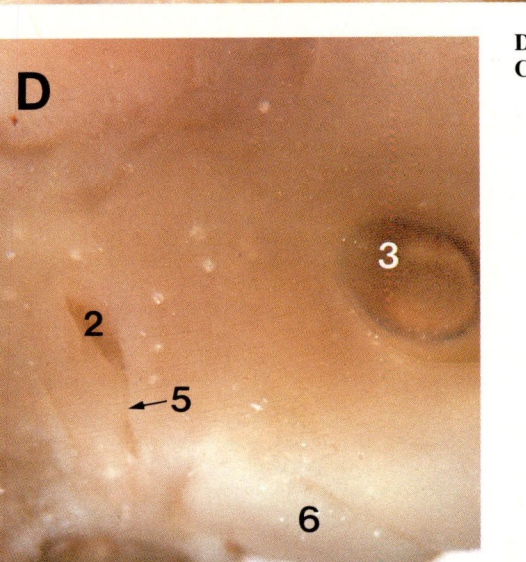

D. Same embryo as in Figure C. (×18)

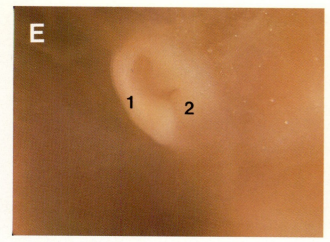

E. Horizon XXII (Day 44–46). 27mmCR (×15.6)

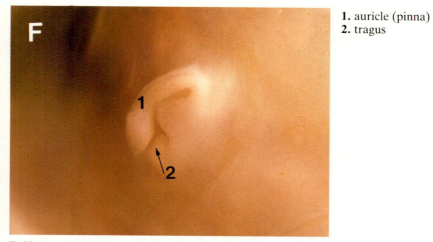

1. auricle (pinna)
2. tragus

F. Horizon XXII (Day 44–46). 27mmCR (×15.6)

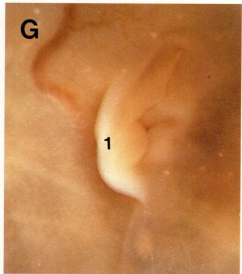

G. Week 8. 35mmCR (×16.2)

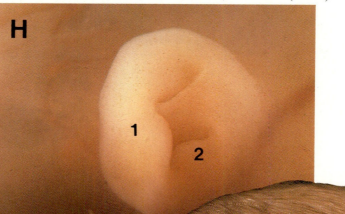

H. Week 9. 48mmCR ♂
(×15.6)

K. Week 24. Origins of the ear. The continuous line encloses the area derived from the first arch, the broken line encloses the area derived from the second arch. 228mmCR ♂ (×1.8)

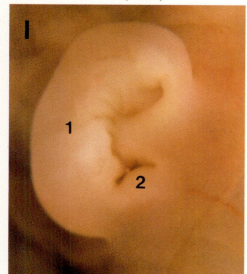

I. Week 13. 95mmCR ♂ (×8.1)

J. Week 15. 130mmCR ♀ (×4.1)

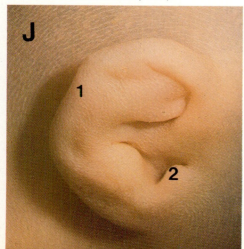

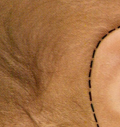

K

Ear: internal

The otic placodes are ectodermal thickenings (with a possible contribution of neuroectoderm) on the hindbrain region immediately caudal to the acousticofacial mass which sink below the surface and form vesicles (otocysts) (Week 4). The otocysts give rise to the membranous labyrinth of the inner ear.

Inner ear

A hollow diverticulum which will form the endolymphatic duct and sac appears on the upper medial aspect of the otocyst. The upper and lower parts of the otocyst enlarge to form two areas: the utricular (vestibular) and saccular (cochlear) divisions; the constriction between them forms the utriculosaccular duct. Three circular pouches arise from the utricular part and their central walls fuse and are resorbed. Their peripheral walls remain as the semicircular ducts. The lateral canal lies horizontally, the superior canal lies in the frontal plane, the posterior canal initially lies in a frontal plane, and then swings through 90° to lie sagitally. The superior and posterior canals share the *crus commune* into the utricular part of the otocyst.

The saccular part of the otocysts divides into two regions: an upper expanded part which will form the saccule while the lower coils two and a half times to form the cochlear duct. The constriction separating the saccule and cochlear duct is the *ductus reuniens*.

The epithelium in six regions modifies to neuroepithelium; a crista in the ampulla of each semicircular duct, two maculae one each in the utricle and saccule, and the organ of Corti along the duct of the cochlea.

The geniculate ganglion of the facial nerve separates from the acousticofacial complex; the remaining complex divides into two regions, the vestibular and cochlear (spiral) ganglia. The vestibular ganglion sends processes to the maculae and cristae and the organ of Corti receives processes from the cochlear ganglion.

Mesoderm surrounding the otocyst forms the cartilaginous otic capsule which then disappears immediately adjacent to the otocyst to form the perilymphatic spaces which connect to the subarachnoid space (cochlear aqueduct). The bony (osseous) labyrinth of the middle ear is the remaining ossified otic capsule.

Middle ear

The middle ear forms between the developing inner ear and external auditory meatus.

The tubotympanic recess, which is an endodermal derivative from the first pouch grows between the otocyst and the external auditory meatus. The distal end of the diverticulum expands to form the tympanic cavity. The proximal part forms the auditory or pharyngotympanic (Eustachian) tube. The developing middle ear cavity surrounds the three ossicles (malleus, incus, stapes) their muscles, and the *chorda tympani* nerve so they project into the cavity like a peninsula covered with recess epithelium. The malleus and incus have formed from Meckel's cartilage (first arch) and the stapes from Reichert's cartilage (second arch). The tensor tympani muscle forms from the first arch mesoderm and the stapedius muscle from the second. The muscles are supplied by their arch nerve; the mandibular and facial nerves, respectively.

In the late fetus the tympanic cavity expands and gives rise to the tympanic or mastoid antrum.

- In the neonate the course of the auditory tube is horizontal and enters the pharynx at the junction of the hard and soft palates. By 5 or 6 years of age the opening has shifted up to lie posterior to the inferior concha.

- The majority of the mastoid air cells form after birth. The mastoid process grows primarily between the age of 3 years to puberty.

- In the infant and young child the petrosquamous fissure of the mastoid temporal bone opens directly into the mastoid antrum of the middle ear and is a route for middle ear infection to spread to the meninges.

A. Horizon XXI (Day 42–44). Transverse paraffin wax section of the developing semicircular canals. 24mmCR (×16)

1. cartilagenous otic capsule
2. Eustachian tube
3. hindbrain (medulla)
4. lateral palatine processes
5. semicircular canals
6. tongue

From C.C.H.M.S.

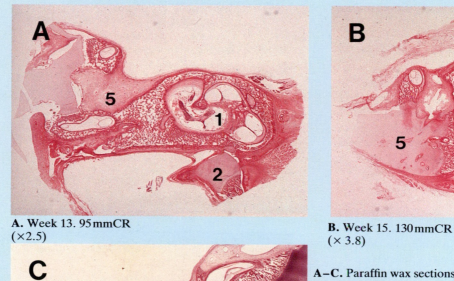

A. Week 13. 95 mm CR (×2.5)

B. Week 15. 130 mm CR (×3.8)

A and B *from C.C.H.M.S.*

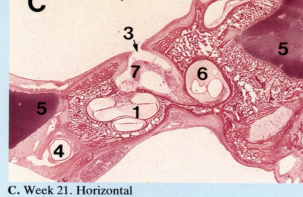

A–C. Paraffin wax sections of the developing ear.

1. cochlea
2. first arch derivatives
3. internal auditory meatus
4. internal carotid artery
5. petrous temporal bone
6. vestibule
7. vestibulocochlear (VIII) nerve

C *from Dr J. Wakely*

C. Week 21. Horizontal section through the left ear. (×3.8)

A. Neonatal incus and stapes. (×5.6)

1. incus
2. stapes

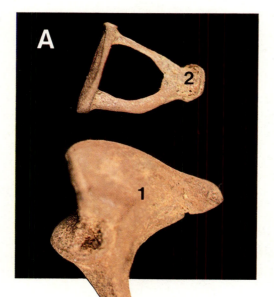

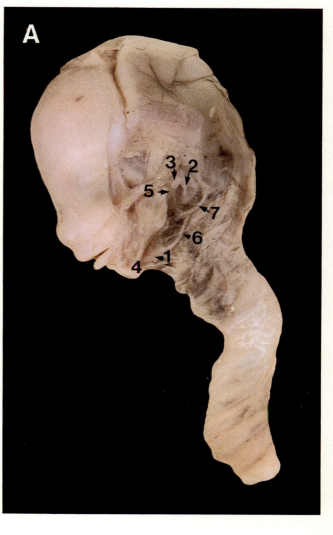

A. Week 13–14. The head and neck dissected to show elements of the first and second branchial arches. (×2.1)

1. hyoid bone
2. incus
3. malleus
4. mandible
5. Meckel's cartilage
6. stylohyoid ligament
7. tympanic ring

From R.F.H.S.M.

Pharynx

Branchial arches and grooves

Early in Week 4 a series of paired swellings appear on either side of the mid-line in the future head and neck region. They are present both externally and internally. These branchial arches support the cranial foregut region or pharynx. The foregut extends from the oral membrane to the entry of the bile duct. At the end of Week 4 six pairs of branchial arches are present, the last two being rudimentary. The fifth arch may be absent. Each arch is separated from the next by a branchial groove or cleft. The external appearance is similar to gills and gill slits in a fish. There are six arches, the first is also known as the mandibular arch and the second as the hyoid arch. The first arch is divided into two processes; one forms the mandible, the second contributes to the maxilla. The second arch contributes to the hyoid bone and the adjacent area. Each arch is covered by ectoderm externally, foregut endoderm internally, and has a core of mesoderm. Neural crest cells migrate into each arch and surround the mesodermal core. The mesoderm and the neural crest will form muscles, skeletal and connective tissues. Each arch also contains an artery, a cartilaginous bar and a nerve which has grown from the brain.

During Week 5 the hyoid arch overgrows the third and fourth arches to form the cervical sinus. Gradually the grooves and the cervical sinus become less recognizable and the neck is smooth.

Branchial arch muscles form striated muscles in the head and neck.

The branchial arch nerves are: first – trigeminal, second – facial, third – glossopharyngeal, fourth – superior laryngeal branch of vagus, sixth – recurrent laryngeal branch of vagus.

Branchial arch artery derivatives (see Blood vessels).

Branchial arch cartilage derivatives (see Skull).

Pharyngeal pouches

The foregut endoderm lines the inner aspect of the branchial arches as they bulge into the pharynx. Each arch is separated from the next by a groove or cleft called a pharyngeal pouch. In the pouch the endoderm contacts the ectoderm of the branchial groove to form the branchial membrane. The first pouches are clearly defined, while the fifth is rudimentary or absent.

The first dorsal pouch forms the tubotympanic recess (tympanic cavity, mastoid antrum and the Eustachian tube); the second dorsal pouch forms the palatine tonsil. The ventral parts of the first and second pouches are obliterated by tongue formation. The third dorsal pouch forms the inferior parathyroids, while the ventral third pouch forms the thymus gland. The fourth dorsal pouch gives rise to the superior parathyroids and the fourth ventral pouch to the ultimobranchial body.

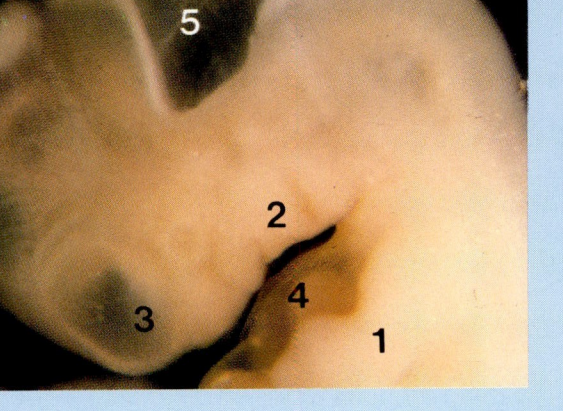

From C.C.H.M.S.

From L.H.S.M.

From L.H.S.M.

A. Horizons XI and XII (Day 24–27). The pharyngeal region. 4 mm CR (×39)

1. aortic arch
2. branchial arch (two)
3. branchial groove
4. dorsal aorta
5. mandibular prominence (process)
6. maxillary prominence (process)
7. neural crest
8. optic vesicle
9. pharyngeal pouch
10. prosencephalon (diencephalon)
11. stomodeum
12. thyroid diverticulum

B. Horizon XVII (Day 34–36). The pharyngeal region. 12 mm CR (×7.7)

1. arm bud (left)
2. branchial arches
3. forebrain
4. heart
5. hindbrain

C. Horizon XIV (Day 28–30). Transverse section of the pharyngeal region. 7 mm CR (×32)

1. aortic arch (two)
2. branchial arch (three)
3. branchial arch (one)
4. branchial arch (two)
5. branchial groove (one)
6. cervical plexus
7. cervical sinus
8. ependymal layer of the spinal cord
9. hypoglossal nerve (XII)
10. neurohypophysis
11. mandibular process
12. marginal layer of spinal cord
13. maxillary process
14. myotome
15. optic cup
16. spinal ganglion
17. sternocleidomastoid, trapezius premuscle mass
18. stomodeum
19. third ventricle

D. Horizon XIV (Day 28–30). Transverse section of the pharyngeal region. 7 mm CR (×33)

Neck

By approximately the end of Week 8, the embryo has developed a neck. This is the result of partial extension of the head.

● An important feature of neck development is the associated descent of the heart.

● Extension of the head is important in palate formation during Week 8–10.

● At birth, the neck and trunk musculature are not sufficiently developed to support the large head which should be supported when lifting the infant.

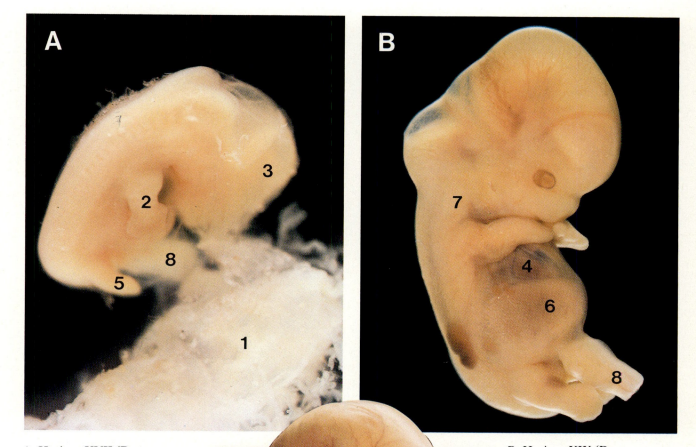

A. Horizon XVII (Day 34–36). 12 mmCR (×6.3)

B. Horizon XIX (Day 38–40). 20 mmCR (×5.2)

A–C. Development of the neck.

1. amnion and chorion
2. arm
3. brain
4. heart
5. leg
6. liver
7. neck
8. umbilical cord

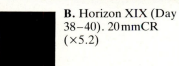

C. Week 13. 92 mmCR ♀ (×1.2)

Thyroid

During Week 3 to 4 a median endodermal thyroid diverticulum appears in the floor of the pharynx opposite the first and second pharyngeal pouches. This bilobed solid diverticulum is in close contact with the aortic sac and as the sac migrates caudally during neck development the thyroid migrates to its position in the neck. During migration its stalk is drawn out to form the thyroglossal duct and its original site marked on the tongue as the *foramen cecum*. The distal portion of the duct forms the pyramidal lobe of the thyroid, while the remaining duct disappears during Week 5.

By Week 7 the gland has reached its site in the neck. The ultimobranchial body (fourth pharyngeal pouch) fuses with the thyroid and gives rise to parafollicular or 'C' cells in the thyroid. These cells are neural crest derivatives and store and secrete calcitonin to regulate calcium levels in body fluids. The original solid endodermal mass is infiltrated by vascular mesoderm which breaks the endoderm into plates and by Week 10 the plates have formed cells grouped around a follicle lumen.

Colloid appears in the follicles during Week 11 and thyroxine by Week 8.

● Occasionally remnants of the mid-line thyroglossal duct persist and may give rise to aberrant thyroid tissue, sinuses, cysts and fistulae.

● A lingual thyroid is not uncommon.

Parathyroids

The superior parathyroid glands develop from the fourth pharyngeal pouch endoderm. The inferior parathyroid glands develop from the third pharyngeal pouch endoderm. Their primordia appear as buds whose cells form the chief cells while vascular mesoderm infiltrates the bud to form the capillary network.

The fourth pharyngeal pouch gives rise to the thyroid gland as well as to the superior parathyroid glands which are found on the posterior surface of the thyroid. The third pharyngeal pouch gives rise to the thymus gland as well as the inferior parathyroid glands and as the thymus gland migrates the inferior parathyroids are carried caudally to a final position on the posterior thyroid surface inferior to the superior parathyroids.

During Week 12 parathyroid hormone is produced.

● Between birth and puberty the parathyroids double in size.

A–F. Thyroid development. View of the ventral (front) surface.

1. common carotid artery
2. cricoid cartilage
3. inferior thyroid veins
4. isthmus of thyroid
5. lobe of thyroid gland
6. sternocleidomastoid muscle

A. Horizon XVIII (Day 36–38). The early thyroid. View of the right side. 14 mmCR (×19.8)

1. mandibular prominence
2. thorax
3. thymus primordia
4. thyroid primordium

B. Horizon XIX (Day 38–40). 20 mmCR (×19.8)

C. Week 9. 50 mmCR ♀ (×19.8)

1. chin
2. cricoid cartilage
3. inferior thyroid veins
4. isthmus of thyroid
5. lobe of thyroid gland
6. omohyoid muscle
7. sternocleidomastoid muscle
8. thyroglossal duct

D. Week 12. Viewed from the left and front. 85 mmCR ♀ (×10.2)

E. Week 13. 97 mmCR ♂ (×5.3)

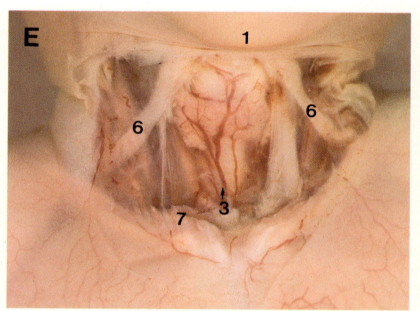

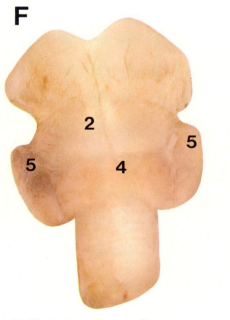

F. Week 13. 101 mmCR ♀ (×6.1)

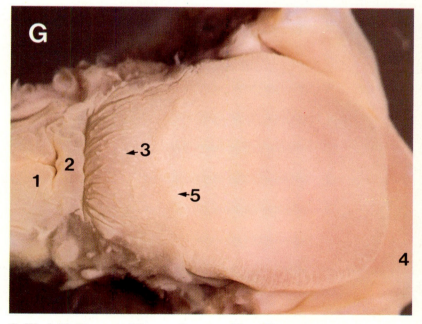

G. Week 13. Dorsum of the tongue to illustrate the *foramen cecum*. 100 mmCR ♀ (×5.4)

1. arytenoid swelling
2. epiglottis
3. *foramen cecum*
4. lip
5. vallate papillae

Thymus

The thymus develops when two bilateral masses from the third pharyngeal pouch fuse in the mid-line. This fused endodermal mass and the adjacent mesoderm are infiltrated by lymphoid stem cells by Week 10. Endodermal cells form the Hassall corpuscles and cytoreticulum.

After Week 10 young lymphocytes from the thymus circulate in the blood stream and 'seed' the spleen, lymph nodes and Peyer's patches where they multiply.

The thymus is prominent and occupies a large part of the superior mediastinum.

● In the neonate the most common form is a bilobar thymus though it may be trilobar or have no definite lobulation.

● The maximum size is around 12 years in females and 14 years in males.

● After puberty the thymus becomes infiltrated with fat and in old age is present as a small mass of fibrous tissue.

A–H. Ventral view of the developing thymus.

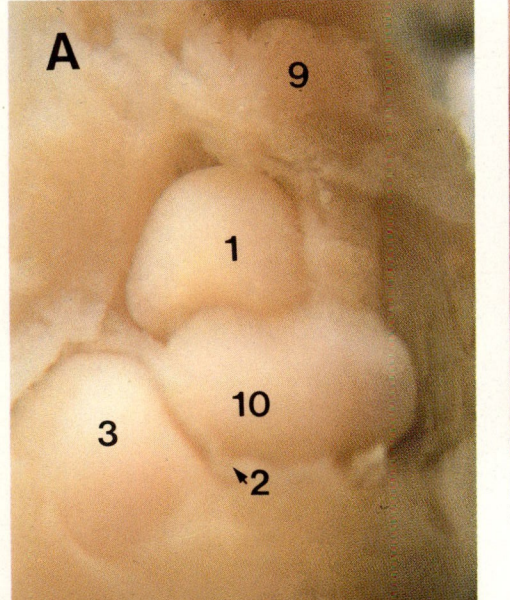

A. Horizon XVII (Day 34–36). 12mmCR (×16)

1. atrium
2. diaphragm
3. liver
4. lung (right)
5. pericardium
6. phrenic nerve
7. rib
8. sympathetic chain
9. thymus
10. ventricle

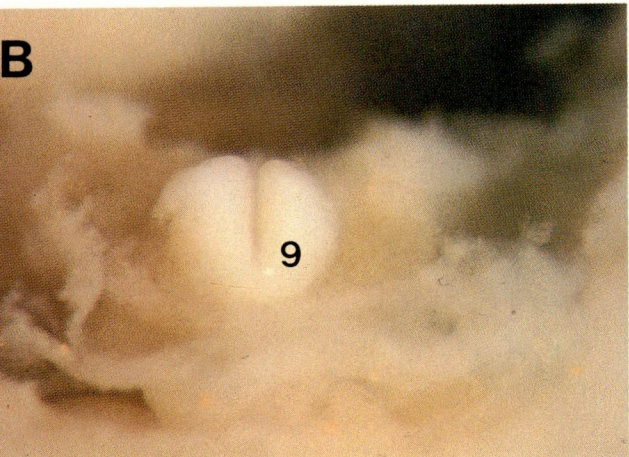

B. Horizon XVIII (Day 36–38). 14mmCR (×33.8)

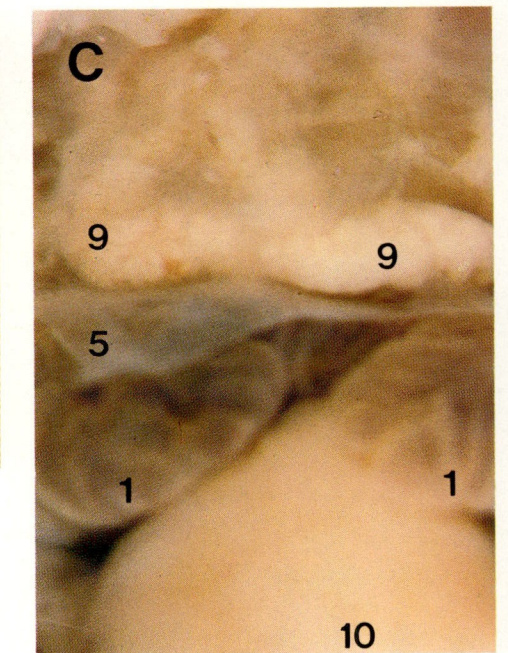

C. Week 9. 48mmCR (×16)

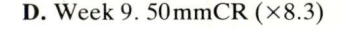

D. Week 9. 50mmCR (×8.3)

E. Week 10. 57mmCR ♂ (×8)

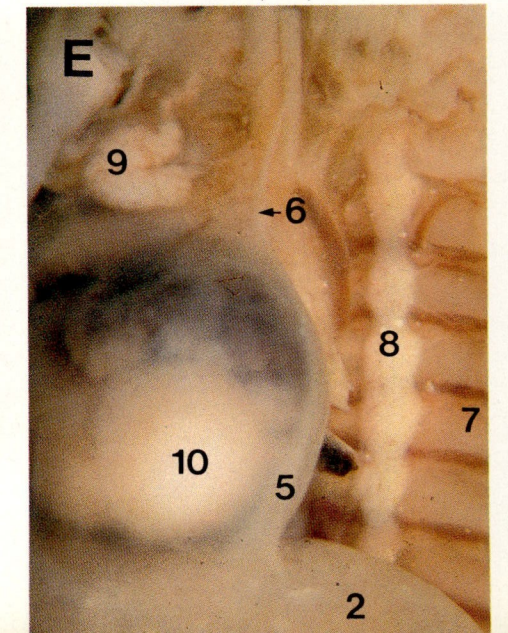

F. Week 11. 62 mmCR ♂
(×17)

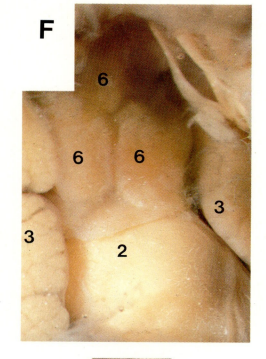

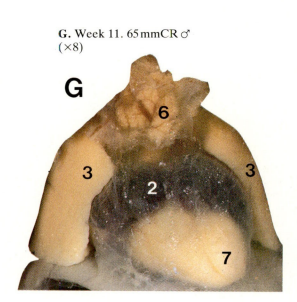

G. Week 11. 65 mmCR ♂
(×8)

1. anterior interventricular branch of left coronary artery and great cardiac vein
2. atrium
3. lung
4. pericardium
5. rib
6. thymus
7. ventricle

H. Week 15. 123 mmCR ♀
(×5)

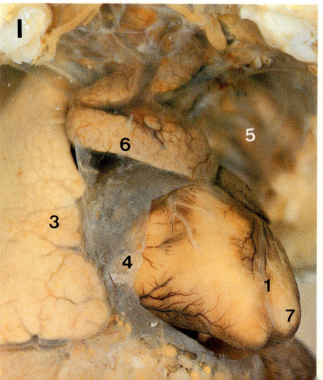

I. Week 17. View of the right side of the developing thymus. 152 mmCR ♂ (×2.7)

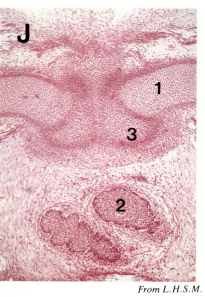

J. Horizon XXIII (Day 46–48). Transverse section through the developing manubrium sterni and thymus gland. 28 mmCR (× 72)

1. clavicle
2. thymus
3. two sternal bars of manubrium sterni

From L.H.S.M.

Thorax

General body plan

The early trunk and abdomen (Week 6) are dominated by the appearance of the heart and liver. As the fetus develops these two organs decrease in size relative to the rest of the body.

● At birth the right side of the liver is larger than the left side due to preferential growth.

A–J. Changes in dissected specimens of the thorax and abdomen.

1. arm
2. diaphragm
3. head
4. heart
5. intestine
6. leg
7. liver
8. lung
9. mesonephros
10. stomach
11. umbilical cord

A–C. Lateral view.

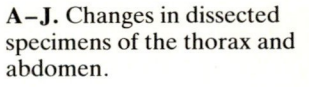

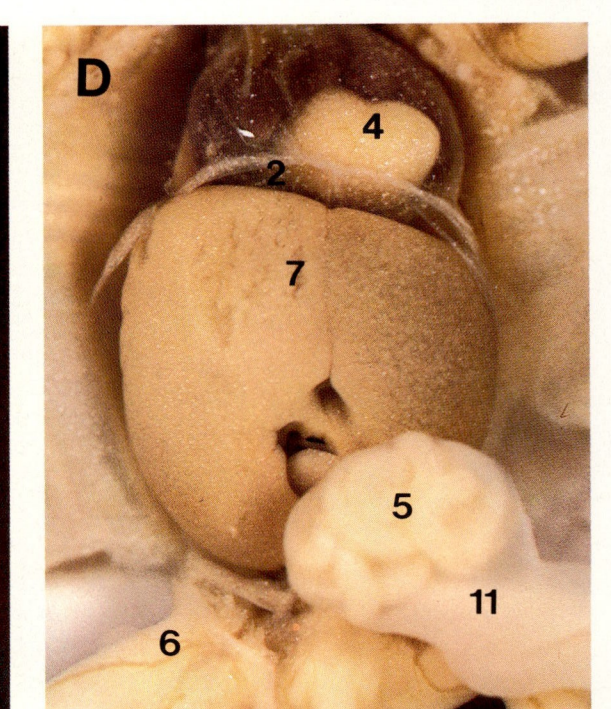

A. Horizon XVII (Day 34–36). 12 mm CR (×8.4)

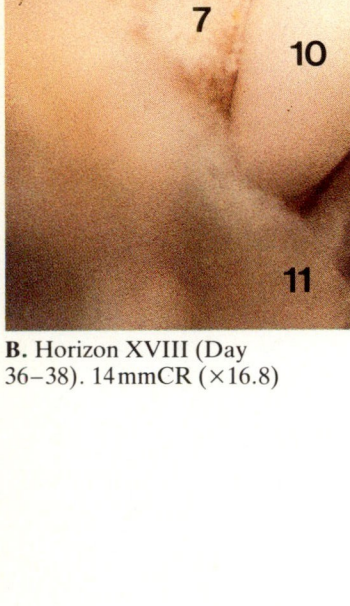

B. Horizon XVIII (Day 36–38). 14 mm CR (×16.8)

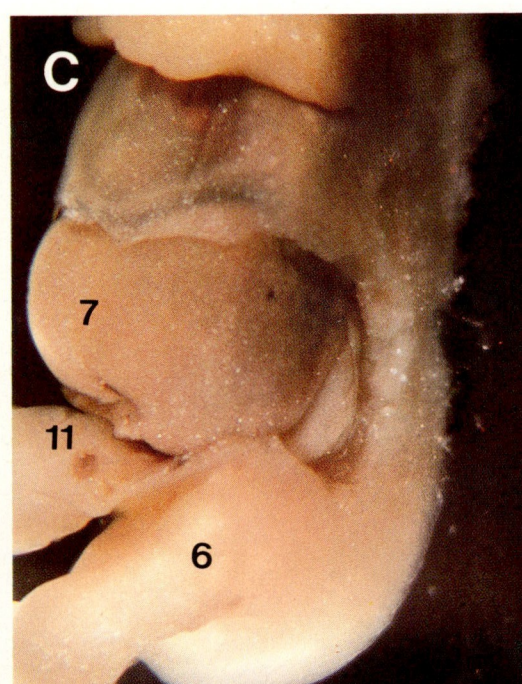

C. Horizon XIX (Day 38–40). 20 mm CR (×7.8)

D. Week 8. 34 mm CR (×6)

D–J. Ventral view.

E. Week 9. 48 mm CR ♂ (×4)

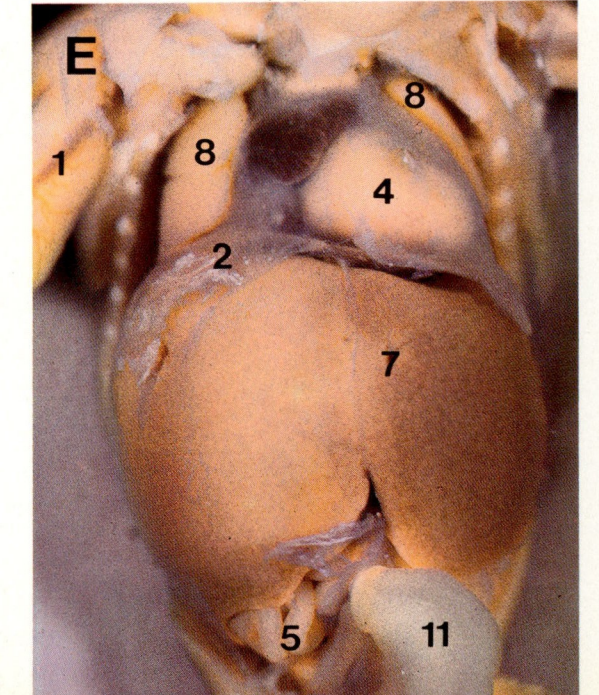

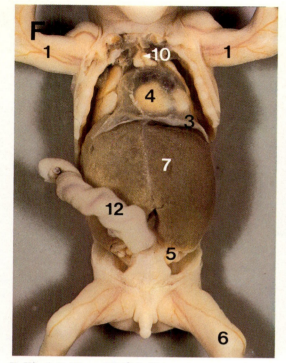

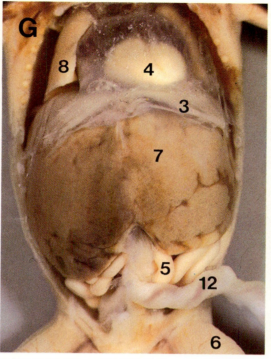

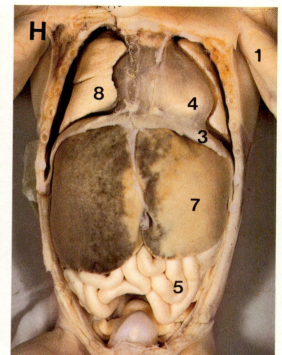

F. Week 9. 50 mmCR ♀ (×2)

G. Week 11. 65 mmCR ♂ (×3.2)

H. Week 13. 92 mmCR ♀ (×1.9)

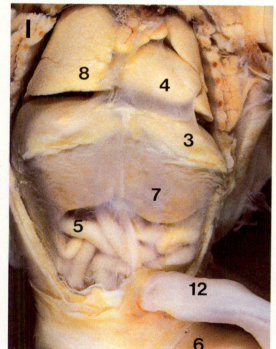

1. arm
2. brain
3. diaphragm
4. heart
5. intestine
6. leg
7. liver
8. lung
9. nose
10. thymus
11. tongue
12. umbilical cord
13. vertebral column

I. Week 13. 101 mmCR ♀ (×1)

A. Week 22. A median sagittal section to illustrate the position of vital organs. 159 mmCR (×1.2)

From R.F.H.S.M.

J. Week 18. 152 mmCR ♂ (×1.1)

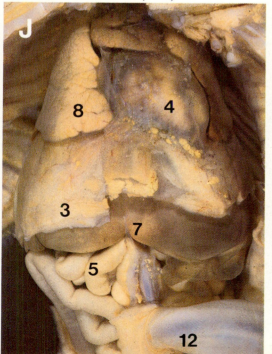

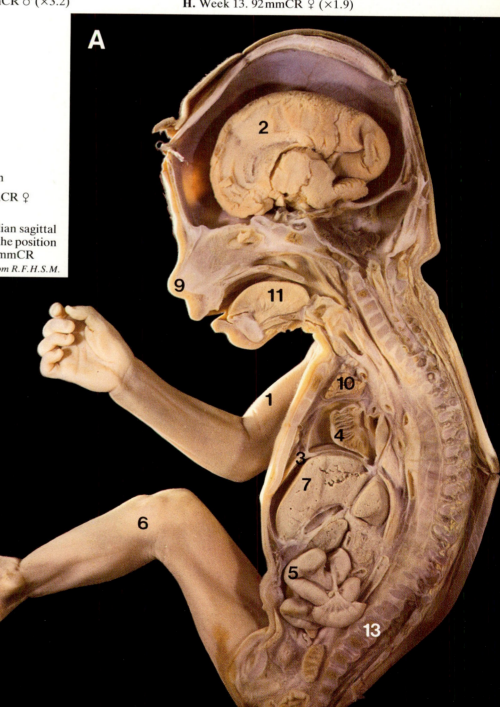

Heart

The heart develops from splanchnopleuric mesoderm which forms a horseshoe-shaped area in the anterior part of the embryonic disc. Two mid-line endothelial tubes form (Day 18–19) from this region and fuse to form a single heart tube at Day 22. The two umbilical veins open into the caudal (venous) end of the heart tube while the two primitive aortae open from the cephalic (arterial) end. The surrounding splanchnopleuric mesoderm condenses to form the myoepicardial mantle. Between the heart tube and mantle tube connective tissue forms cardiac jelly which develops into subendocardial tissue. The inner tube will form the endocardium while the outer tube will form the myocardium and epicardium. As the head fold forms, the heart tube comes to lie dorsal to the coelom and ventral to the gut. A dorsal mesentery (mesocardium) suspends the heart. Later a passage (the transverse sinus) forms through this dorsal mesocardium.

The heart tube divides into bulges: these in cephalic to caudal order are bulbus cordis, primitive ventricle and atrium. The truncus arteriosus is soon recognizable cranial to the bulbus cordis and is continuous with the aortic sac. The sinus venosus appears inferior to the atrium and has two horns each formed by the confluence of one common cardinal, one umbilical and one vitelline vein.

As the heart tube continues to grow, a 'U' shaped bulboventricular loop forms from the primitive ventricle and the bulbus cordis bulges to the left and cranially. As the loop forms, the atrium is carried cephalic to the bulboventricular loop and comes to lie closely apposed to it. The sinus venosus is carried cranially to lie dorsal to the atrium. The primitive atrium expands to the right and left. The division between the bulbus cordis and ventricle is lost and a single ventricular chamber is formed.

The heart begins to contract by Day 22 and an ebb and flow circulation is established. By the end of Week 4 the circulation is unidirectional. The heart is divided internally between Week 4 and 5.

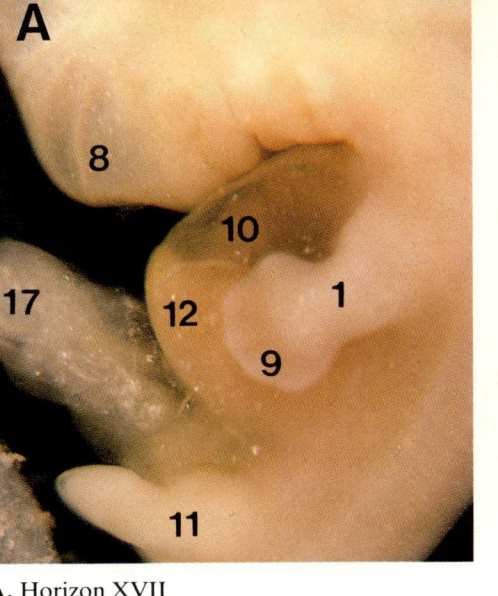

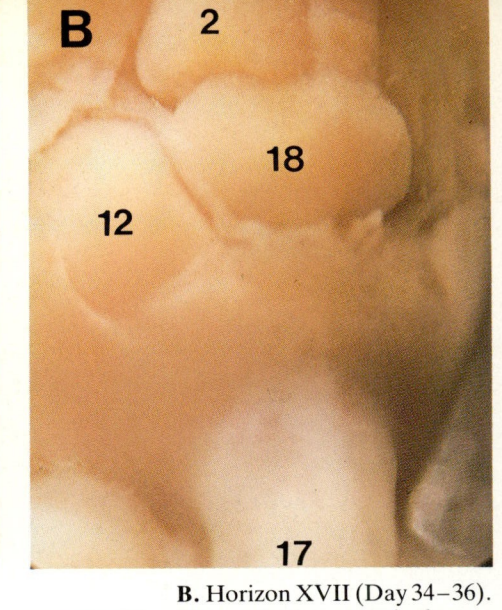

A. Horizon XVII (Day 34–36). The heart *in situ*. Viewed from the left. 12mmCR (×8.4)

B. Horizon XVII (Day 34–36). The ventricles are a single chamber. Viewed from the ventral surface. 12mmCR (×16.8)

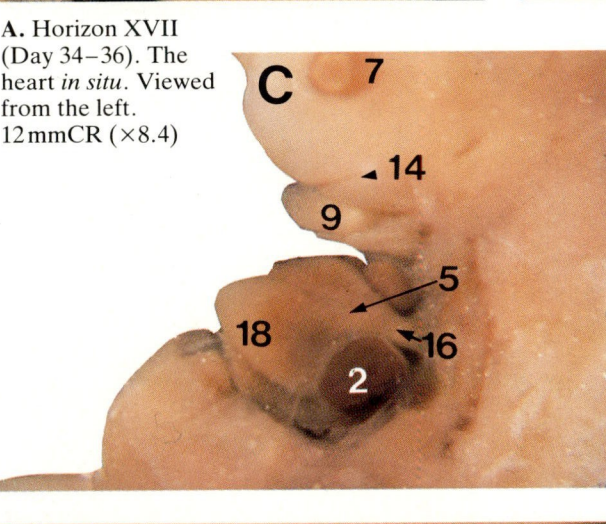

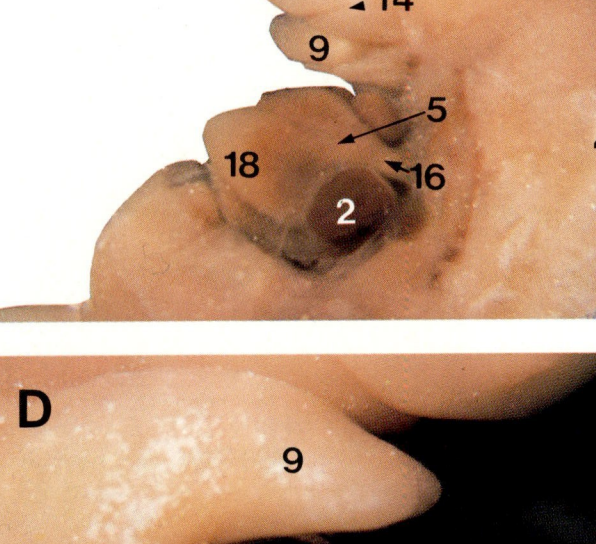

C. Horizon XIX (Day 38–40). Two ventricles are present. Viewed from the left. The left arm has been removed. 20mmCR (×8.4)

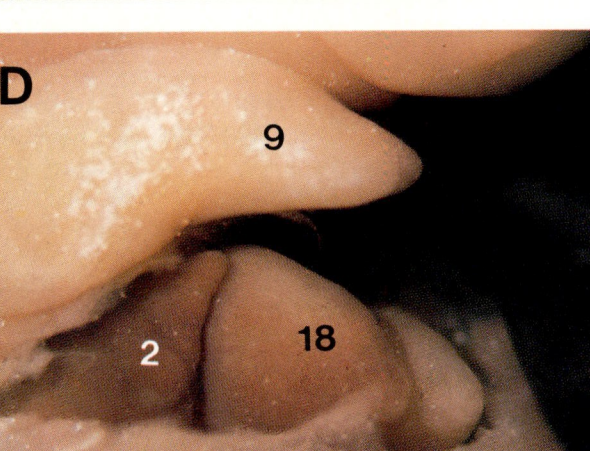

D. The same embryo as in Figure **C**. View of the right side. (×16)

A–F. External features of the developing heart.

1. arm bud
2. atrium
3. auricular appendage
4. back
5. bulbus cordis
6. common carotid artery
7. eye
8. forebrain
9. hand plate (paddle)
10. heart
11. leg bud
12. liver
13. lung
14. mouth
15. pulmonary trunk
16. truncus arteriosus
17. umbilical cord
18. ventricle

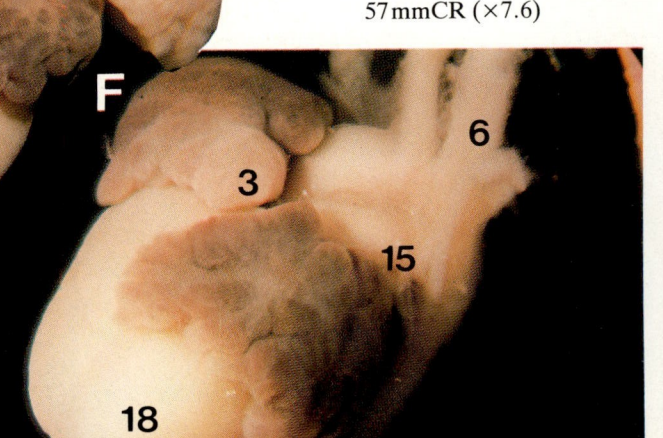

E. Week 9. The heart and lungs dissected from the specimen. View of the ventral surface. 48mmCR (×7.6)

F. Week 10. The dissected heart viewed from the left. 57mmCR (×7.6)

A. A series of developing hearts from the ventral surface. (×4)
Small: Week 9. 48 mm CR
Middle: Week 13. 92 mm CR ♀
Large: Week 15. 123 mm CR ♀

1. aorta
2. atrium
3. auricle
4. great cardiac vein and anterior interventricular artery
5. pulmonary trunk
6. superior vena cava
7. ventricle

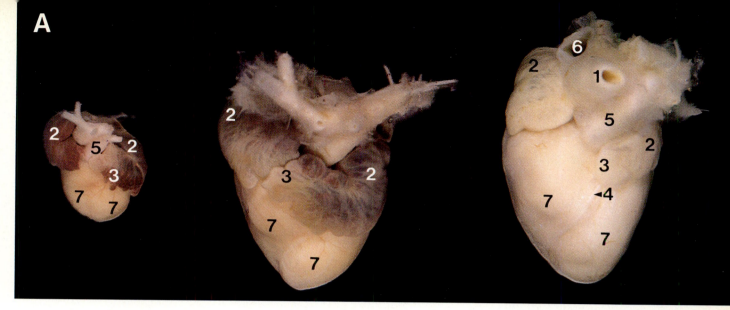

A and B. Week 10. The heart *in situ* with pericardium and following its removal. 56 mm CR

1. auricle
2. diaphragm
3. liver
4. lung
5. pericardium
6. thymus
7. ventricle

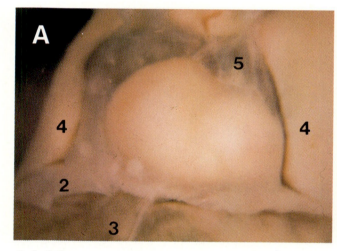

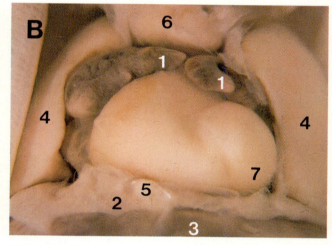

A. (×3.2)

B. (×3.2)

A and B. Week 13. The blood supply to the heart's external surface. 92 mm CR ♀ (×9)

1. auricle
2. coronary sinus
3. great cardiac vein and anterior interventricular artery
4. inferior vena cava
5. middle cardiac vein
6. posterior vein of the left ventricle
7. pulmonary vein
8. ventricle

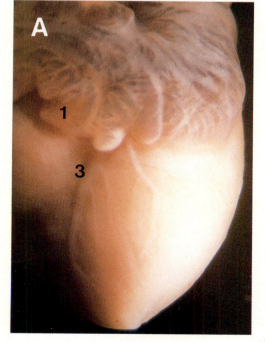

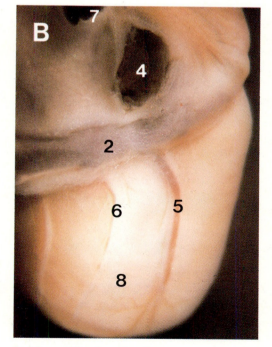

A. View of the ventral surface.

B. View of the dorsal surface.

Atrium

Partition of atrioventricular canal. Endocardial cushions form in the atrioventricular canal on the dorsal and ventral walls. During Week 5 the cushions grow toward each other, fuse (atrioventricular cushion) and divide the canal into right and left halves.

Partition of primitive atrium. The sinus venosus opens into the future right atrium. Right and left venous valves form on either side of the sinus venosus opening and two valves fuse cephalic to the sinus venosus as the septum spurium. In Week 6 a mid-line crescent-shaped septum, septum primum, forms on the dorsal atrial wall. This septum grows toward the ventral wall, completely dividing the primitive atrium into two atria and fusing with the atrioventricular cushion. As septum primum approaches the cushion, the opening (foramen primum) becomes progressively smaller. As the septum primum fuses with the left side of the cushion foramen primum disappears and the foramen secundum forms in the septum primum near its dorsal margin.

At the end of Week 5, the septum secundum appears on the ventrocranial wall and grows in a crescent shape toward the dorsocaudal wall between the septum primum and the septum spurium. This septum is an incomplete partition leaving an opening, the foramen ovale. The septum primum degenerates at its dorsal point of origin and the remainder of the septum forms the valve of the foramen ovale.

Sinus venosus. All venous blood enters the right atrium through the sinus venosus which has equally-sized right and left horns. During Week 4 the right horn enlarges and the left horn becomes a tributary which will form the coronary sinus. These changes are the result of two left-to-right shunts of blood (see Circulatory system: Blood vessels). As the atrium grows it incorporates the right sinus venosus into its dorsal wall. The right anterior and common cardinal veins form the superior vena cava, the right vitelline vein the terminal part of the inferior vena cava, the right umbilical vein regresses and disappears. The greater part of the atrium is derived from the sinus venosus and is smooth walled. The primitive atrium forms the auricle and has musculi pectinati in its walls.

The septum spurium and upper part of the right venous valve together form the crista terminalis. The lower part of the right venous valve forms the valves of the inferior vena cava and coronary sinus.

The single pulmonary vein opens into the left atrium. As the atrium grows it incorporates the pulmonary vein and its four tributaries (two to each lung) into its walls. This part of the atrium is smooth-walled, while the part derived from the primitive atrium has musculi pectinati in its walls.

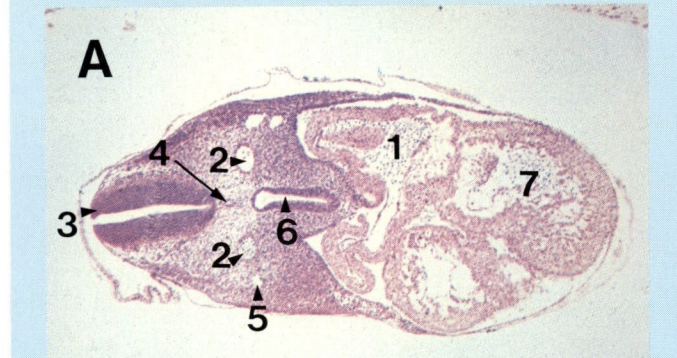

From C.C.H.M.S.

A. Horizons XI and XII (Day 24–27). Transverse section through the early heart. 4 mmCR (×100)

1. atrium
2. dorsal aorta
3. neural tube
4. notochord
5. precardinal vein
6. tracheoesophageal tube
7. ventricle

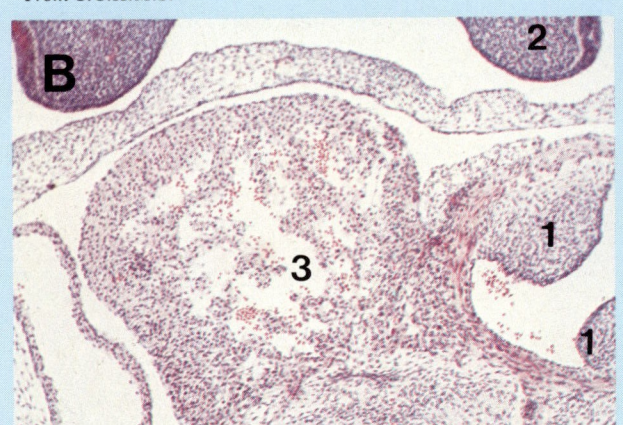

B. Horizon XVI (Day 32–34). Transverse section through the early ventricle. 10 mmCR (×167)

1. conus swellings
2. medial nasal prominence
3. ventricle

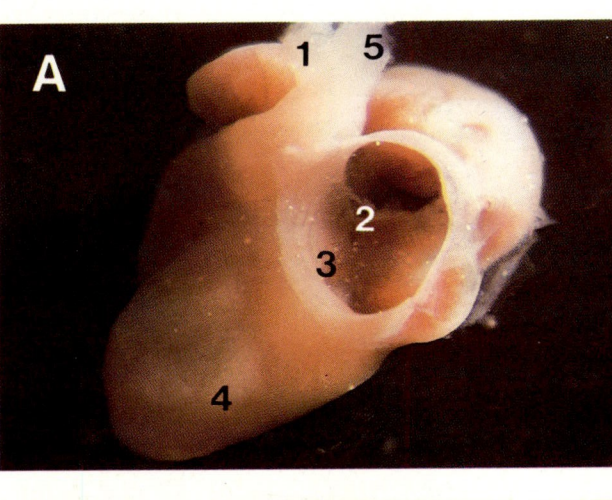

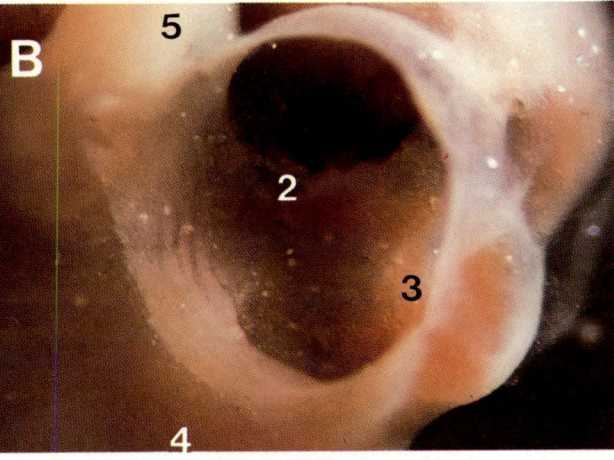

A and B. Horizon XIX (Day 38–40). The septum primum viewed through the opened left atrium. 20 mmCR ♀

1. aorta
2. developing septum primum
3. left atrium with fused endocardial cushions
4. left ventricle
5. pulmonary trunk

A. (×8.4)

B. (×16)

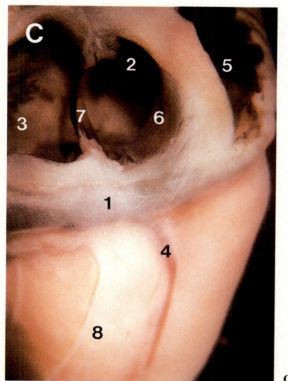

C and D. Week 13. The left atrium opened on the dorsal (back) surface to illustrate the septae. The area between the two septa has been artificially enlarged. 92 mm CR ♀

1. coronary sinus
2. foramen ovale (enlarged)
3. left atrium
4. middle cardiac vein
5. right atrium
6. septum secundum
7. septum primum
8. ventricle

C. (×9.5)

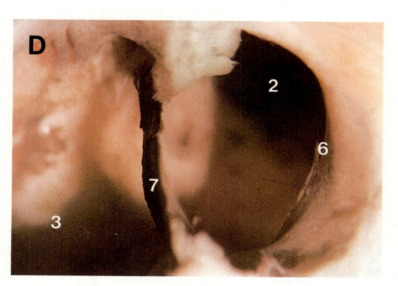

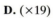

D. (×19)

Ventricle

Partition of primitive ventricle. The primitive ventricle is divided into right and left halves by an interventricular septum arising from the floor near the apex of the primitive ventricle. This crescent-shaped septum grows cranially toward the atrioventricular cushion. An interventricular foramen between the edge of the interventricular septum and fused endocardial cushions disappears during Week 7 when the right bulbar ridge, left bulbar ridge and atrioventricular cushion tissue fuse.

Ventricular walls. A sponge-work of muscle bundles is formed some of which form trabeculae carneae, others papillary muscles and chordae tendineae.

Partition of bulbus cordis and truncus arteriosus. During Week 5 two ridges appear opposite to one another in the bulbus cordis and truncus arteriosus which spiral inferiorly toward the heart. These ridges fuse (spiral septum) in the mid-line and divide the bulbus cordis and truncus arteriosus into two vessels, the aorta and the pulmonary trunk. The bulbus cordis is eventually incorporated into the ventricles, the infundibulum into the right ventricle, and the aortic vestibule into the left ventricle.

Cardiac valves. The semilunar valves of the aorta and pulmonary trunk form from three subendocardial swellings. These swellings hollow out and form cusps. The tricuspid and mitral valves form similarly.

Conducting system. The sinu-atrial node forms in the right wall of the sinus venosus and is incorporated into the right atrium. Cells from the left wall of the sinus venosus are incorporated into the interatrial septum and, with cells from the atrioventricular canal region, are known as the atrioventricular node and bundle of His.

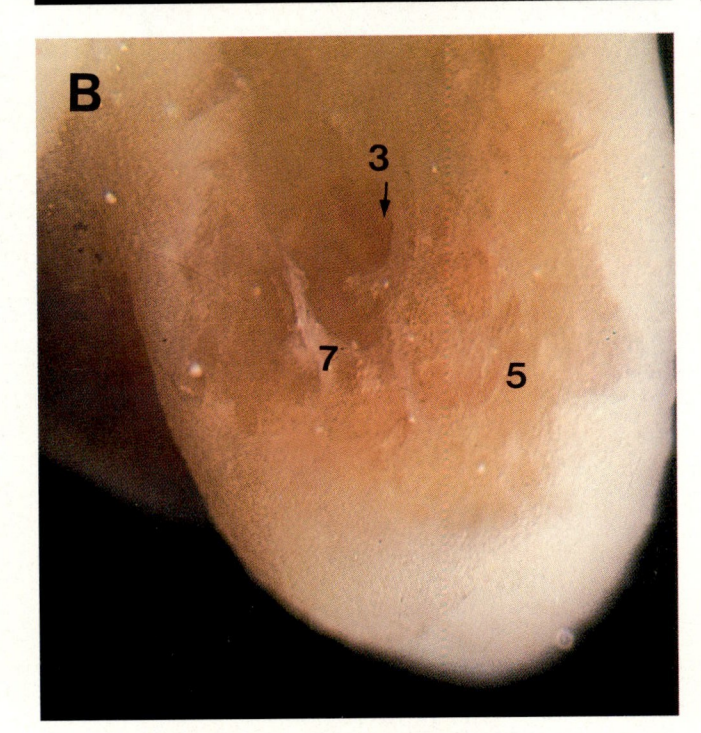

A and B. Horizon XIX (Day 38–40). The ventricle viewed from the left. The wall has been dissected. 20 mmCR

1. aorta
2. auricle
3. interventricular foramen
4. left atrium
5. left ventricle
6. pulmonary trunk
7. trabeculae carneae

A. (×20.4)

B. (×46)

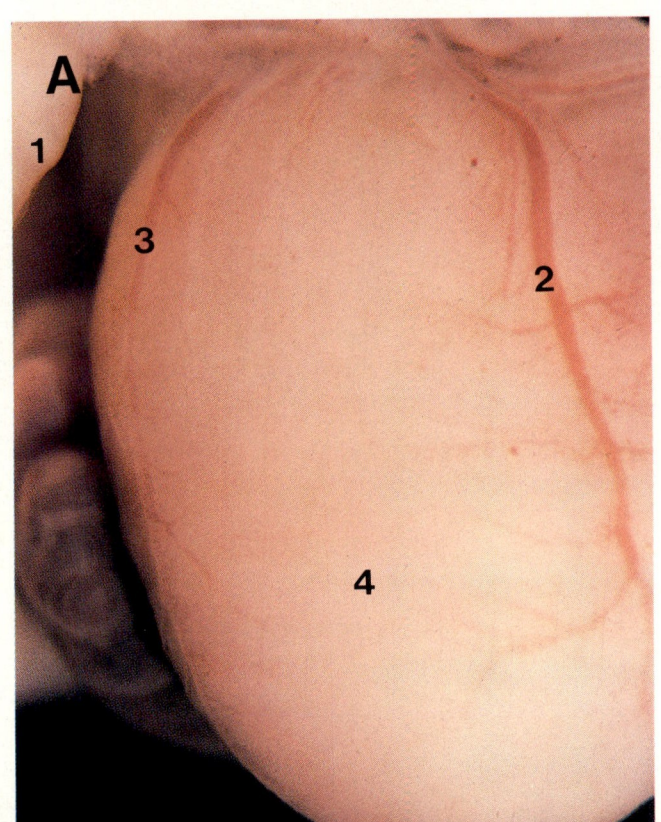

A. Week 9. Blood supply of the dorsal surface of the heart. 48 mmCR ♀ (×23)

1. lung
2. middle cardiac vein and posterior interventricular branch of right coronary artery
3. posterior vein of left ventricle
4. ventricle

Fetal circulation

Oxygenated blood from the placenta returns to the fetus via the umbilical vein, which enters the fetus to become the left umbilical vein.

Some of the oxygenated blood passes through the hepatic sinusoids and some bypasses the liver via the ductus venosus and enters the inferior vena cava where it mixes with venous blood from the fetal lower limbs, pelvis and abdomen. This blood enters the right atrium and is directed toward the foramen ovale by the valve of the inferior vena cava. The lower border of the septum secundum (crista dividens) deflects the flow into two unequal streams. The larger flow passes through the foramen ovale; the lesser flow mixes with the venous return through the superior vena cava and passes through to the right ventricle where it is passed to the pulmonary artery, ductus arteriosus, descending aorta and returns to the placenta via the umbilical arteries. Some is also distributed to the viscera. Little passes to the lungs because of the high pulmonary vascular resistance.

The main stream passing through the foramen ovale to the left atrium mixes with any blood returning from the lungs, enters the left ventricle and then the ascending aorta which distributes to the head, neck and upper limbs.

Changes at birth

At birth the foramen ovale, ductus arteriosus, ductus venosus, umbilical arteries and umbilical vein become no longer functional.

With the interruption to placental circulation, there is a drop in blood pressure in the inferior vena cava and right atrium. As the lungs are aerated and the pulmonary blood flow greatly increased, the pressure in the left atrium is greater than in the right atrium. This increased pressure presses the septum primum against the septum secundum and closes the foramen ovale.

The ductus arteriosus constricts at birth as do the umbilical arteries. The cord is usually not tied for a minute or two to allow blood in the placenta to return to the neonate via the umbilical vein.

Later the ductus arteriosus, ductus venosus and the umbilical vessels are occluded by proliferation of endothelial and fibrous tissue.

The umbilical vein is discernible as the ligamentum teres which usually retains a reduced but patent lumen even in the adult.

The umbilical arteries remain distally as the medial umbilical ligaments and proximally remain patent and give off the superior vesical arteries.

The ligamentum venosum is the remnant of the ductus venosus.

In the heart the septum primum forms the floor of the fossa ovalis, the lower margin of the septum secundum forms the annulus ovalis.

The ductus arteriosus forms the ligamentum arteriosum. The ductus is obliterated by tissue by the end of the third month after birth.

A. Week 15. 123 mm CR ♀ (×3.9)

B. Week 18. 152 mm CR ♂ (×4)

A and B. The ductus arteriosus viewed from the left. Left lung removed.

1. arch of aorta
2. auricular appendage of the heart
3. common carotid artery
4. descending aorta
5. ductus arteriosus
6. intercostal vessels
7. left subclavian artery
8. right lung
9. sympathetic trunk
10. thymus gland
11. trachea
12. ventricle of the heart

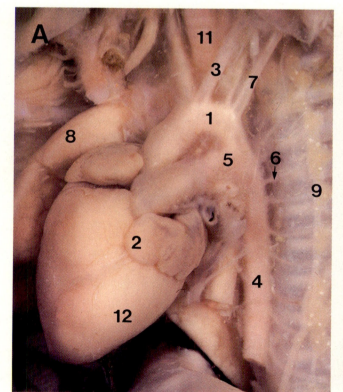

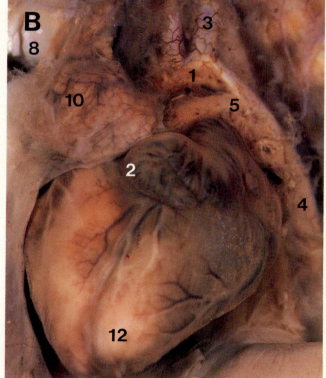

Circulatory system

Blood and blood vessels

The first blood and blood vessels develop from angioblasts (mesoderm) on the yolk sac, connecting stalk and in the chorion during Horizon VI (Day 13–15). In Week 3 small groups of angioblasts form blood islands in the yolk sac and body stalk. In each island spaces appear and the central cells form nucleated primitive red blood cells and the peripheral ones the vascular endothelium of the blood vessels. Later several islands join together to form vessels. Mesoderm surrounding the vessels will form the connective tissue and muscular elements of the vessels.

As blood islands are established in the liver (Week 5), spleen (Week 10) and bone marrow (Week 9–12) the extra-embryonic hemopoietic supply disappears (Week 6). After birth only the bone marrow normally continues as an hemopoietic organ.

Fetal blood does not coagulate until Week 10–12. Before the end of Week 3 two endothelial heart tubes form similarly, fuse to form a single heart tube and by Day 20 have linked up with the blood vessels of the embryo, allantois and yolk sac. By the end of Week 3 the cardiovascular system is established and the heart is contracting from the sinus venosus. By the end of Week 4 the contractions have established a unidirectional flow.

Blood returns to the heart from the embryo via the anterior and posterior common cardinal veins, from the placenta via the umbilical veins and from the yolk sac via the vitelline veins. All three vessels on each side join at the septum transversum and enter the heart.

Blood leaves the heart to the body via the aortic arches to the paired dorsal aortae which form a single vessel posteriorly, to the placenta via the umbilical arteries and to the yolk sac via the vitelline arteries.

- While the neonatal kidney adjusts functionally during the first week after birth the blood urea is slightly high.

- Fetal hemoglobin predominates at birth.

Arteries

Each branchial arch is supplied by an artery arising from the aortic sac and passing to its respective right or left aorta. The arteries are not all present at the same time; the first two degenerate before the last appears and the fifth is rudimentary. By Horizon XIV (Day 28–30) the dorsal aortae are extended cranially to form the internal carotids and from the sixth arch artery a branch called the pulmonary artery supplies each lung bud. The first and second arch arteries develop into the maxillary and stapedial arteries respectively.

Carotid arteries. The common carotids form from the third aortic arches. Where the third and fourth arch arteries are connected to one another by sections of aortae these segments disappear to leave the original third arch arteries to form the proximal internal carotids and the aortae to form the distal portions. The internal carotids give off anterior and middle cerebral branches and an ophthalmic branch to the optic vesicle. The external carotids may receive a contribution from the roots of the first arch arteries.

Umbilical arteries. At birth the umbilical arteries become non-functional but remain patent at the proximal end where each has a superior vesical branch to supply the bladder.

Vitelline arteries. The vitelline arteries disappear and a new vessel forms a single superior mesenteric artery supplying the midgut. Later, the celiac artery will form to supply the foregut and the inferior mesenteric to supply the hindgut.

Intersegmental arteries. There are approximately 30 pairs of intersegmental arteries arising from the dorsal aortae. They pass successively between the somites. In the neck they join together to form the vertebral artery. In the thorax and abdomen they are retained as the intercostal arteries and lumbar arteries respectively. The right seventh intersegmental artery contributes to the right subclavian while the left seventh intersegmental artery forms the left subclavian of the adult. The fifth lumbar arteries with the umbilical arteries form the common iliac arteries.

Pulmonary trunk. As the spiral ridges divide the truncus arteriosus (see Heart) two vessels are formed; the pulmonary trunk and the ascending aorta. As this division extends into the aortic sac, the sixth arch artery connects to the pulmonary trunk and the remaining vessels to the aorta.

Aorta. The left half of the truncus arteriosus forms the ascending aorta; the fourth arch artery forms the arch of the aorta and the left dorsal aorta forms the descending aorta. The distal part of the sixth arch artery forms the ductus arteriosus (see Changes at birth).

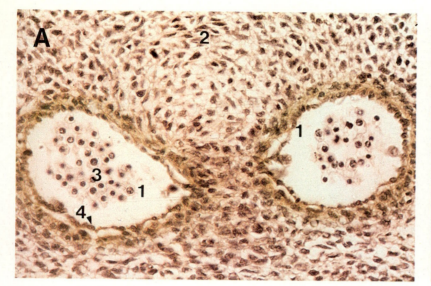

A. Horizon XV (Day 31–32).
Transverse section of the two
dorsal aortae with blood cells.
7mmCR (×610)

From L.H.S.M.

1. aorta
2. mesoderm
3. nucleated red blood cells
4. vascular endothelium

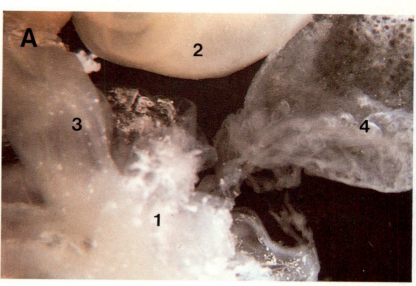

A. Horizon XVII (Day
34–36). Yolk sac of the early
embryo. 12mmCR (×9.6)

1. amnion
2. forebrain
3. umbilical cord
4. yolk sac

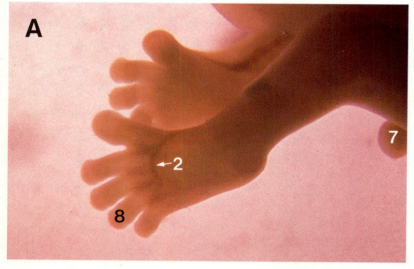

A. Week 8. The dorsal venous
arch of the foot. 34mmCR
(×9.6)

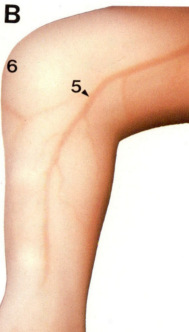

B. Week 9. Great saphenous
vein of the leg. 48mmCR
(×9.2)

A–C. Blood vessels
developing in the limbs. Note
the thin layer of skin over the
vessels.

1. dorsal carpal arch
2. dorsal venous arch of foot
3. dorsum of hand
4. finger (minimus)
5. great saphenous vein
6. knee
7. phallus
8. toes

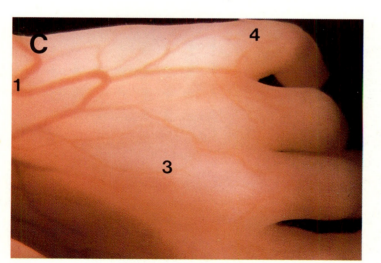

C. Week 13. Dorsal carpal
arch. 95mmCR (×9.2)

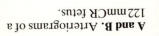

A and B. Arteriograms of a 122 mmCR fetus.

1. abdominal aorta
2. anterior tibial
3. axillary
4. basilar
5. brachial
6. common carotid
7. deep palmar arch
8. dorsalis pedis
9. external carotid
10. external iliac
11. femoral
12. heart
13. internal carotid
14. lung
15. middle cerebral
16. popliteal
17. posterior tibial
18. radial
19. right pulmonary
20. subclavian
21. superior mesenteric
22. ulnar
23. umbilical
24. vertebral

A. Anteroposterior view.
(×1.8)

From Mr R. H. Watts

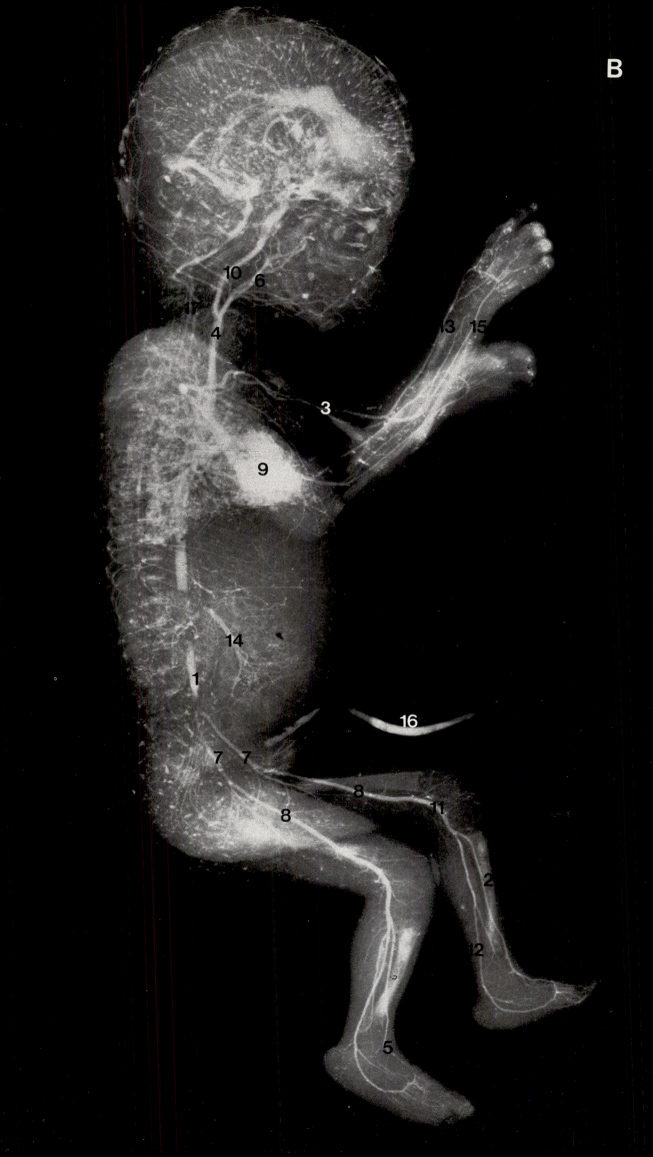

1. abdominal aorta
2. anterior tibial
3. brachial
4. common carotid
5. dorsalis pedis
6. external carotid
7. external iliac
8. femoral
9. heart
10. internal carotid
11. popliteal
12. posterior tibial
13. radial
14. superior mesenteric
15. ulnar
16. umbilical
17. vertebral

B. Lateral view. (×1.8)

From Mr R.H. Watts

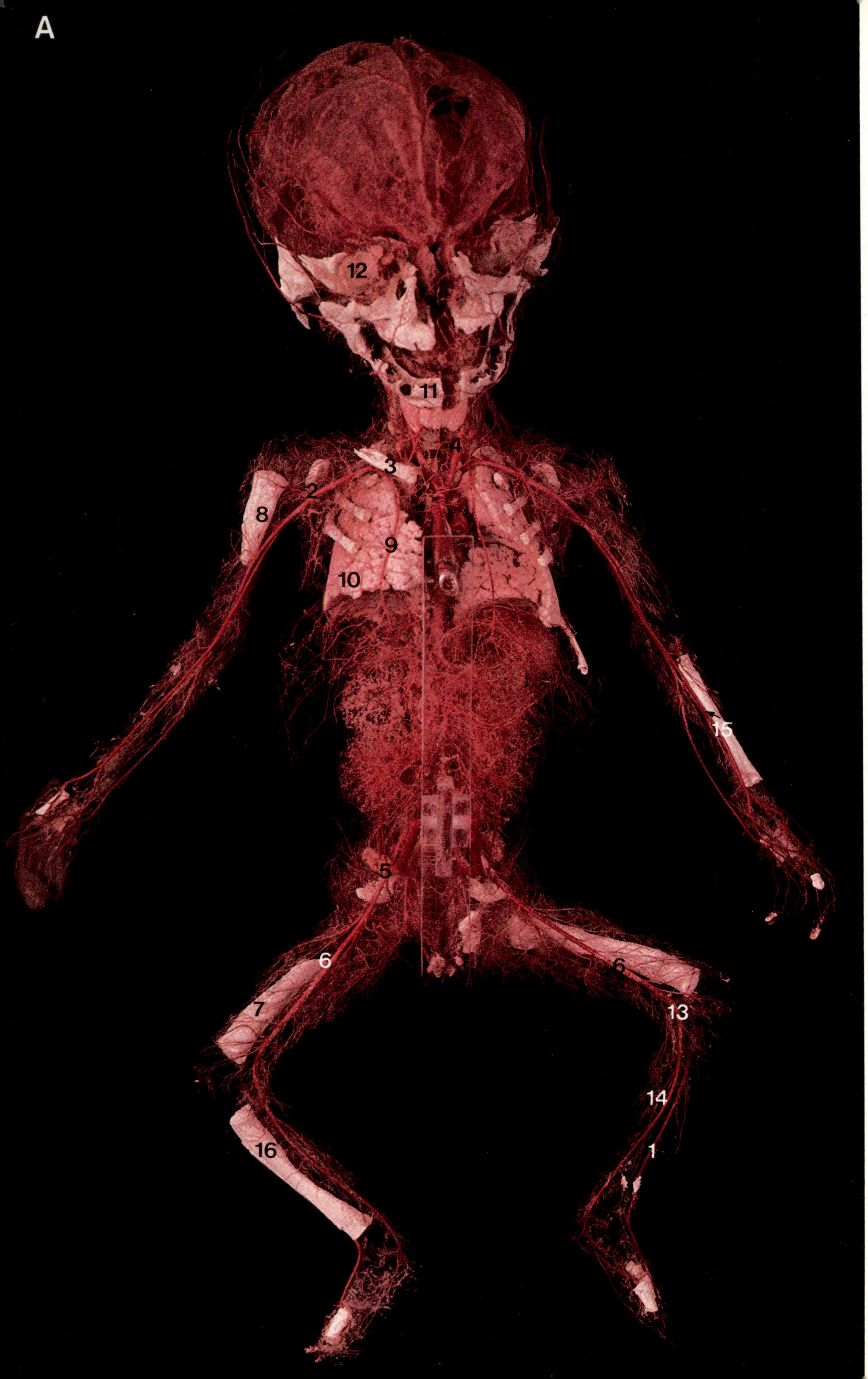

A. Cast of the arterial supply of the fetus. (×1)

1. anterior tibial
2. axillary
3. clavicle bone
4. common carotid
5. external iliac
6. femoral
7. femur (broken) bone
8. humerus (broken) bone
9. internal thoracic
10. lung
11. mandible bone
12. orbit bones
13. popliteal
14. posterior tibial
15. radial
16. tibia bone

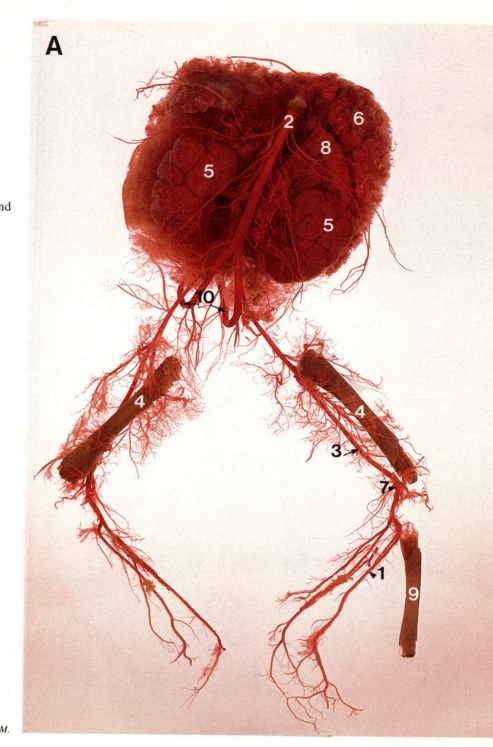

A. Resin cast of the arterial supply of the kidneys and lower limbs. Viewed from behind. (×1.2)

1. anterior tibial artery
2. aorta
3. femoral artery
4. femur
5. kidney
6. liver
7. popliteal artery
8. suprarenal (adrenal) gland
9. tibia
10. umbilical arteries

From R.F.H.S.M.

Veins

Anterior cardinal veins. Blood drains from three plexi in the head into the anterior (pre-) cardinal veins. The superficial vessels of the plexi form dural venous sinuses and the deep vessels form the cerebral veins.

Common cardinal veins. The anterior and posterior cardinal veins join to form the common cardinal veins lying in the septum transversum and opening into the sinus venosus. The right common cardinal vein forms the superior vena cava, while the left becomes a tributary of the coronary sinus.

Posterior cardinal veins. The posterior cardinal veins drain the body walls, spinal cord and mesonephros. They are largely obliterated by the mesonephros pressing against them and are replaced by a new pair of subcardinal veins. These lie medial to the mesonephros and connect with the subcardinal anastomosis.

A new channel (subcardinal vitelline anastomosis) forms to connect the stump of the right vitelline vein to the subcardinal vein. This channel together with the right subcardinal, sacrocardinal segment and right vitelline forms the inferior vena cava.

Finally the supracardinals appear, become broken up in the region of the kidneys, unite by an anastomosis and form the azygos and hemiazygos vessels. The root of the azygos vein forms from the right posterior cardinal vein.

Umbilical and vitelline veins. On each side the umbilical and vitelline veins pass through the septum transversum and enter the sinus venosus. Where the vessels cross the septum transversum they become invested by the liver cords and form hepatic sinuses. Caudal to this region the right umbilical vein atrophies in Week 6. Cranial to the liver sinusoids the right and left umbilical veins and the left vitelline vein atrophy. Blood from the placenta flows via the left umbilical vein into the septum transversum where a shunt, the ductus venosus, connects the flow to the right vitelline vein which has enlarged to form the hepatocardiac channel.

At birth the placental flow ceases and the left umbilical vein becomes the ligamentum teres whilst the ductus venosus becomes the ligamentum venosum. The hepatic sinusoids drain into the right hepatocardiac channel which forms the terminal part of the inferior vena cava.

Portal vein. Caudal to the liver three sets of vessels develop to connect the two vitelline veins. The cranial and caudal anastomosing vessels pass ventrally and the middle passes dorsally to the duodenum. The portal vein forms when the left vitelline vein disappears between the cranial and middle anastomoses and the right vitelline vein disappears between the middle and caudal anastomoses. The intrahepatic portion of the portal vein forms from hepatic sinusoids derived from the vitelline vein.

The vitello-intestinal duct and caudal parts of the vitelline vein degenerate concomitantly.

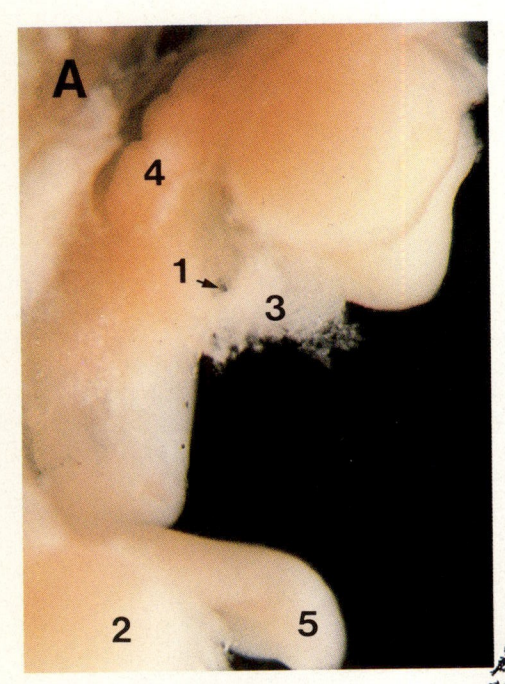

A. Horizon XVIII (Day 36–38). The developing inferior vena cava viewed from the right. 14mmCR (×16.5)

1. developing inferior vena cava
2. leg bud (right)
3. liver cords (liver dissected off)
4. lung bud
5. midgut herniation

C. Week 10. The blood vessels dissected out of the developing liver viewed from the dorsal (back) surface. 60mmCR (×8.1)

1. caudate lobe
2. ductus venosus
3. left lobe
4. portal sinus
5. portal vein
6. quadrate lobe
7. right lobe
8. umbilical vein

B. A resin cast of the blood supply to the developing liver. (×1.4)

1. common iliac veins
2. inferior vena cava
3. kidney
4. left hepatic vein
5. left lobe of liver
6. portal vein
7. right hepatic vein
8. right lobe of liver

From R.C.S.E.

Lungs

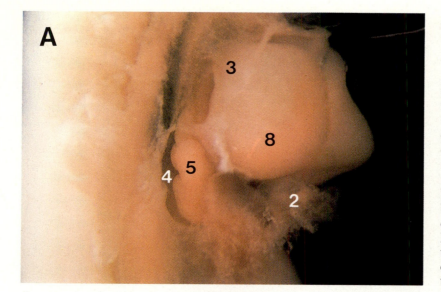

A. Horizon XVIII (Day 36–38). Right lung viewed *in situ*. 14mmCR (×18.9)

A–G. Development of the lungs.

1. left main bronchus
2. liver cords
3. pericardium
4. pleural membrane
5. right lung
6. right main bronchus
7. trachea
8. ventricles of the heart
9. inferior lobe ⎫
10. superior lobe ⎬ left lung
11. inferior lobe ⎫
12. middle lobe ⎬ right lung
13. superior lobe ⎭

B. The lung buds shown in Figure **A** dissected from the embryo. The lungs already show the adult pattern of lobes. (×36)

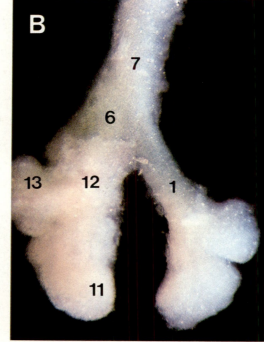

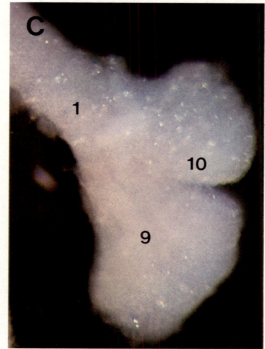

C. The left lung in Figure **B** at a higher magnification. (×72)

A respiratory diverticulum forms in the floor of the pharynx at Day 26. Two endodermal lung buds grow from the caudal end of this diverticulum (Day 28) and are surrounded by splanchnic mesoderm. These two components will form the lung. The cephalic end of the diverticulum will form the trachea. During Week 5 the smaller left lung bud divides into two lobes and the right into three lobes which correspond with the main bronchi and lobes of the adult lung. The right main bronchus is more vertical than the left early in development. The lung resembles a gland at this stage. Each bronchus then subdivides several times (Week 24) to form a bronchial tree. The original columnar epithelium has become stretched to form cuboidal and then squamous epithelium.

Respiratory movements occur before birth which draw amniotic fluid into the lungs. Fluid from the lungs and tracheal glands is also present in the airways.

At birth the first breath must overcome the elastic resistance of the lungs themselves and the surface tension of the fluid in the lungs. The alveoli near the bronchi dilate, while those at the periphery expand by Day 3 to 4 of postnatal development. The neonate has one eighth to one sixth of the adult number of alveoli. Alveoli continue to form until approximately 8 years of age.

- A natural 'detergent' or surfactant is secreted in the lungs at Week 23–28 and can reduce the surface tension of the fluids which line the airways. Hyaline membrane disease, which is associated with a deficiency or absence of surfactant, is a common cause of death in infants born before Week 32. Thyroxine stimulates surfactant production.

- The fluid-filled lungs of a stillborn infant will sink at autopsy when placed in water. Lungs of an infant which has drawn breath will float. This fact may be of medico-legal importance.

- After birth a foreign body is more likely to enter the right main bronchus than the left because of the more vertical direction of the right bronchus.

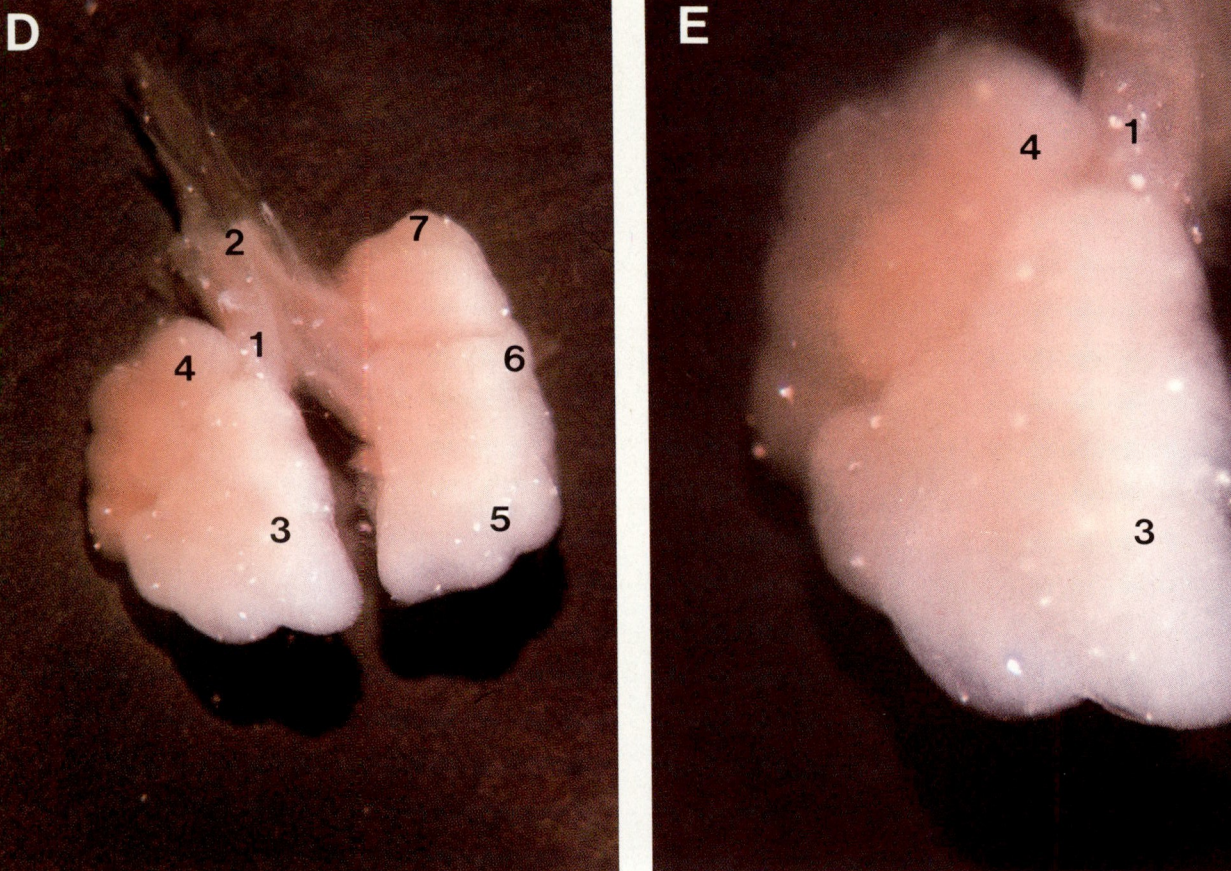

D. Horizon XIX (Day 38–40).
Dissection of early lung
viewed from the back (dorsal)
surface. 20mmCR (×21.9)

1. left main bronchus
2. trachea
3. inferior lobe ⎫
4. superior lobe ⎭ left lung
5. inferior lobe ⎫
6. middle lobe ⎬ right lung
7. superior lobe ⎭

E. The left lung in Figure **D** at
a higher magnification viewed
from the back. (×45.6)

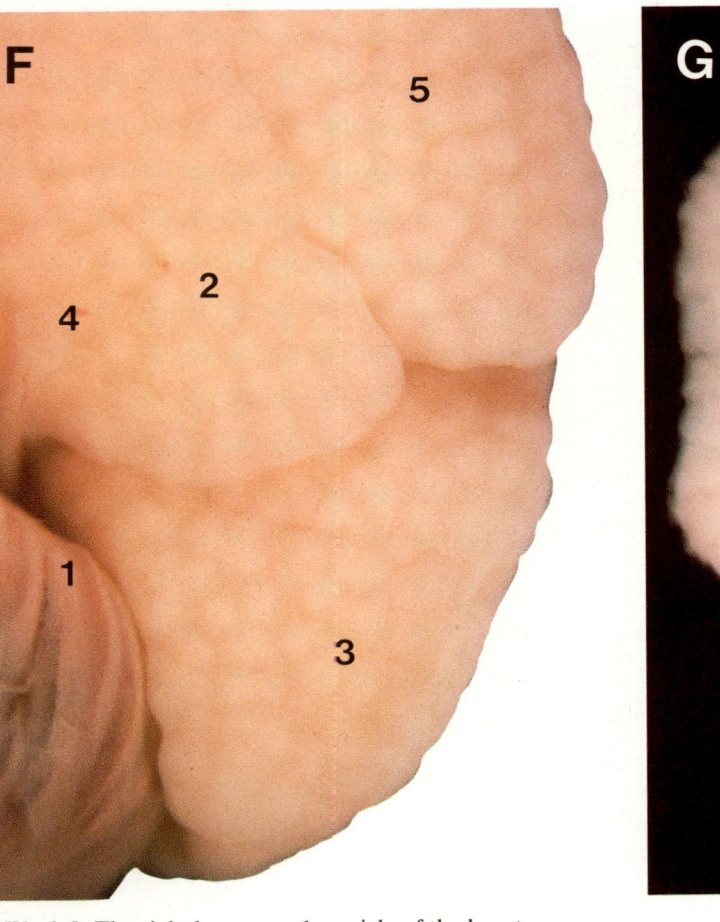

G. Week 10. The left lung
viewed from the costal surface
56mmCR (×10.8)

1. inferior lobe
2. superior lobe

F. Week 9. The right lung
viewed from the
diaphragmatic surface. Note
the lobules. 48mmCR ♀
(×21.9)

1. auricle of the heart
2. lobules
3. inferior lobe ⎫
4. middle lobe ⎬ right lung
5. superior lobe ⎭

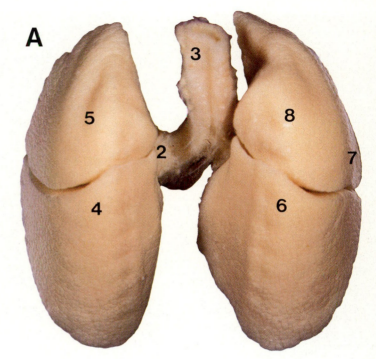

A. Week 13. Lungs viewed from the back (dorsal) surface 92 mm CR ♀ (×4.1)

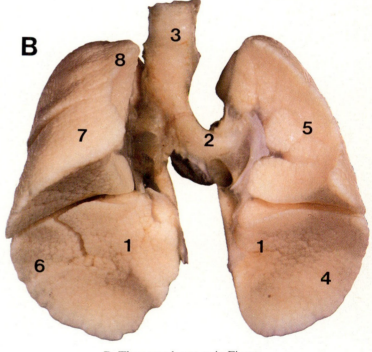

B. The same lungs as in Figure A viewed from the ventral and diaphragmatic surface. (×4.1)

1. diaphragmatic surface
2. left main bronchus
3. trachea
4. inferior lobe } left lung
5. superior lobe }
6. inferior lobe ⎫
7. middle lobe   ⎬ right lung
8. superior lobe ⎭

A. Development of the lungs as viewed from the back (dorsal) surface. (×5.4)
Week 9. The smallest lungs. 48 mm CR ♂
Week 10. The largest lungs. 60 mm CR ♀

1. left main bronchus
2. trachea
3. superior lobe } left lung
4. inferior lobe }
5. inferior lobe ⎫
6. middle lobe   ⎬ right lung
7. superior lobe ⎭

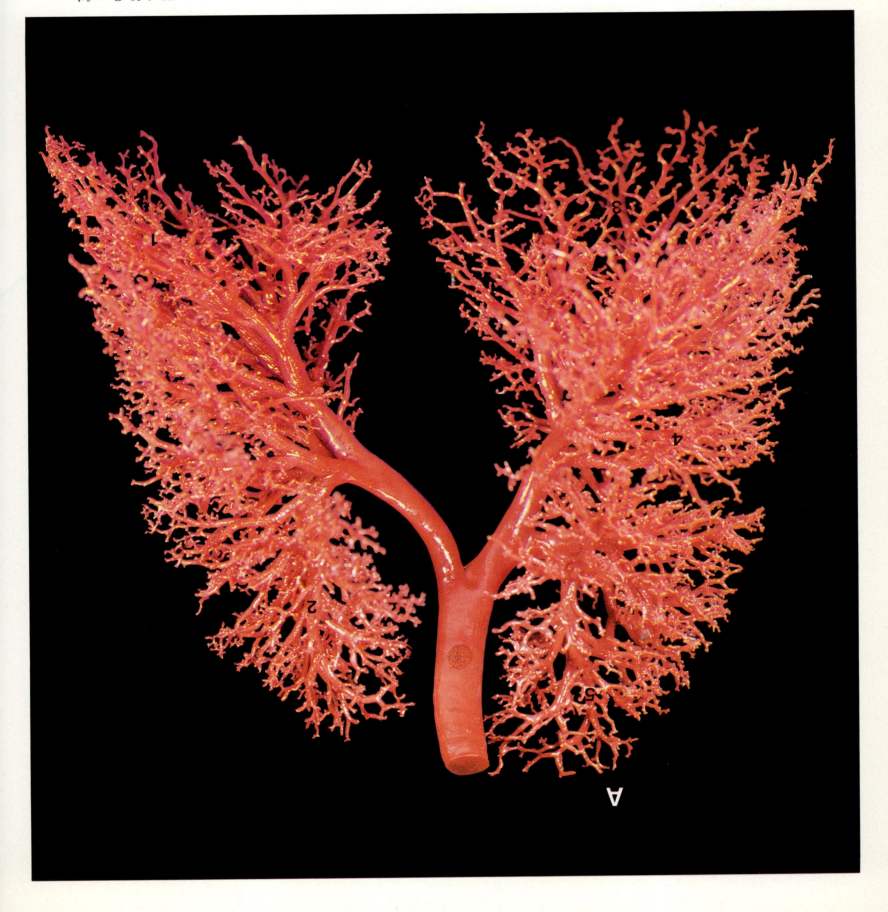

From R.C.S.E.

A. Week 30. Cast of the
bronchial tree viewed from the
front (ventral) surface.
(×2.5)

left lung { 1. inferior lobe
2. superior lobe

right lung { 3. inferior lobe
4. middle lobe
5. superior lobe

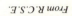

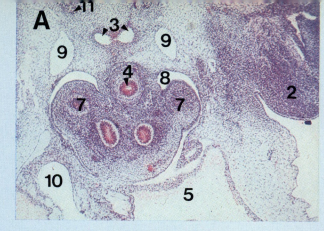

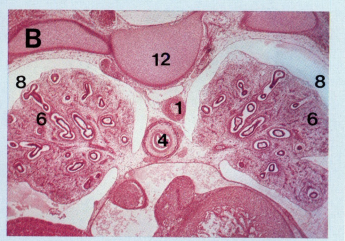

A. Horizon XVI (Day 32–34).
Lung buds. 10 mmCR (×88)

From L.H.S.M.

B. Horizon XXIII (Day
46–48). 28 mmCR (×33)

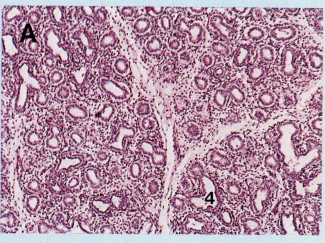

A–C. Early development of
the lung.

1. aorta
2. arm bud
3. dorsal aortae
4. esophagus
5. left atrium
6. lung
7. lung bud
8. pleural cavity
9. posterior cardinal vein
10. sinus venosus
11. sympathetic trunk
12. vertebral body

C. Week 8. Sagittal
section.
35 mmCR (×26)

From Mr G. Bottomley

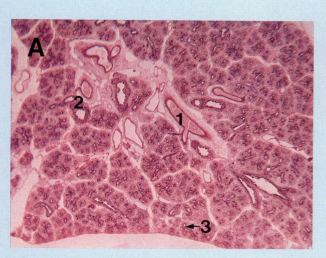

1. blood vessels
2. bronchi
3. bronchioles
4. early airways

A. Week 13. The lung
resembles a gland. 101 mmCR
♀ (×104)

A. Week 20. The lung more
closely resembles the neonate
lung. (×16)

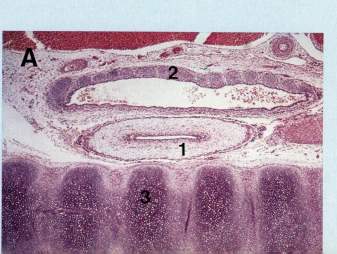

A. Horizon XXIII (Day
46–48). Longitudinal section
of the trachea. 29 mmCR
(×42)

1. esophagus
2. trachea
3. vertebral body

Diaphragm

The diaphragm has several origins: the sternal and costal parts from the septum transversum and small contributions from the thoracic wall (costal), and a dorsolateral part of the pleuro-peritoneal membrane.

The dorsal mesentery contributes to the area between the esophagus and aortic hiatus. Ventral to the esophageal hiatus the septum transversum contributes a small area. The remaining lumbar area of the diaphragm is from mesoderm around the aorta and in the dorsal body wall.

The muscles of the diaphragm form (Day 32) primarily from the fourth cervical myotome which invades the septum transversum. The phrenic nerve (C3,4,5) is carried with the septum transversum as it migrates caudally.

The liver and the enlarging pleural cavities cause the diaphragm to be dome-shaped.

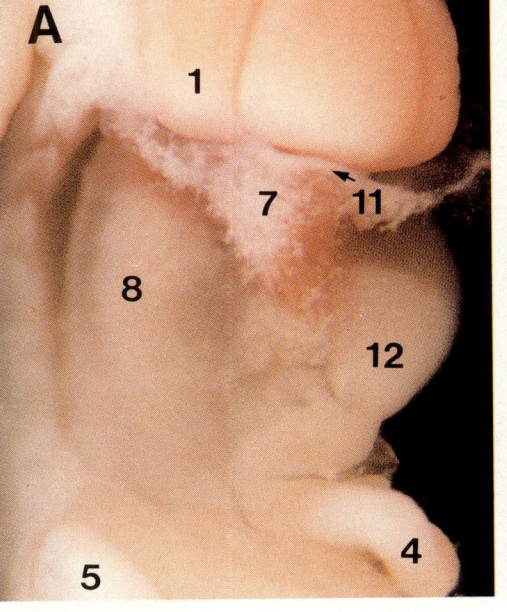

A. Horizon XVIII (Day 36–38). 14 mmCR (×17)

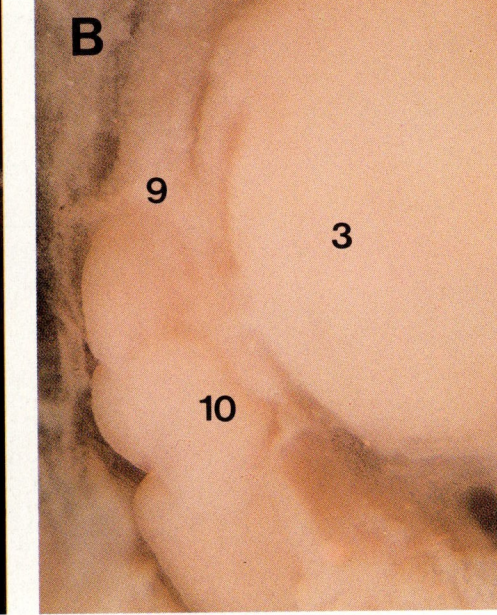

B. Horizon XVIII (Day 36–38). 14 mmCR (×34)

A–D. Contributions to the early diaphragm.

1. atrium
2. cactus needle
3. heart
4. intestine
5. leg bud
6. liver
7. liver removed
8. mesonephros
9. pleuroperitoneal membrane
10. right lung bud
11. septum transversum
12. stomach

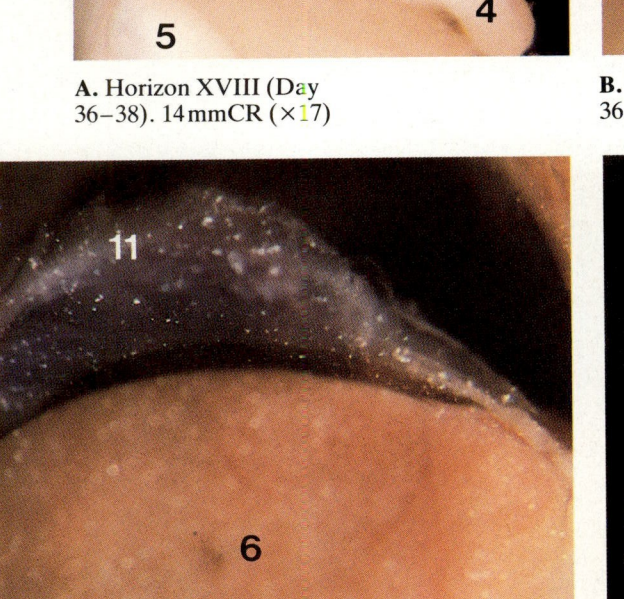

C. Horizon XIX (Day 38–40). The liver viewed from the left side. 20 mmCR (×18)

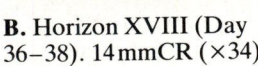

D. Same embryo as in Figure C. The liver has been removed. No muscle is present yet. (×18)

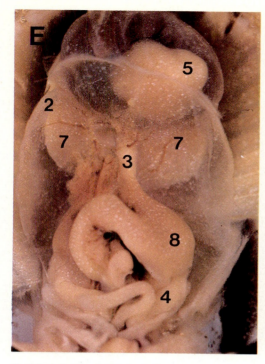

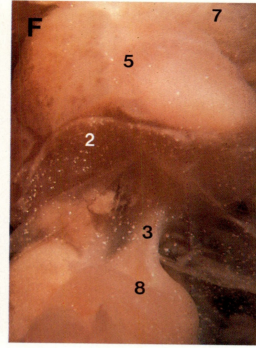

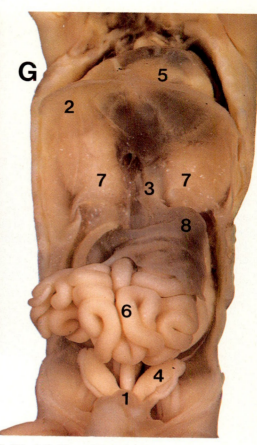

E. Week 8. 34 mmCR (×5.3)

F. Week 8. 40 mmCR (×8.4)

E–G. Diaphragm viewed from below.

1. bladder
2. diaphragm
3. esophagus
4. gonad
5. heart
6. intestine
7. lung
8. stomach

G. Week 9. 50 mmCR (×5.6)

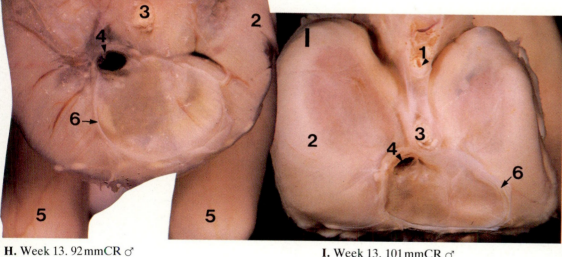

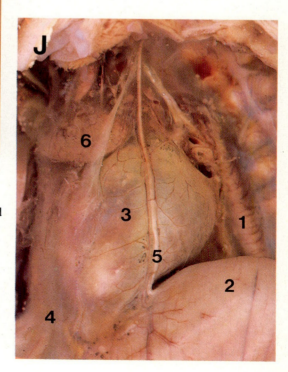

H. Week 13. 92 mmCR ♂ (×2.8)

I. Week 13. 101 mmCR ♂ (×1.5)

H and I. Diaphragm viewed from above.

1. aorta
2. diaphragm
3. esophagus
4. inferior vena cava
5. leg
6. pericardium
7. spinal cord
8. vertebral body

J. Week 18. Phrenic nerve and the diaphragm viewed from the left. Left lung removed. 152 mmCR (×2.7)

1. aorta
2. diaphragm
3. heart
4. pericardium
5. phrenic nerve
6. thymus

121

Abdomen

Body wall

Initially the anterior abdominal wall is a thin layer of epithelium and mesoderm over the developing organs.

Muscles are formed from myotomes which are originally on the back (dorsal) and migrate as two sheets around the body on to the ventral surface.

In Week 8 the two sheets fuse in the midline and their join is marked as the linea alba.

A–D. Body wall. View of the abdomen from the cephalic aspect.

1. arm
2. genital tubercle
3. head
4. leg bud (leg)
5. linea alba
6. ribs
7. tail
8. umbilical cord

A. Horizon XVII (Day 34–36). 12 mmCR (×17)

B. Horizon XXII (Day 44–46). 27 mmCR (×8.4)

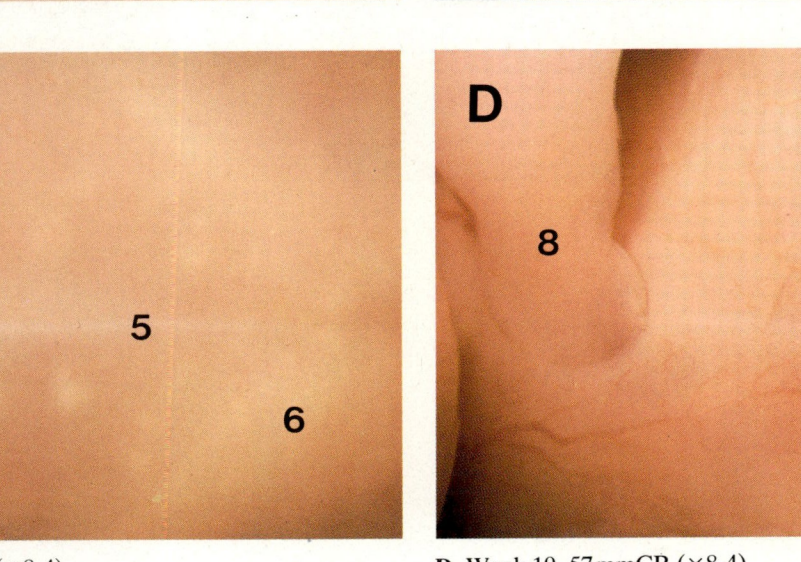

C. Week 9. 46 mmCR (×8.4)

D. Week 10. 57 mmCR (×8.4)

A. Horizon XVIII (Day 36–38). 14mmCR (×17)

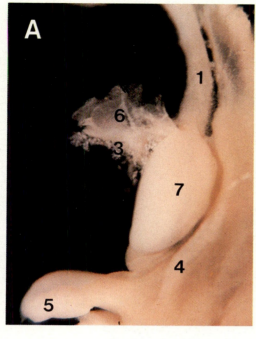

A–D. Development of the esophagus. Viewed from the left.

1. esophagus
2. greater omentum
3. liver cords (liver removed)
4. mesonephros
5. midgut herniation
6. septum transversum
7. stomach

Esophagus

The esophagus and trachea are separated as the respiratory diverticulum is pinched off caudally.

The esophagus is a short endodermal tube (Week 4) (see Yolk sac) surrounded by mesoderm which will condense to form the muscle and submucosal layers. By Week 7 the esophagus has elongated owing to the ascent of the pharynx. The endoderm of the tube proliferates and almost obliterates the lumen, later (Week 8) it recanalizes. The lining of the esophagus is ciliated at Week 11 and loses most of its cilia by Week 28.

- The mainly striated muscle of the upper esophagus forms from the caudal branchial arches and is supplied by the vagus nerve. The mainly non-striated muscles of the lower esophagus develop from the splanchnic mesoderm.

- The esophagus of the neonate may have patches of ciliated columnar cells which disappear rapidly after birth.

- The upper end of the esophagus of the neonate is at the level of C4–C6 and the lower end is at the level of T9. These levels are approximately two vertebrae higher than in the adult.

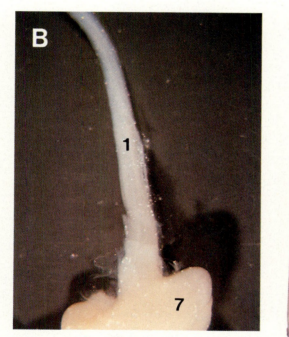

B. Week 8. Viewed from the front. 40mmCR (×8.4)

C. Week 17. 150mmCR ♀ (×3)

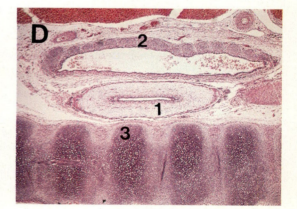

D. Horizon XXIII (Day 46–48). Sagittal section of the developing esophagus. 29mmCR (×36)

1. esophagus
2. trachea
3. vertebral body

Stomach

At Week 4 the foregut caudal to the esophagus forms a spindle-shaped dilatation which descends into the abdomen by Week 6 to 7. During this descent the stomach broadens and the greater curvature forms on the more rapidly growing dorsal border. The stomach rotates through 90° (Week 5) along its longitudinal axis so that the original left side of the stomach becomes the ventral surface and the right side the dorsal surface.

The stomach is suspended dorsally by a mesentery, the dorsal mesogastrium. Ventrally the septum transversum thins to form the ventral mesogastrium.

After rotation of the stomach the dorsal mesogastrium elongates and hangs from the greater curvature as the greater omentum. The lesser sac is the space between the large double-layered greater omentum and the entrance to the lesser sac is the epiploic foramen. The spleen develops in the sheet of the dorsal mesogastrium.

At Week 7 mucosal pits are present and by Week 14 gastric glands begin to bud off from the pits. Rennin is present in Week 18.

- The stomach of the neonate has a capacity of 30–35 ml, it increases to 100 ml by the end of the first month.

- The musculature of the fetal stomach contracts during development (Week 11) but does not have true peristaltic activity.

Spleen

The spleen develops from mesoderm in the dorsal mesentery of the stomach. A number of mesodermal masses fuse by Week 6 to 7 to form the spleen and lymphoblasts produce lymphocytes. By Week 13–20 megakaryocytes, myeloblasts and erythroblasts are present in the spleen and hemopoiesis reaches a peak.

- In the neonate the long axis of the spleen is usually vertical or oblique.

- Accessory spleens are a common anomaly and usually occur in the greater omentum.

- A functioning thymus in the fetus and the development of the white pulp of the spleen are directly related.

- The spleen produces lymphocytes throughout life.

124

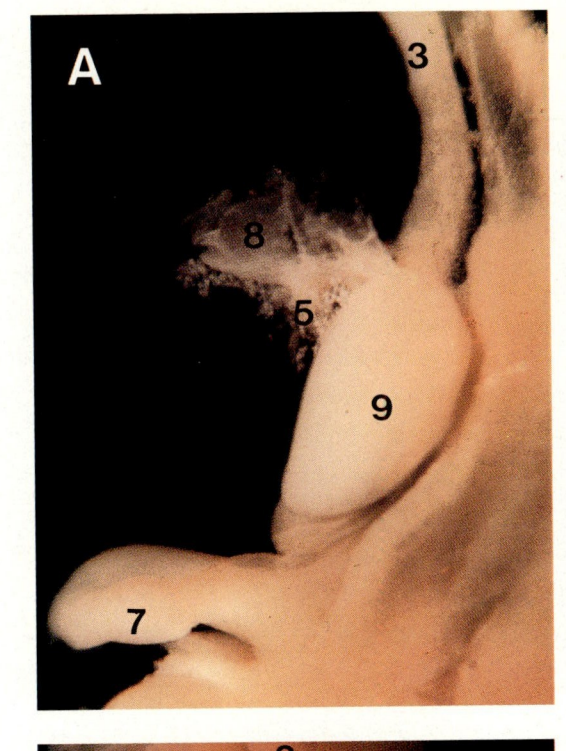

A–C. Horizon XVIII (Day 36–38). Early development of the stomach. 14 mm CR (×17)

1. cactus needle
2. dorsal mesentery
3. esophagus
4. leg bud
5. liver cords (liver removed)
6. mesonephros
7. midgut herniation
8. septum transversum
9. stomach

A. View from the left.

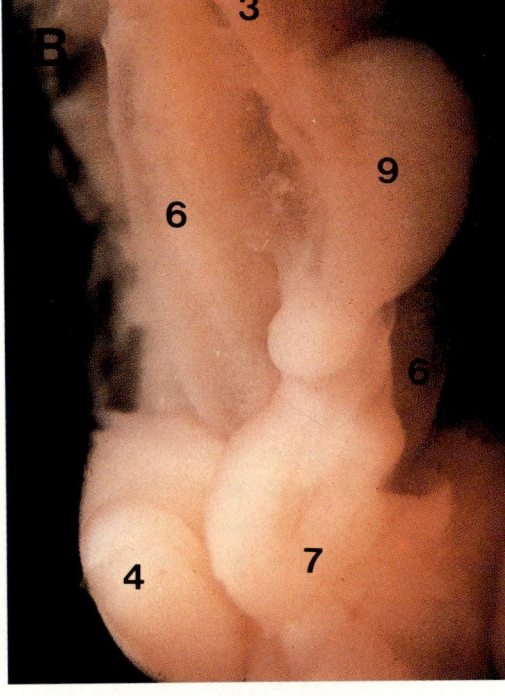

B. View from the ventral surface.

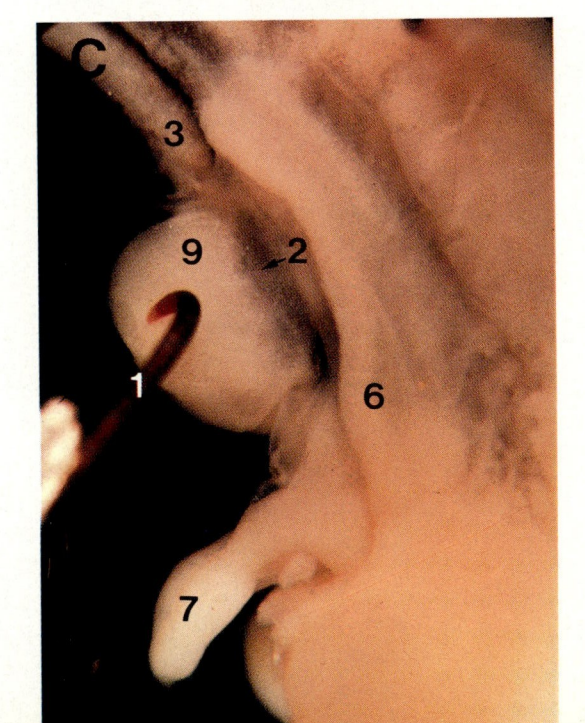

C. View from the left.

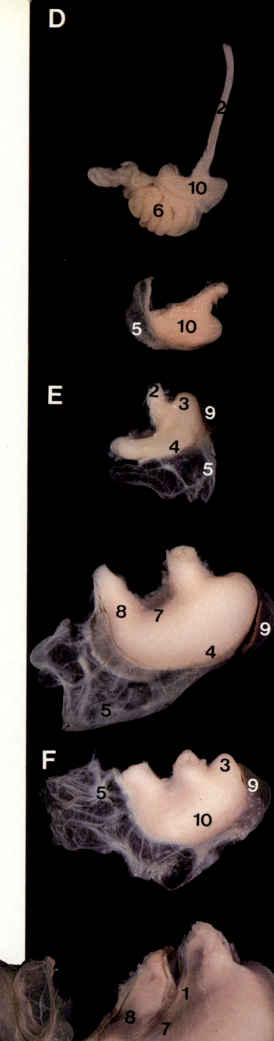

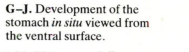

D–F. Development of the stomach and spleen viewed from the front.

1. cardia
2. esophagus
3. fundus
4. greater curvature
5. greater omentum
6. intestine
7. lesser curvature
8. pyloric antrum
9. spleen
10. stomach

G–J. Development of the stomach *in situ* viewed from the ventral surface.

1. bladder
2. diaphragm
3. gonad
4. intestine
5. kidney
6. liver
7. pin head (dressmaking)
8. spleen
9. stomach
10. suprarenal (adrenal) gland

G. Horizon XIX (Day 38–40). 20 mmCR (×17)

D. Week 8. Smallest specimen. 40 mmCR (×3.2) Largest specimen. 48 mmCR (×3.2)

H. Week 10. 57 mmCR (×8.6)

E. Week 11. Smallest specimen. 65 mmCR (×3) Week 13. Largest specimen. 92 mmCR (×3)

F. Week 15. Smallest specimen. 123 mmCR (×2) Week 18. Largest specimen. 152 mmCR (×2)

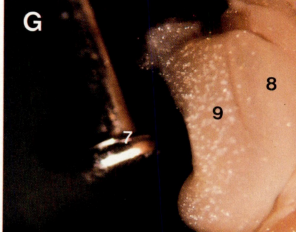

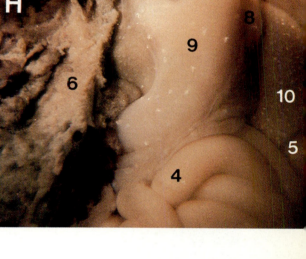

I. Week 11. 65 mmCR (×3.7)

J. Week 15. 123 mmCR (×3)

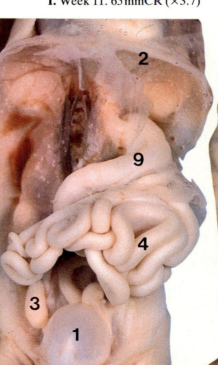

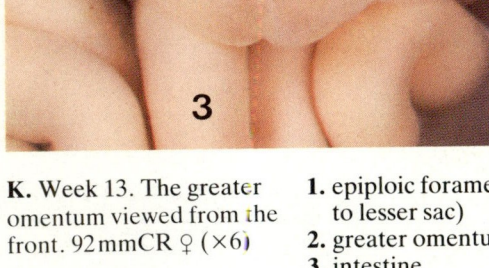

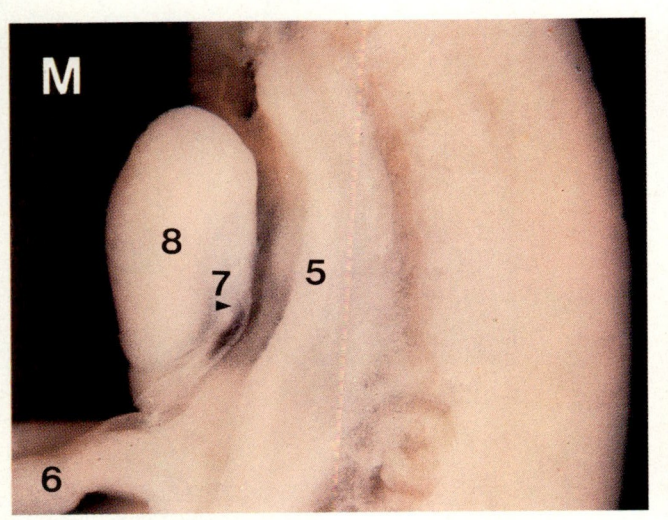

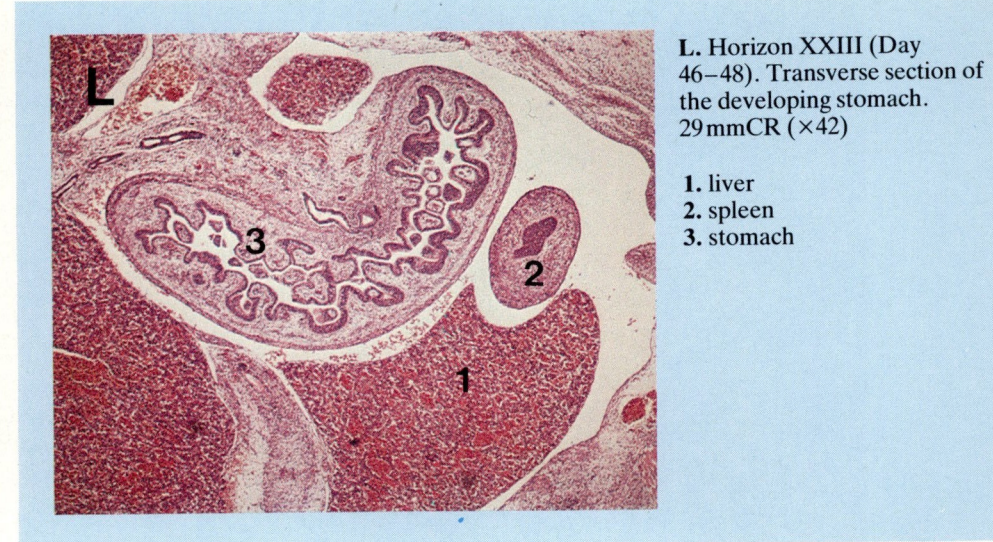

K. Week 13. The greater omentum viewed from the front. 92 mmCR ♀ (×6)

1. epiploic foramen (entrance to lesser sac)
2. greater omentum
3. intestine
4. stomach

L. Horizon XXIII (Day 46–48). Transverse section of the developing stomach. 29 mmCR (×42)

1. liver
2. spleen
3. stomach

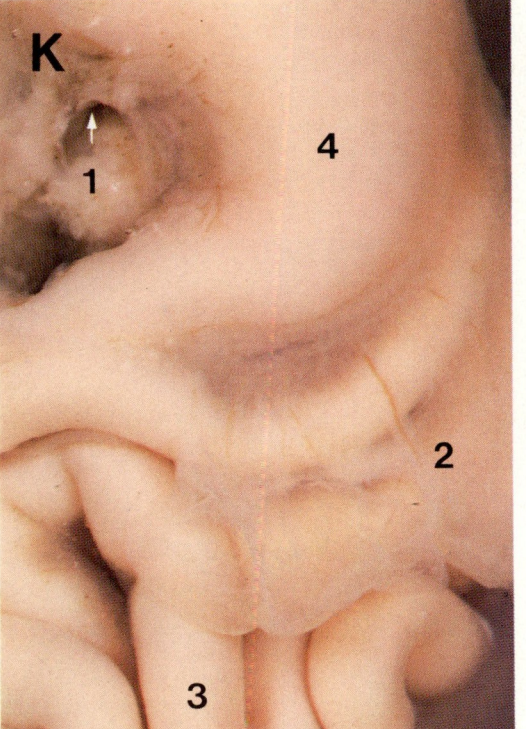

M. Horizon XVIII (Day 36–38). 14 mmCR (×16)

M–O. Splenic development viewed from the left side.

1. body wall
2. greater omentum
3. intestine
4. kidney
5. mesonephros
6. midgut herniation
7. spleen
8. stomach
9. suprarenal (adrenal) gland

N. Horizon XIX (Day 38–40). The spleen has been reflected medially. 20 mmCR (×16)

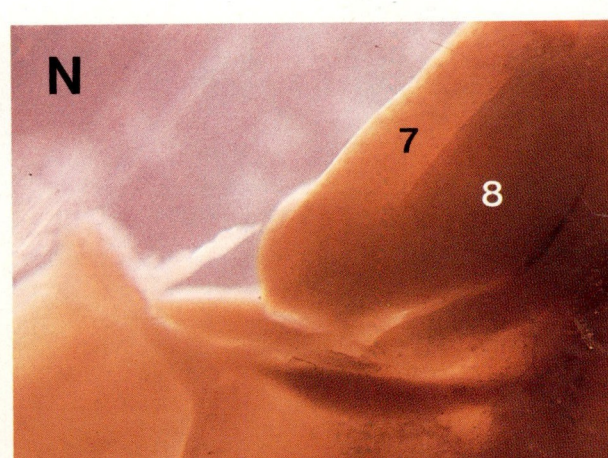

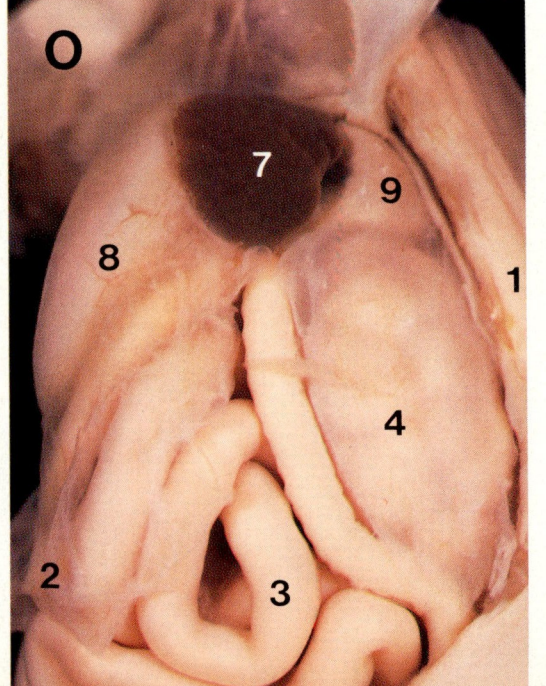

O. Week 13. 92 mmCR ♀ (×3.8)

Pancreas

A. Horizon XVIII (Day 36–38). Early pancreas viewed from the left side. The left leg bud and liver have been removed. 14mmCR (×16.5)

1. abdomen
2. body wall
3. genital tubercle
4. gonadal ridge
5. mesonephric kidney
6. midgut herniation
7. pancreas primordium (dorsal)
8. stomach

The pancreas forms during Week 5–8 from two endodermal buds of the foregut caudal to the stomach, a large dorsal bud appears first followed by a smaller, ventral bud. The ventral bud arises on the ventral duodenum at the site of the common bile duct. When the gut rotates (Week 5) the ventral bud is carried medially (clockwise) to fuse with the dorsal bud in the dorsal mesogastrium. Their ducts also anastomose.

The dorsal bud forms part of the head, neck, body and tail of the pancreas, and the ventral bud part of the head and uncinate process. The duct of the ventral bud and a distal part of the dorsal bud duct form the main pancreatic duct and the proximal part of the dorsal duct becomes the smaller accessory duct.

The parenchyma, acini and the islets of Langerhans are endodermal in origin, while the septa and the connective tissue covering are mesodermal. Their development (Week 12) is similar to salivary gland formation.

● Insulin is formed from Week 20.

● There are relatively more islets of Langerhans in the neonate than in the adult.

A and B. Horizon XIX (Day 38–40). The dorsal and ventral pancreatic buds are in contact. Viewed from the right side. 20mmCR

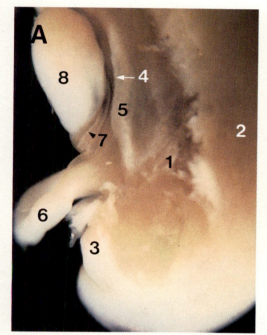

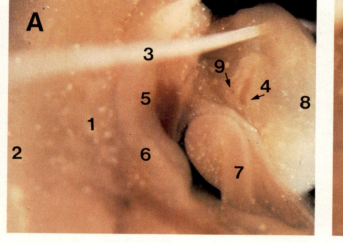

A. (×16.5)

1. abdomen
2. body wall
3. cactus needle
4. dorsal pancreas
5. gonadal ridge
6. mesonephric kidney
7. midgut
8. stomach
9. ventral pancreas

B. Higher magnification of the embryo in Figure A. (×34.4)

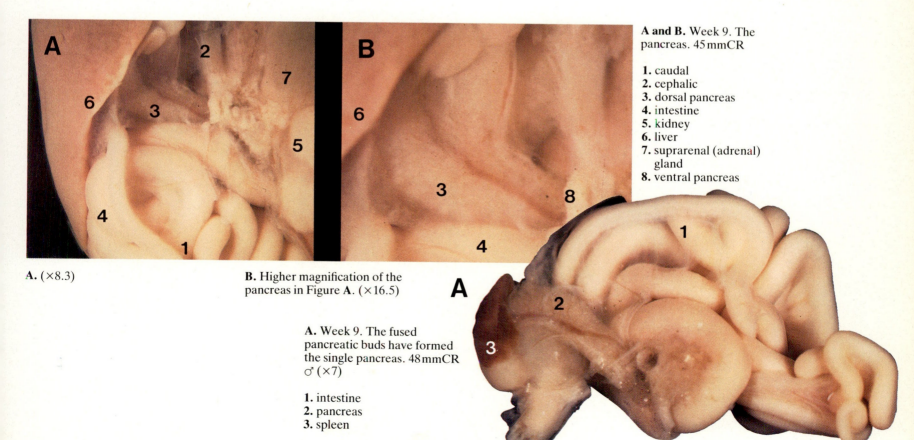

A. (×8.3)

B. Higher magnification of the pancreas in Figure A. (×16.5)

A and B. Week 9. The pancreas. 45mmCR

1. caudal
2. cephalic
3. dorsal pancreas
4. intestine
5. kidney
6. liver
7. suprarenal (adrenal) gland
8. ventral pancreas

A. Week 9. The fused pancreatic buds have formed the single pancreas. 48mmCR ♂ (×7)

1. intestine
2. pancreas
3. spleen

Liver

In Week 4 the liver forms as an endodermal outgrowth (hepatic diverticulum) from the foregut. It penetrates the splanchnic mesoderm of the septum transversum. The hepatic diverticulum then divides (Week 5) into right and left branches and columns of endodermal cells (liver cords or parenchyma) grow out into the surrounding mesoderm. Sinusoids are formed as the invading liver cells anastomose around spaces present in the septum transversum. The mesoderm forms the connective and hemopoietic tissue, the Kupffer cells and the fibrous capsule of the liver. The bile duct system forms when the terminal branches of the right and left hepatic buds canalize.

Originally the right and left lobes are of equal size, but the right lobe becomes much larger after Week 6 due to relative growth changes. The caudate and quadrate lobes form from the right lobe (Week 6). The liver occupies most of the abdominal cavity at Week 6.

As the liver enlarges, the yolk sac regresses and hemopoiesis occurs in the liver at Week 6, reaches a peak at Week 12–24, but ceases at birth.

Lymphocyte formation occurs in the liver at Week 10, but ceases by birth. Coagulation factors are produced in the liver after Week 10–12.

Bile is produced in Week 13–16.

● Large reserves of carbohydrates are laid down in the liver and skeletal muscle before birth to provide a source of energy for the infant until suckling is well established (around the third day after birth).

Gallbladder

In Week 4 the gallbladder is a solid endodermal outgrowth in continuity with the liver diverticulum. The outgrowth enlarges rapidly and during Week 7 it canalizes, and forms a sac. The stalk becomes the cystic duct connected to the duodenum via the common bile duct.

Initially the gallbladder is in the mid-line, but it becomes more peripheral.

Bile pigment is secreted at Week 13–16 and colours the colonic contents (meconium) green.

● The neonatal gallbladder is more embedded in the liver substance than in the adult and the fundus often does not extend beyond the margin of the liver.

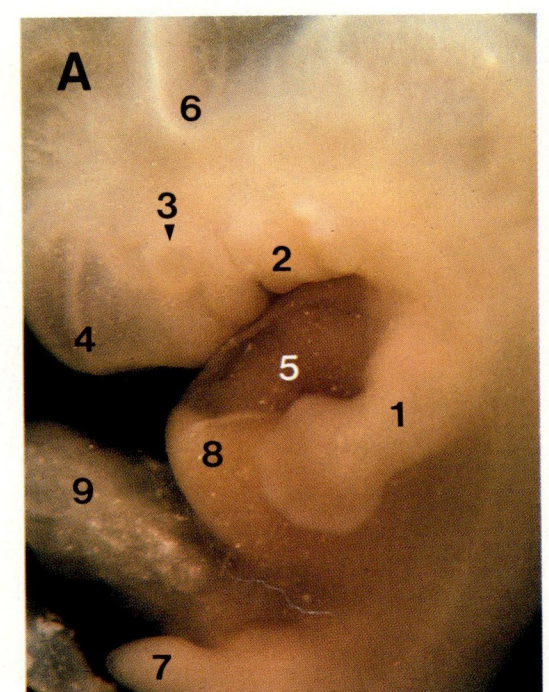

A. Horizon XVII (Day 34–36). Early liver development viewed from the left side. 12 mmCR (×8.7)

1. arm bud and hand plate (paddle)
2. branchial arch
3. eye
4. forebrain
5. heart
6. hindbrain
7. leg bud
8. liver
9. umbilical cord

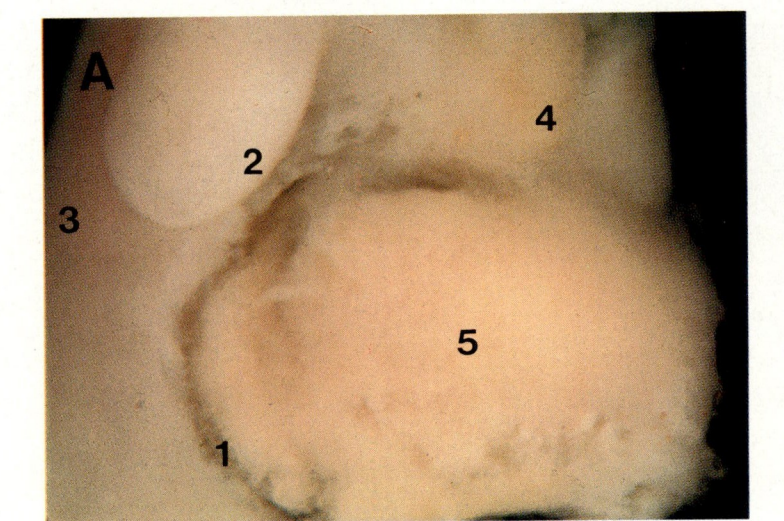

A. Horizon XVIII (Day 36–38). The liver viewed from the right and front. The skin has been removed. 14 mmCR (×17.4)

1. abdominal cavity
2. arm bud (right)
3. back
4. heart bulge
5. liver

A–D. The early liver.

1. arm bud and hand plate with finger rays
2. back
3. eye
4. heart
5. hepato-cardiac veins (vitelline veins)
6. leg bud and foot paddle
7. liver bulge
8. mandibular prominence
9. maxillary prominence
10. midgut herniation
11. septum transversum
12. umbilical cord

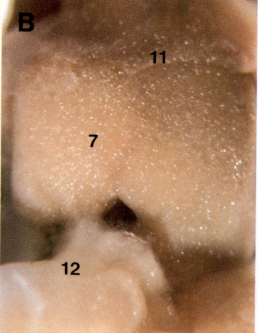

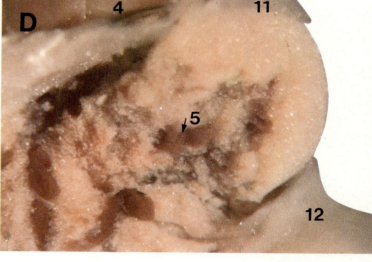

A. Horizon XIX (Day 38–40). The liver viewed from the right and front. 20mmCR (×8.9)

B. Higher magnification of the liver in Figure **A**. The anterior abdominal wall has been dissected off. View from the front. (×17.7)

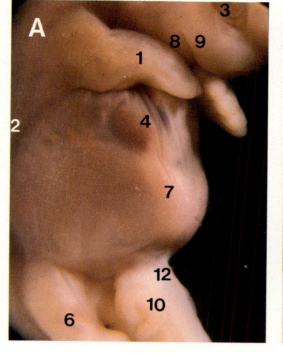

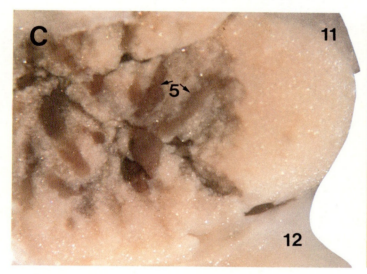

C. The liver in Figure **A** dissected from the right side. Note the hepato-cardiac veins. (×17.7)

D. Further dissection of the liver in Figure **A**. (×17.7)

A and B. Horizon XVIII (Day 36–38). The liver.

1. arm bud (left)
2. back
3. body wall
4. leg bud
5. liver cords
6. stomach
7. umbilical cord

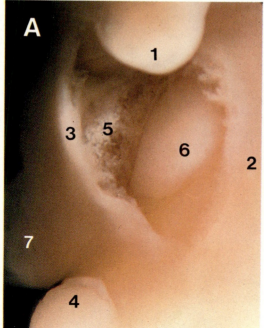

A. Viewed from the left side. Note the liver trabeculae. 14mmCR (×17.7)

B. Higher magnification of the liver in Figure **A**. (×37)

A–C. Transverse paraffin wax sections of the developing liver.

1. body wall
2. diaphragm
3. esophagus
4. liver
5. lungs
6. rib
7. tributary of hepatic vein
8. spinal cord
9. stomach
10. umbilical vein
11. vertebral body

A. Horizon XIV (Day 28–30). 7 mmCR (×71)

B. Horizon XXIII (Day 46–48). 28 mmCR (×11)

C. Higher magnification of the liver posterior to the section in Figure B. (×28)

A–C from L.H.S.M.

A and B. Full term fetus. Two transverse sections through the upper abdomen.

1. anterior abdominal wall
2. kidney
3. large intestine
4. liver
5. small intestine
6. spleen
7. stomach
8. vertebral body

A. Specimens viewed from above (the superior surface). (×0.6)

B. The same specimens viewed from below (the inferior surface). (×0.6)

A and B from R.F.H.S.M.

A and B. Liver development. The dissected livers are viewed from the ventral surface.

1. falciform ligament
2. left lobe
3. right lobe
4. umbilical vein

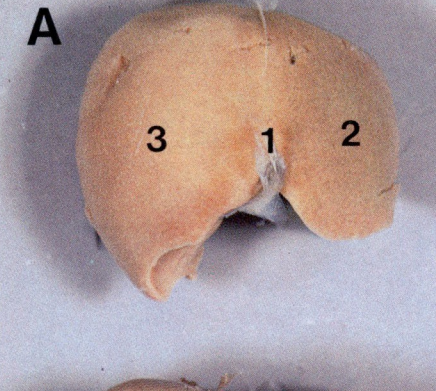

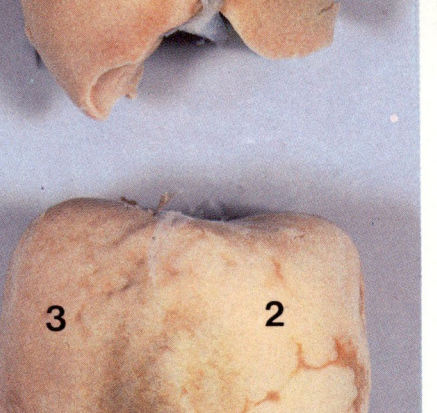

A. Week 9. Smallest liver. 48 mmCR ♀ (×3.1)
Week 11. Largest liver. 65 mmCR ♂ (×3.1)

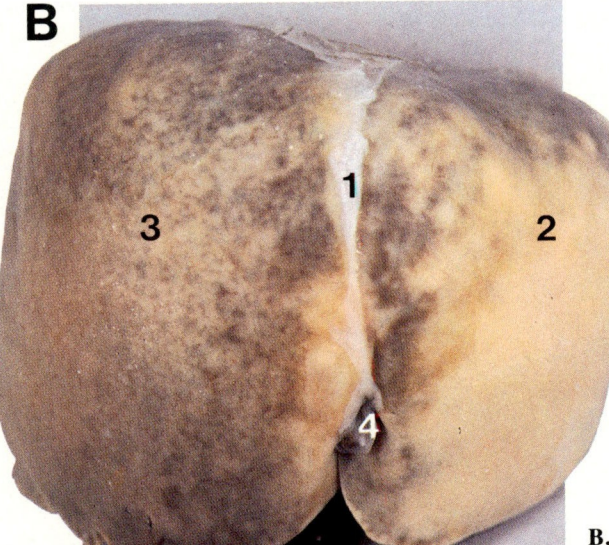

B. Week 13. 92 mmCR ♀ (×2.8)

A and B. The course of the umbilical vein in the falciform ligament and in the liver.

1. diaphragm
2. intestine
3. kidney
4. liver
5. lung
6. pericardium
7. stomach
8. suprarenal (adrenal) gland
9. umbilical cord

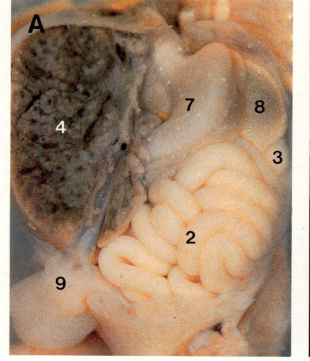

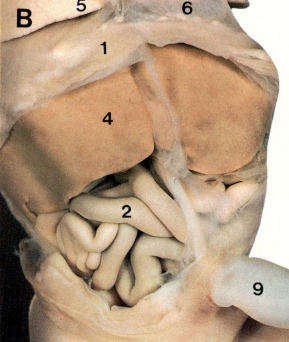

A. Week 10. The anterior (ventral) surface of the liver has been removed. 57 mm CR ♂ (×5.3)

B. Week 13. 101 mm CR ♀ (×2.3)

A. Week 10. Smallest liver. 57 mm CR ♂ (×3.1)

B. Week 11. Largest liver. 65 mm CR ♂ (×2)

A–D. Posterior (dorsal) surface of the liver.

1. bare area
2. caudate lobe
3. colic impression
4. esophageal groove
5. gallbladder
6. gastric impression
7. left lobe of liver
8. ligamentum teres and falciform ligament
9. porta hepatis
10. quadrate lobe
11. renal impression
12. right lobe of liver

C. Week 13. 92 mm CR ♀ (×2.5)

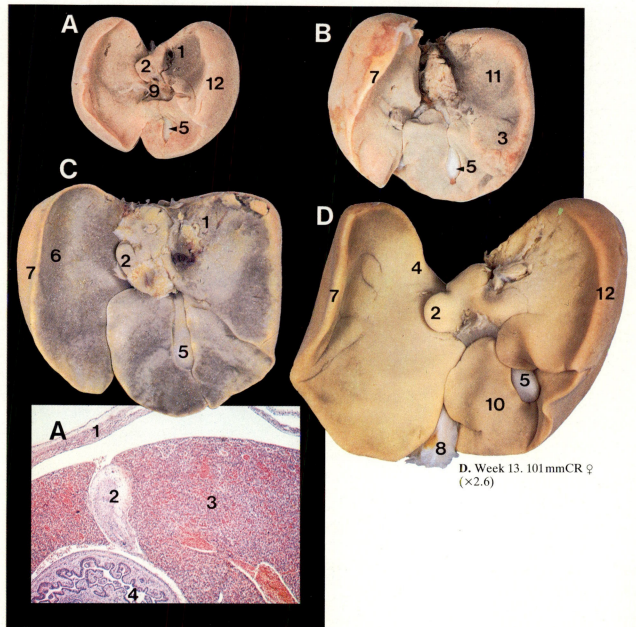

D. Week 13. 101 mm CR ♀ (×2.6)

A. Horizon XXIII (Day 46–48). Transverse section of the liver. 29 mm CR (×35)

1. anterior abdominal wall
2. gallbladder
3. liver
4. stomach

Midgut rotation

In Week 4 the early intestine is a straight tube (see Yolk sac) and then in Week 5 and 6 it grows to form a single loop supplied centrally by the superior mesenteric artery. Two landmarks are present on the loop: the yolk stalk and the cecal diverticulum which marks the join between the small and large intestine. The yolk stalk is at the apex of the loop dividing it into two parts; a cranial or proximal limb and a caudal or distal limb. The early abdomen (Week 6) is occupied primarily by the liver and the rapidly growing intestine occupies an extra-embryonic position in the umbilical cord. The proximal limb of the intestine grows very rapidly and forms several coils while the distal limb grows very slowly. As the opening into the umbilical cord is narrow, rotation occurs in the apex region. The yolk stalk connection to the intestine shrinks and breaks, the distal intestinal coil rotates 90° anticlockwise so the cecal diverticulum (and distal limb) is carried toward the right hand side of the body. The cecum and appendix are differentiating from the cecal diverticulum as the intestine returns (reduction) to the larger abdominal cavity (Week 10). The proximal limb of the intestine returns first (Week 8) and passes behind the superior mesenteric artery. The majority returns at Week 9. The returning intestine rotates another 180° anticlockwise so the appendix and cecum lie near the right lobe of the liver. Later as they descend into the right iliac fossa the proximal part of the colon forms the ascending colon and hepatic flexure.

As the intestines reach their adult positions their mesenteries are pressed against the posterior abdominal wall where all the mesenteries are retained except that of the midgut duodenum and the ascending colon. The duodenum (except for the first 25 mm in the adult) and the ascending colon are retroperitoneal.

The proximal limb will form the 5.5–6.0 m of adult small intestine (duodenum, jejunum and upper part of ileum). The distal limb which will form the large intestine is less in diameter than that of the small intestine until Week 18.

During Week 6 and 7 the epithelial lining of the duodenum proliferates and almost fills the lumen, but it is quickly re-established.

Villi appear in Week 8 and the intestinal mucosa absorbs fluid from the amniotic fluid. The glands of Lieberkuhn appear at the base of the villi toward the end of Week 12 and Brunner's glands (duodenal) shortly afterwards. Lymph nodes and Peyer's patches are present from Week 18–20. Elastic tissue is primarily in the blood vessel walls. The musculature is poorly developed and peristalsis is weak and discontinuous.

- Meckel's diverticulum is the persistence of the yolk stalk connection to the umbilical cord.

- The neonatal intestine is sterile at birth but a bacterial flora is quickly acquired.

- The intestinal musculature is poorly developed at birth and the intestinal wall thin. In the first few months elastic tissue increases greatly in the walls.

A. Horizon XVII (Day 34–36). The midgut is beginning to herniate into the umbilical cord. Viewed by transmitted light from the right side. 12 mmCR (×7.8)

1. arm bud
2. back
3. eye (right)
4. heart
5. leg bud
6. liver
7. midgut herniation
8. tail
9. umbilical cord

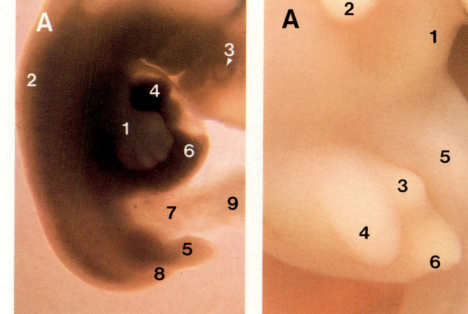

A. Horizon XVII (Day 34–36). The midgut herniating into the umbilical cord. 12 mmCR (×15.6)

1. abdomen
2. arm bud (right)
3. genital tubercle
4. leg bud
5. midgut herniation
6. tail
7. umbilical cord

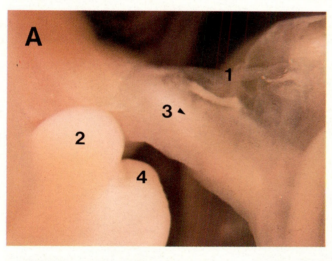

A. Horizon XVIII (Day 36–38). Midgut herniation. 14 mmCR (×15.9)

1. amnion
2. leg bud
3. midgut herniation
4. tail

A. Horizon XVIII (Day 36–38). Midgut herniation. Viewed from the left side. The left leg bud and liver have been removed. 14 mmCR (×15.4)

1. back
2. genital tubercle
3. mesonephric kidney (left)
4. midgut herniation (umbilical cord removed)
5. stomach
6. tail

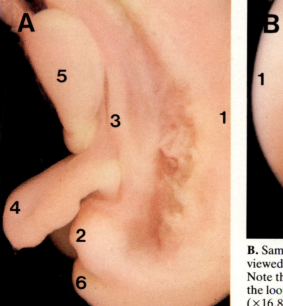

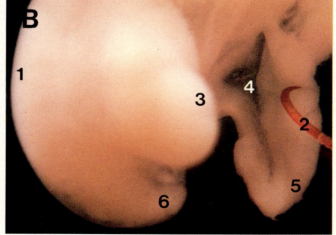

B. Same embryo as in Figure **A** viewed from the right side. Note the dorsal mesentery in the loop of the midgut. (×16.8)

1. back
2. cactus needle
3. leg bud
4. mesentery
5. midgut
6. tail

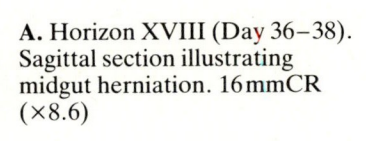

A. Horizon XVIII (Day 36–38). Sagittal section illustrating midgut herniation. 16 mmCR (×8.6)

1. brain
2. genital tubercle
3. heart
4. liver
5. lung
6. mandible
7. midgut herniation
8. nose

From C.C.H.M.S.

A–C. Midgut herniation viewed from the right.

1. abdomen
2. arm
3. elbow
4. finger
5. foot
6. knee
7. leg (right)
8. midgut herniation
9. rib
10. toe
11. umbilical cord

A. Horizon XIX (Day 38–40). 20 mmCR (×17.4)

B. Horizon XXII (Day 44–46). 27 mmCR (×8.7)

C. Week 8. 34 mmCR (×8.7)

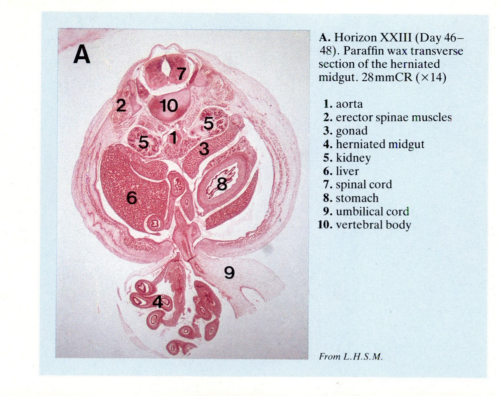

A. Horizon XXIII (Day 46–48). Paraffin wax transverse section of the herniated midgut. 28 mmCR (×14)

1. aorta
2. erector spinae muscles
3. gonad
4. herniated midgut
5. kidney
6. liver
7. spinal cord
8. stomach
9. umbilical cord
10. vertebral body

From L.H.S.M.

A and B. Midgut herniation dissected from the umbilical cord.

1. appendix
2. esophagus
3. knee
4. leg
5. liver
6. small intestine
7. stomach
8. umbilical cord

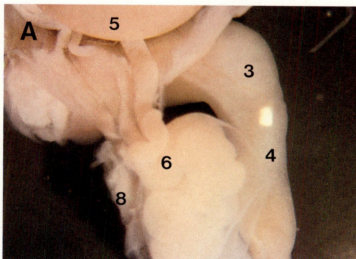

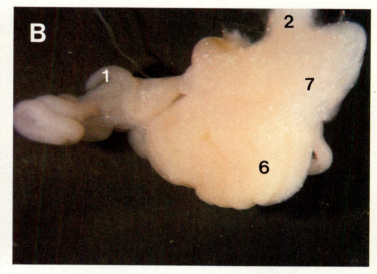

A. Week 8. The anterior abdominal wall and right leg have been removed. 32 mmCR (×8.9)

B. Week 8. 40 mmCR (×8.9)

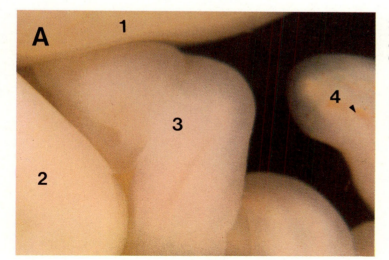

A. Week 10. Midgut herniation has returned to the enlarged abdominal cavity. 60 mmCR ♀ (×8.9)

1. abdomen
2. leg
3. umbilical cord
4. umbilical vessels

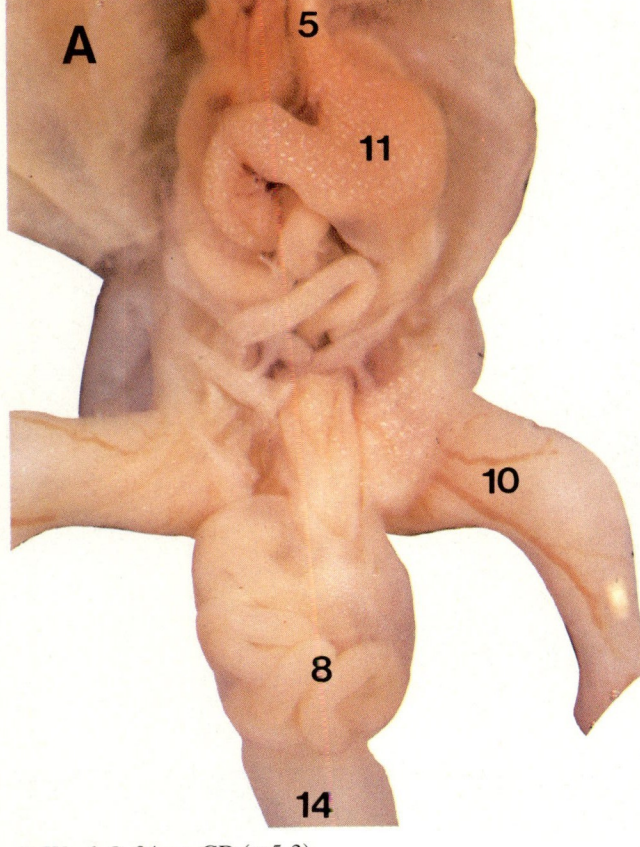

A. Week 8. 34 mm CR (×5.3)

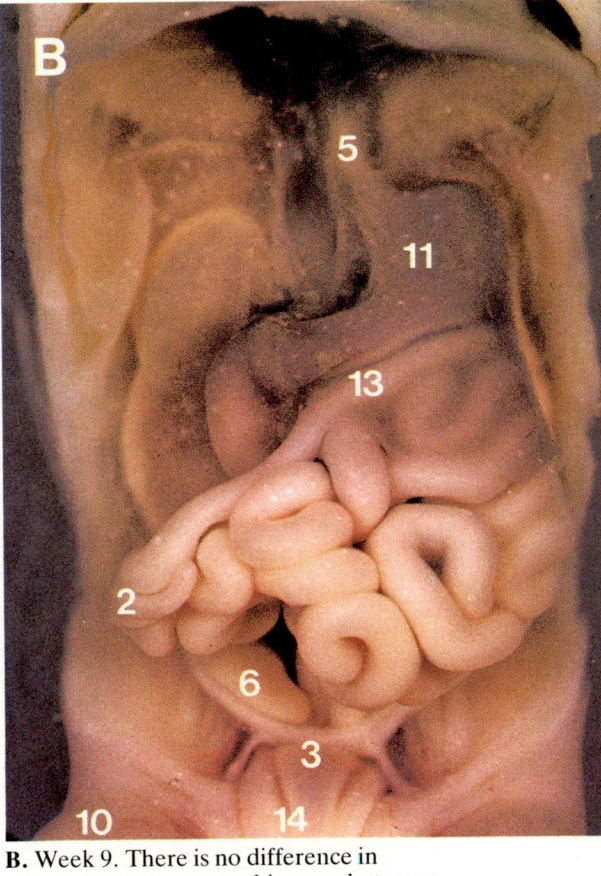

A–F. Return of the midgut to the abdominal cavity and the position of the intestine. Viewed from the front. The liver has been removed.

1. anterior abdominal wall
2. appendix
3. bladder
4. diaphragm
5. esophagus
6. gonad
7. greater omentum
8. herniated midgut
9. kidney
10. leg
11. stomach
12. suprarenal (adrenal) gland
13. transverse colon
14. umbilical cord

B. Week 9. There is no difference in external appearance at this stage between small and large intestines. 50 mm CR ♀ (×6.1)

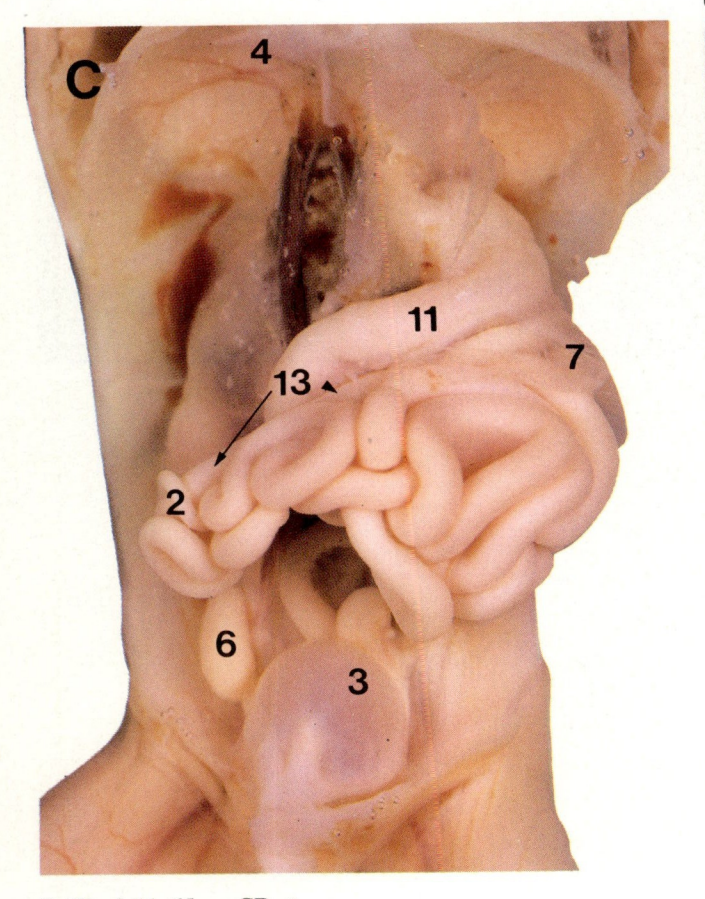

C. Week 11. 65 mm CR ♂ (×4.5)

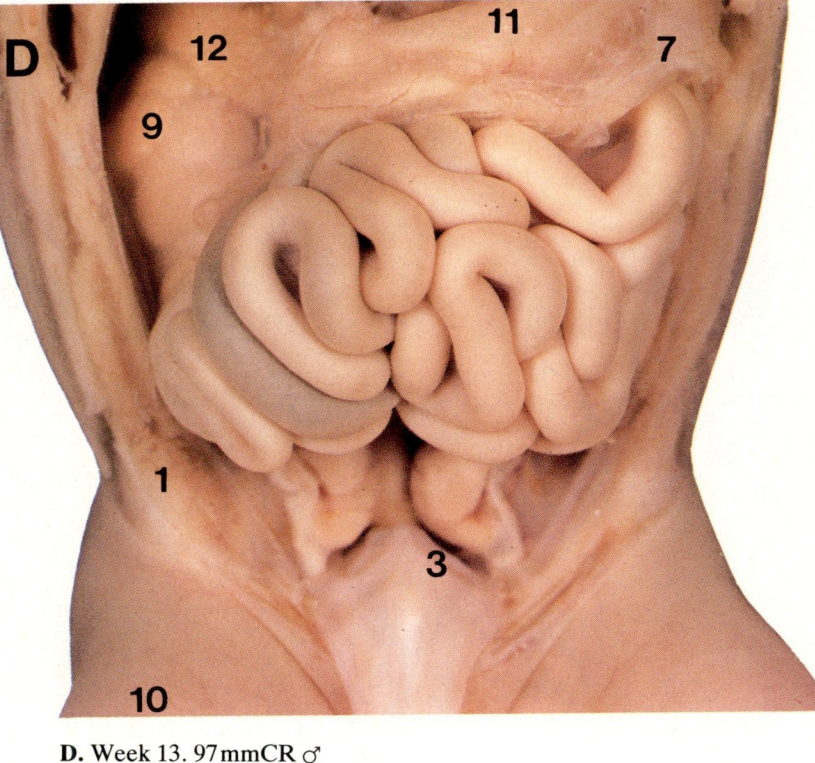

D. Week 13. 97 mm CR ♂ (×3.6)

1. anterior
   abdominal wall
2. diaphragm
3. esophagus
4. greater
   omentum
5. kidney
6. leg
7. site of hepatic
   flexure
8. stomach
9. suprarenal
   (adrenal) gland
10. transverse colon
11. umbilical cord

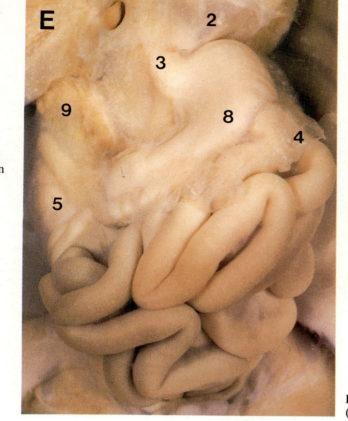

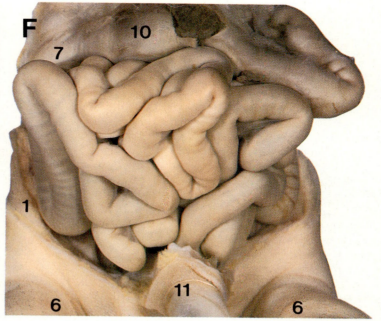

F. Week 18. 152 mm CR ♂
(×2.2)

E. Week 15. 123 mm CR ♀
(×3.4)

A. Week 9. Intestinal villi.
50 mm CR (×33)

1. villi

B. Week 10. Villi fill the
intestine. 60 mm CR ♀ (×15.6)

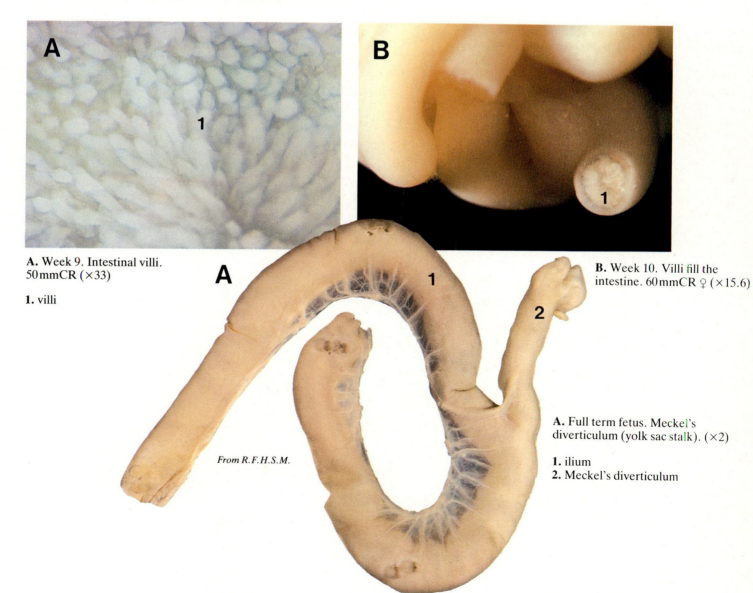

From R.F.H.S.M.

A. Full term fetus. Meckel's
diverticulum (yolk sac stalk). (×2)

1. ilium
2. Meckel's diverticulum

Hindgut

The midline hindgut is continuous with the caudal midgut and ends in the primitive cloaca (see Yolk sac). The allantois lies anterior to the anterior cloaca. In Week 6 the urorectal septum divides the cloaca and cloacal membrane into two parts: the rectum, anal canal and anal membrane, and the urogenital sinus and urogenital membrane. The perineal body forms where the septum fuses with the cloacal membrane. Mesoderm proliferates around the anal membrane and causes the proctodeum (or anal pit) to form. In Week 8 the membrane ruptures and the anal canal communicates with the amniotic cavity.

The hindgut moves to the left as the midgut coils return to the abdominal cavity. It gives rise to the distal part of the transverse colon, the descending and sigmoid colon, the rectum, and the upper part of the anal canal, and part of the urogenital system.

The inferior mesenteric artery supplies the hindgut.

The mesentery of the descending colon fuses with peritoneum on the left dorsal abdominal wall and so disappears. The sigmoid colon's mesentery is retained.

The colon has poorly developed tenia coli and the external surface is smooth because it lacks haustra (sacculations) and appendices epiploicae. The colon contains the ingested amniotic fluid and sloughed skin epithelial cells, oral cavity cells, upper respiratory and intestinal tract cells, lanugo hairs, *vernix caseosa*, secretions of the liver, pancreas, gastrointestinal glands, urea, steroids, biliverdin, mucoproteins and mucopolysaccharides. Lipid is absorbed and the remaining contents collect in the colon as meconium after Week 12. At birth the rectum is usually distended with meconium.

- Haustra are formed during the first 6 months.

- Full-term infants defecate within 24 hours of birth.

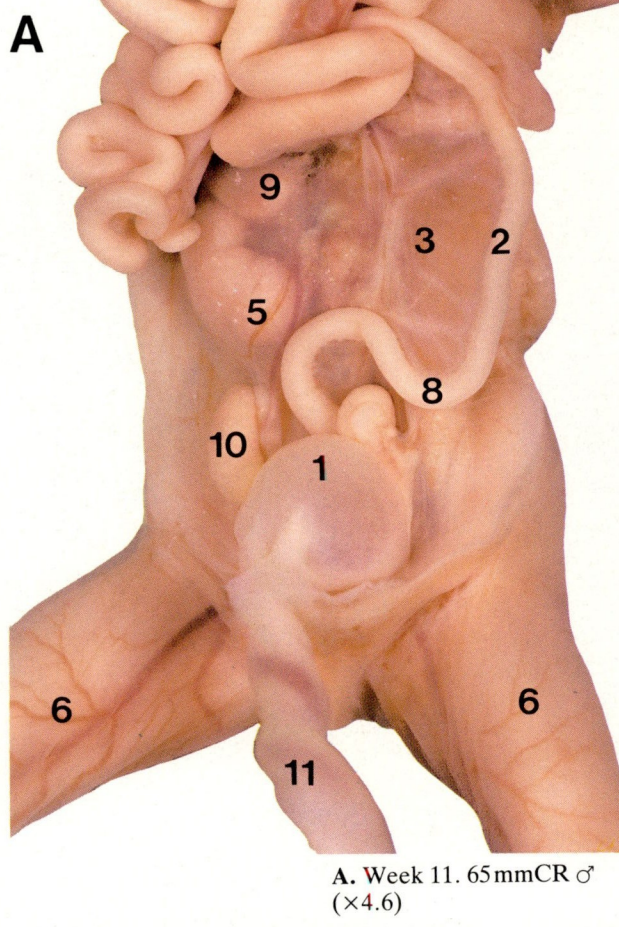

A. Week 11. 65 mmCR ♂ (×4.6)

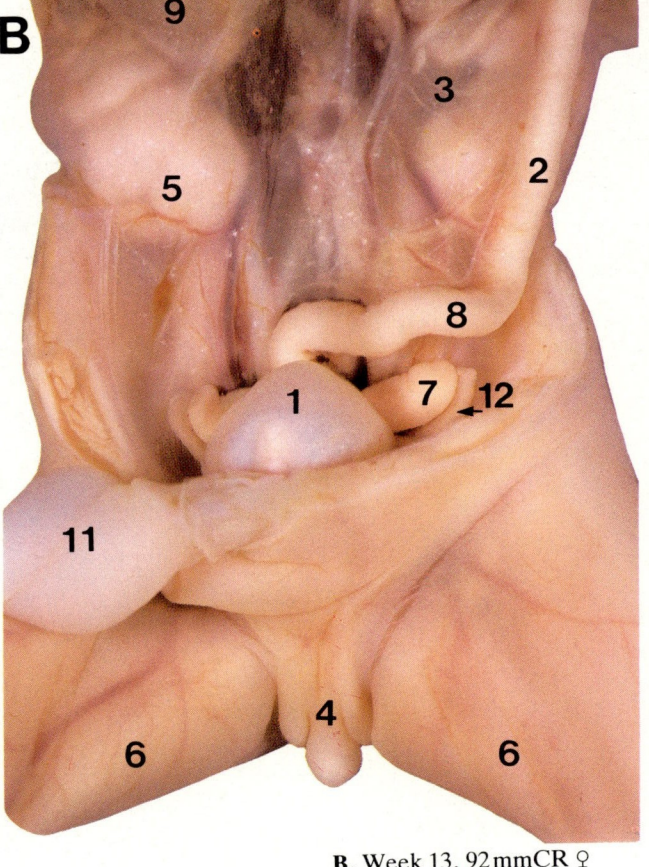

B. Week 13. 92 mmCR ♀ (×3.5)

A–E. Development of the descending colon and rectum. In order not to obscure the view the abdominal organs have been reflected cephalically (superiorly).

1. bladder
2. descending colon
3. descending mesocolon
4. external genitalia
5. kidney
6. leg
7. ovary
8. sigmoid colon
9. suprarenal (adrenal) gland
10. testis
11. umbilical cord
12. uterine (Fallopian) tube

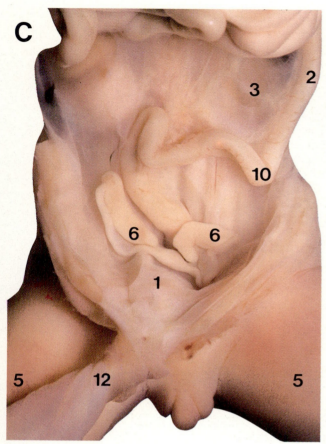

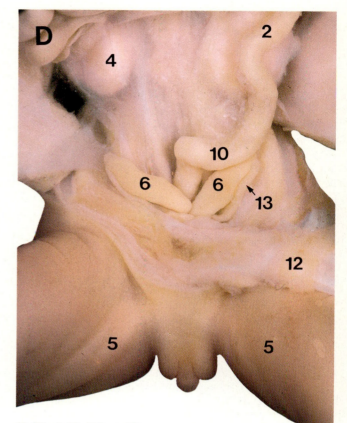

1. bladder
2. descending colon
3. descending mesocolon
4. kidney
5. leg
6. ovary
7. penis
8. rectum (position)
9. scrotum
10. sigmoid colon
11. testis
12. umbilical cord
13. uterine (Fallopian) tube

C. Week 13. 101 mm CR ♀
(×2.8)

D. Week 15. 123 mm CR ♀
(×3.2)

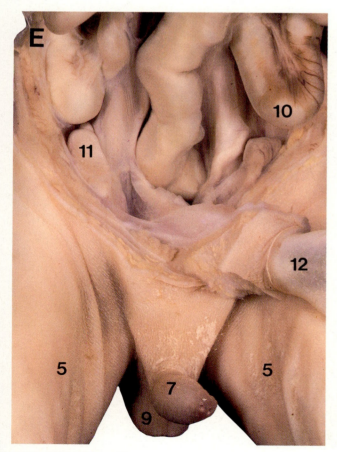

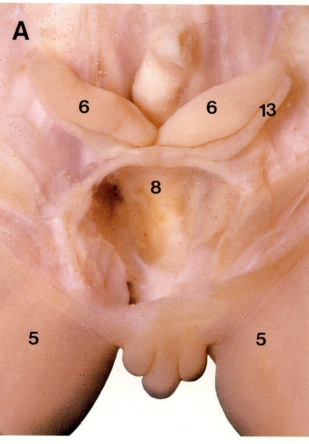

E. Week 18. 152 mm CR ♂
(×2.3)

A. Week 15. The bladder and
part of the uterovaginal
primordium have been
removed to display the
position of the rectum.
123 mm CR ♀ (×4.9)

Cecum and vermiform appendix

The cecal diverticulum is present on the early intestine (Week 6) as a blunt area marking the joining of the small and large intestine. Later (Week 8) as the terminal part of the diverticulum (appendix) does not grow as rapidly as the proximal part (cecum) it forms a long blind sac. As the colon elongates the cecum and appendix descend so that the appendix may lie posterior to the cecum (rectrocecal) or colon (retrocolic) or in a pelvic position.

- The appendix is relatively longer in the neonate in comparison with the adult.
- The cecum is relatively smaller in the neonate than in the adult.
- In the newborn the cecum tapers into the appendix and there is usually no sharp demarcation between the two regions.
- In the neonate the haustra and appendices epiploicae are absent. The haustra develop in the first 6 months after birth.

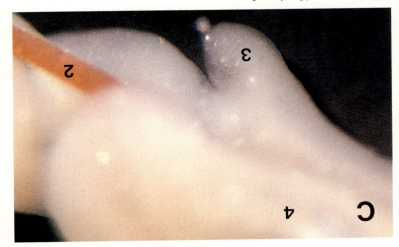

A. Horizon XVIII (Day 36–38). Early cecal diverticulum viewed from the left side. The umbilical cord has been removed. 14 mmCR (×19.8)

1. cecal diverticulum
2. heart
3. leg bud (left)
4. liver removed
5. mesonephric kidney
6. stomach
7. tail

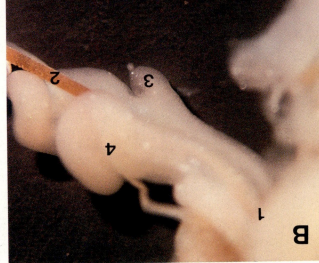

B. Horizon XIX (Day 38–40). Cecal diverticulum viewed from the right side. The umbilical cord has been removed. 20 mmCR (×19.8)

1. abdomen
2. cactus needle
3. cecal diverticulum (with appendix)
4. midgut herniation (umbilical cord removed)

C. Higher magnification of Figure **B**. (×41.3)

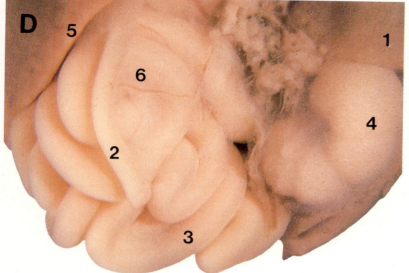

D–G. Further development of the cecum and appendix. Viewed from the dorsal (back) surface.

1. adrenal
2. appendix
3. intestine
4. kidney
5. liver
6. mesentery

D. Week 9. 48 mmCR ♀
(×10.2)

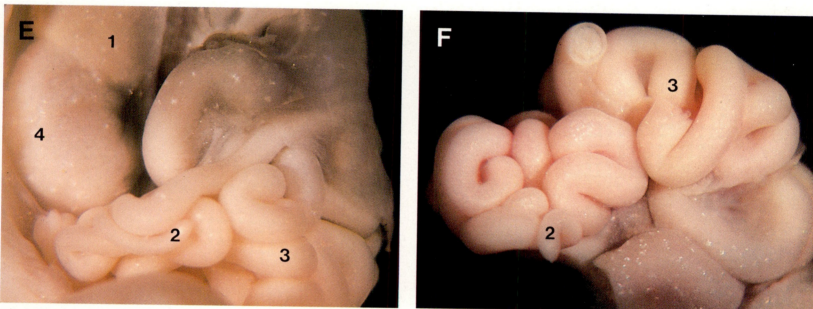

E. Week 10. 60 mmCR ♀
(×20.4)

F. Week 10. 60 mmCR ♀
(×10.2)

G. Week 15. 123 mmCR ♀
(×4.8)

Anal canal

The anal canal has a dual origin: the upper two-thirds from hindgut (supplied by the inferior mesenteric artery) and the lower third (supplied by the internal pudendal artery) from proctodeum (see Hindgut). Approximately where the two join the epithelium changes from columnar to stratified squamous cells and is marked by the pectinate line.

The anal sphincter musculature is well developed at birth.

● If the fetus is anoxic, active peristalsis of the colon and rectum occurs and meconium enters the anal canal. The defecation reflex occurs, the anal sphincter muscles relax and meconium passes into the amniotic fluid.

A–F. Development of the anus.

1. developing anus
2. external genitals
3. genital tubercle
4. leg
5. leg bud
6. tail
7. umbilical cord

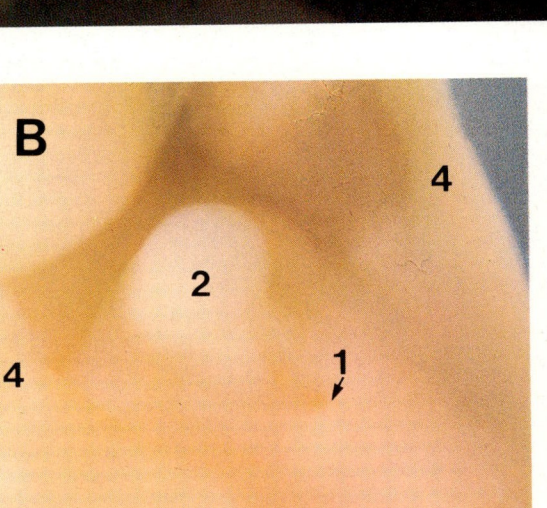

A. Horizon XVIII (Day 36–38). 14 mmCR (×18.3)

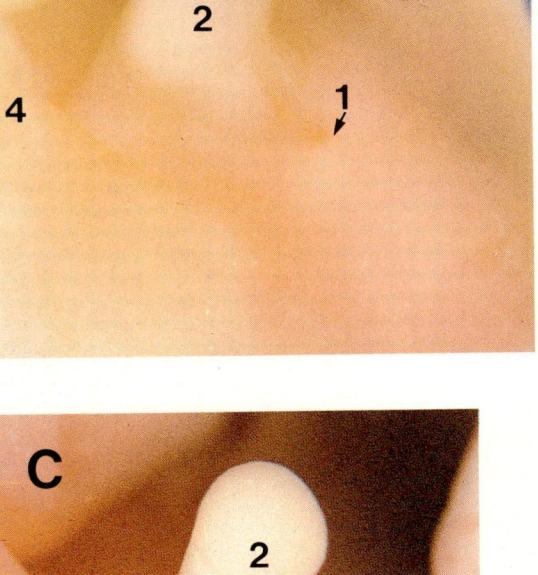

B. Week 8. 32 mmCR (×18.3)

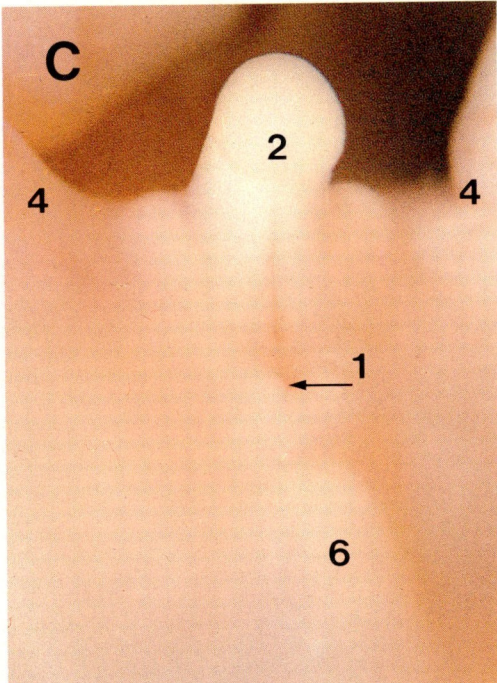

C. Week 8. 34 mmCR (×17)

D. Week 9. 48 mm CR (×18.6)

1. anus
2. buttocks
3. external genitals
4. leg
5. tail

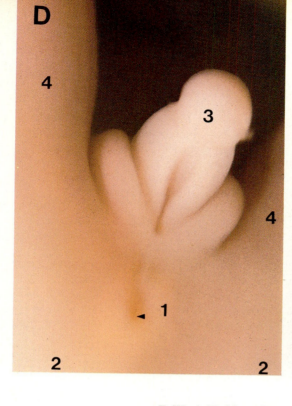

E. Week 10. 56 mm CR ♀ (×18.9)

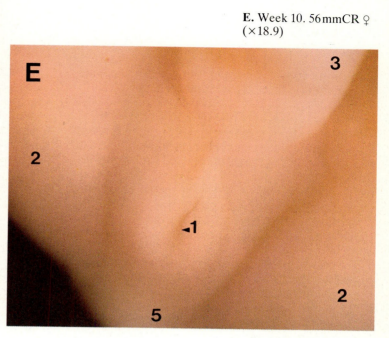

F. Week 12. 85 mm CR ♂ (×9.5)

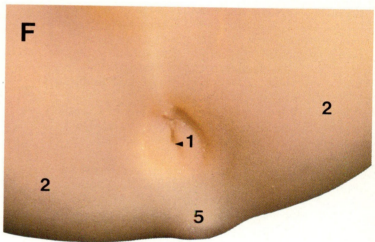

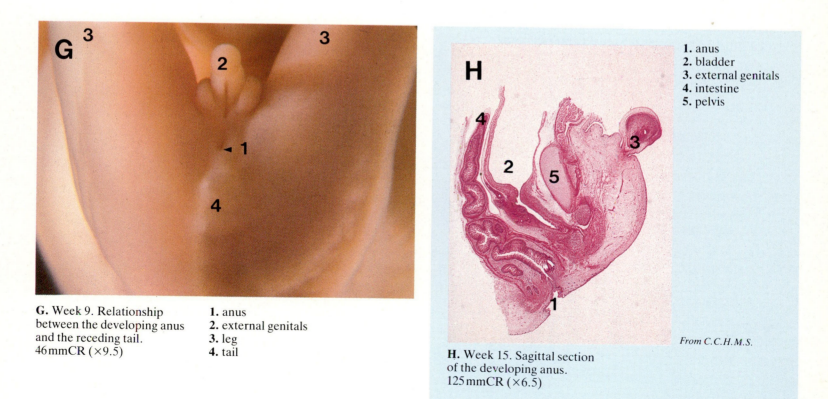

G. Week 9. Relationship between the developing anus and the receding tail. 46 mm CR (×9.5)

1. anus
2. external genitals
3. leg
4. tail

1. anus
2. bladder
3. external genitals
4. intestine
5. pelvis

From C.C.H.M.S.

H. Week 15. Sagittal section of the developing anus. 125 mm CR (×6.5)

143

Kidney

The lower cervical and upper thoracic intermediate mesoderm fuse to form a continuous nephrogenic cord. At Day 23 and 24 the primary excretory duct forms in the dorsal nephrogenic cord at the ninth somite level and as it grows caudally it separates from the nephrogenic cord and becomes hollow. It lies immediately below the ectoderm and turns ventrally to open into the cloaca at Day 28. A diverticulum, the metanephric or ureteric bud, is found where the cord enters the cloaca.

Clusters of cells in the cranial nephrogenic cord form rudimentary and transient nephric tubules: the pronephroi.

The mesonephroi succeeds the pronephroi and form caudally at the L3 level. At one end the 'S' shaped mesonephric tubules open into the primary excretory duct (now the mesonephric duct) and at the other end is found a glomerular capsule with a vascular supply from the aorta. The more cranial tubules atrophy and disappear before the more caudal ones develop. Usually no more than 30–40 tubules are present at one time in an embryo. By the end of Week 6 the mesonephroi together form the mesonephric ridge which is present from the septum transversum to the L3 level. The genital gland forms on its medial aspect. Most of the cranial mesonephroi atrophy and disappear until they remain only at the L1–L3 level.

Derivatives of the remaining tubules are the efferent ductules of the testis and paradidymis in the male and epoophoron and paroophoron in the female.

In the male, the mesonephric duct forms the appendix of the epididymis, vas (ductus) deferens and ejaculatory duct. At the end of Week 13 the seminal vesicle and ampulla of the ductus deferens form at the end of the mesonephric duct. At Week 15 the two areas separate and at Week 24 development of the mesonephric duct is suppressed and they both grow rapidly.

In the female development of the mesonephric duct is suppressed and it forms the longitudinal duct of the epoophoron, appendix vesiculosa and duct of Gartner.

As the metanephric (ureteric) bud grows dorsally from the mesonephric duct in Week 5, its blind end grows into a mass of metanephric mesoderm which forms the metanephric cap. The stalk of the ureteric bud forms the ureter, and gives rise to the pelvis, calyces and collecting tubules. Derivatives of the metanephric cap are the nephrons. Glomerular blood vessels form *in situ* from mesoderm in the glomerular capsule. Urine is formed at Week 8 and is excreted into the amniotic fluid (see Amnion).

Blood supply. The pelvic kidney is supplied by the iliac arteries. As the kidney migrates cephalically it is supplied successively by new aortic branches. Finally at Week 9 it is supplied by the most caudal suprarenal artery (from the aorta) which enlarges to form the renal artery.

- The neonatal kidney is lobulated, but the lobulation is usually lost by 4 to 5 years of age.

- The glomeruli become fully functional about 6 weeks after birth.

- The absence of one kidney (renal agenesis) is relatively common.

- Kidneys containing multiple cysts (polycystic) function poorly. The exact cause of the cysts is uncertain.

A–L. Development of the mesonephric and metanephric kidneys.

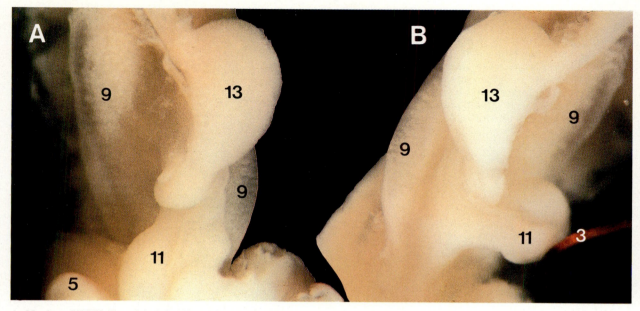

A. Horizon XVIII (Day 36–38). Viewed from the ventral surface. The mesonephric kidney is running the length of the abdomen. The liver has been removed. 14mmCR (×19.8)

B. Same specimen as in Figure **A.** Viewed from the ventral surface. The stomach has been reflected to the right side. (×19.8)

C. View from the left side of the embryo in Figure **A.** (×18.6)

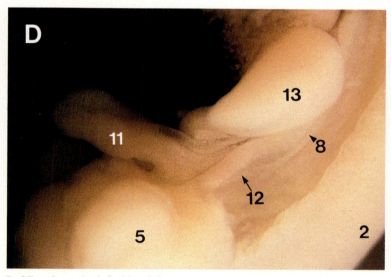

D. View from the left side of the embryo in Figure **A.** (×18.6)

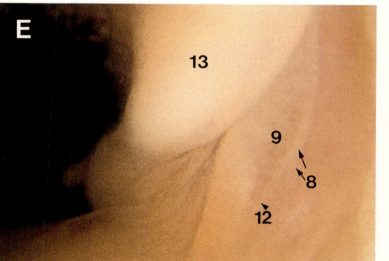

E. Higher magnification of Figure **D.** (×38.8)

1. abdomen
2. back
3. cactus needle
4. heart
5. leg bud
6. liver
7. lung bud
8. mesonephric duct
9. mesonephric tubules
10. metanephric bud
11. midgut
12. paramesonephric duct
13. stomach
14. tail

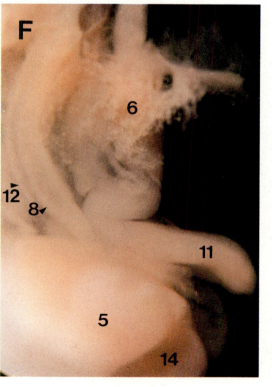

F. View from the right side of the embryo in Figure **A.** (×18)

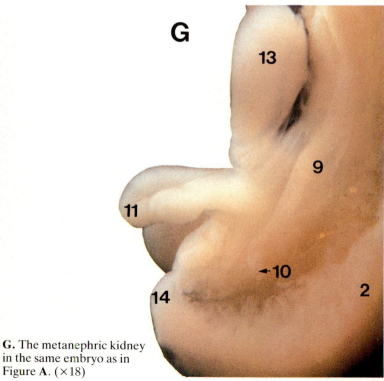

G. The metanephric kidney in the same embryo as in Figure **A.** (×18)

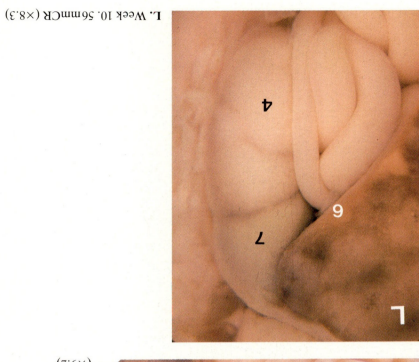

L. Week 10. 56 mm CR (×8.3)

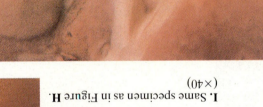

J-L. The metanephric kidney.

K. Week 8. 48 mm CR ♀ (×9.2)

1. bladder
2. gonad
3. intestine (and appendix)
4. kidney (metanephric)
5. leg
6. liver
7. suprarenal (adrenal) gland

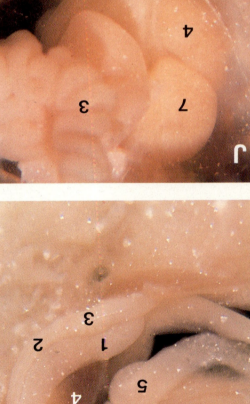

J. Week 8. The intestine has been reflected superiorly. 40 mm CR (×9)

I. Same specimen as in Figure H. (×40)

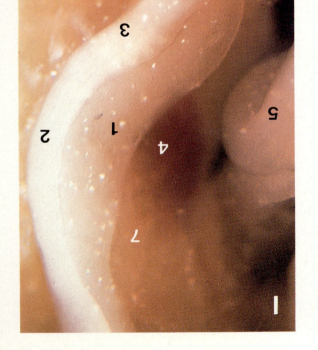

H. Horizon XIX (Day 38–40). The mesonephric kidney degenerating as the metanephric kidney migrates up the posterior abdominal wall to meet the suprarenal (adrenal) gland. Liver removed. Viewed from the left. 20 mm CR (×18.6)

1. gonad
2. mesonephric kidney
3. mesonephric tubules
4. metanephric kidney
5. midgut
6. pancreas
7. suprarenal (adrenal) gland

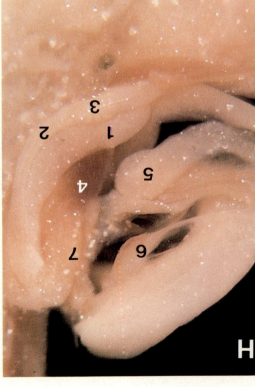

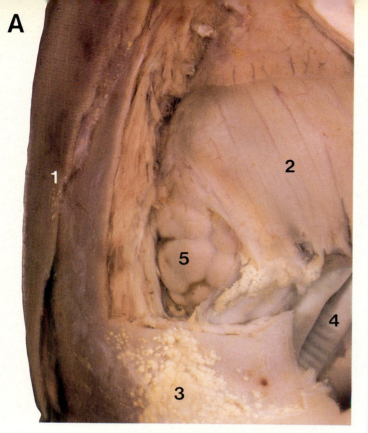

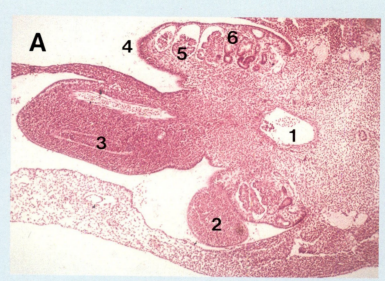

A. Horizon XV (Day 31–32). *From L.H.S.M.*
8 mmCR (×96)

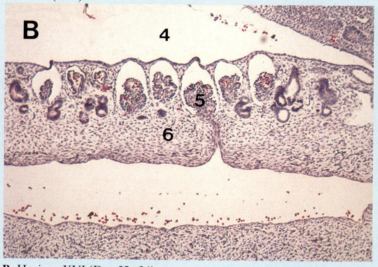

B. Horizon XVI (Day 32–34).
9 mmCR (×120)

A. Week 18. Final position of the fetal kidney. 152 mmCR ♂ (×2)

1. back
2. diaphragm
3. fat
4. intestine
5. kidney

A and B. Increase in size of the metanephric kidney and the suprarenal (adrenal) gland.

1. metanephric kidney
2. suprarenal (adrenal) gland
3. ureter

A. Week 9. View of the ventral surface. Smallest kidney.
48 mmCR ♂ (×18.5)
Week 11. Middle-sized kidney. 65 mmCR ♂ (×2.8)
Week 13. Largest kidney.
101 mmCR ♀ (×2.4)

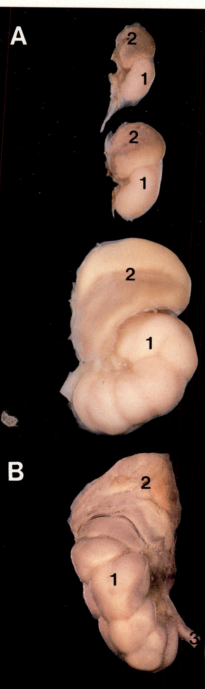

A–C. Transverse paraffin wax sections of the mesonephros in the early embryo.

1. dorsal aortae
2. gonadal ridge
3. hindgut
4. intra-embryonic coelom
5. mesonephric glomerulus
6. mesonephric ridge

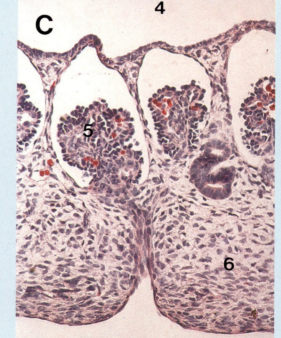

C. Higher magnification of the mesonephric tubules in Figure **B**. (×300)

B. Week 18. Left kidney and suprarenal gland. View of the dorsal surface. 152 mmCR ♂ (×2)

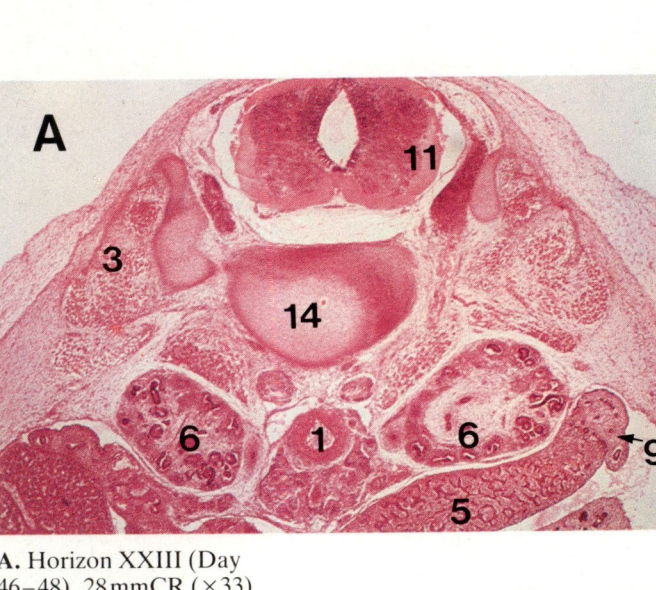

A. Horizon XXIII (Day 46–48). 28 mmCR (×33)

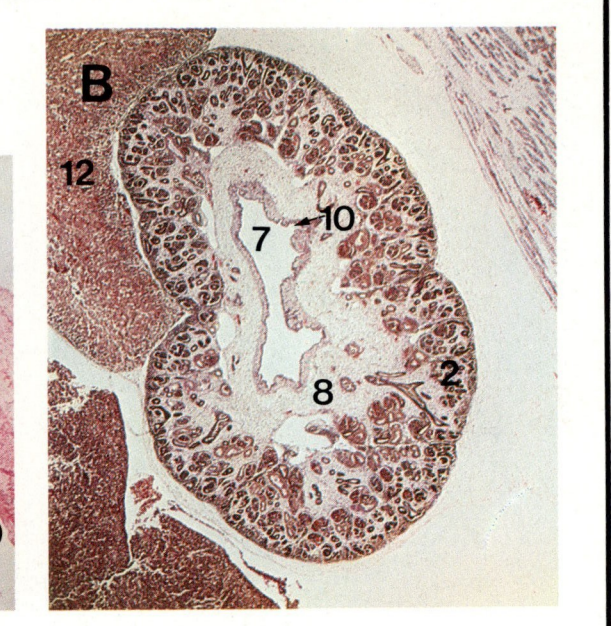

B. Week 8. 35 mmCR (×28)

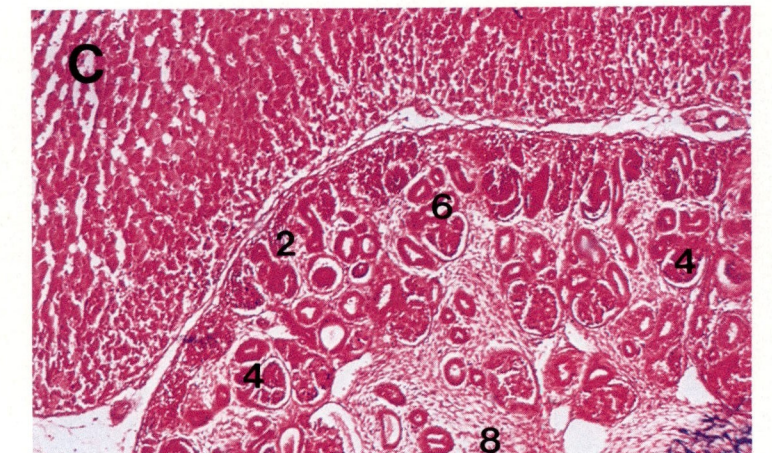

C. Week 8. 35 mmCR (×106)

B and C *from Mr G. Bottomley*

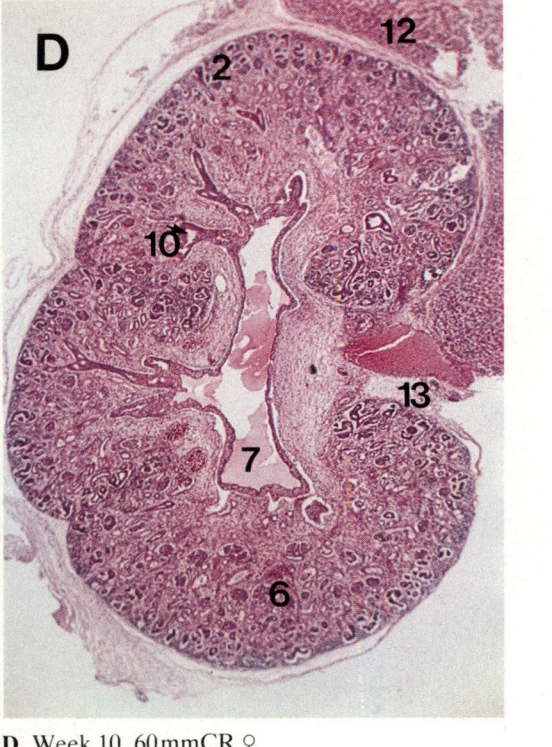

D. Week 10. 60 mmCR ♀ (×28)

A–G. Transverse paraffin wax sections of the metanephric kidney development.

1. aorta
2. cortex
3. erector spinae muscles
4. glomeruli
5. gonad
6. kidney
7. major calyx
8. medulla
9. mesonephros
10. minor calyx
11. spinal cord
12. suprarenal gland
13. ureter
14. vertebral body

1. collecting tubules
2. cortex
3. glomeruli
4. kidney
5. medulla

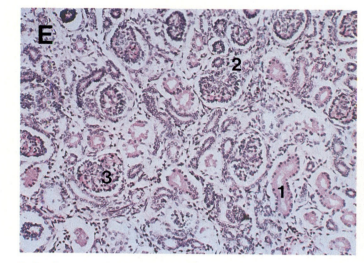

E. Higher magnification of the kidney in Figure **D**. (×112)

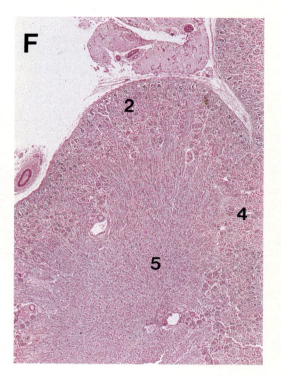

F. Week 18. 152 mmCR ♂ (×28.5)

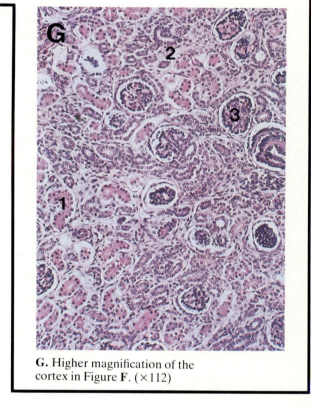

G. Higher magnification of the cortex in Figure **F**. (×112)

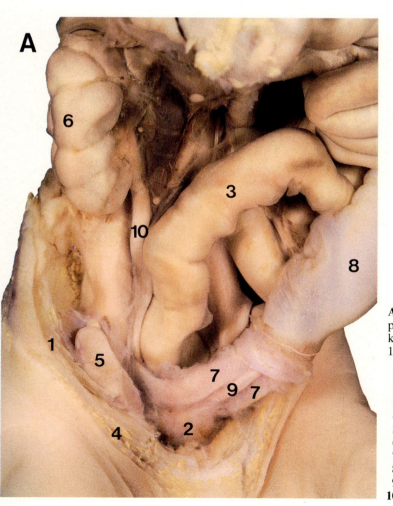

A. Week 18. Relative positions of the ureter, kidney and bladder. 152 mmCR ♂ (×2.5)

1. abdominal wall
2. bladder wall
3. colon
4. fat
5. gonad
6. kidney
7. umbilical artery
8. umbilical cord
9. urachus
10. ureter

Relative position of the kidney

The kidneys form in the pelvic cavity early in Week 5 and migrate cranially onto the posterior abdominal wall. At Day 34–36 they have reached the level of L2.

The renal pelvis which originally faces ventrally rotates to a medial position.

The kidneys rise to meet the suprarenal (adrenal) glands on the posterior abdominal wall.

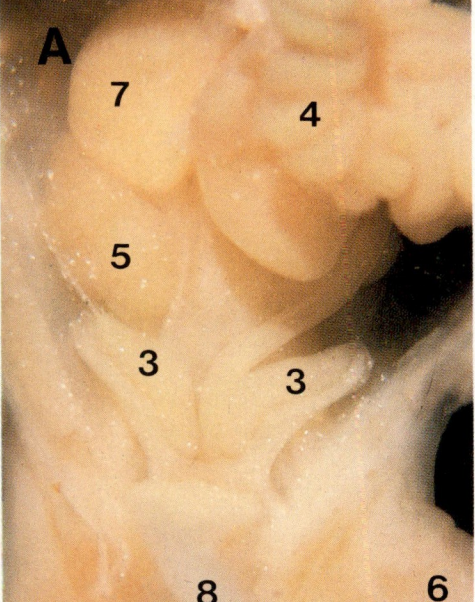

A. Horizon XIX (Day 38–40). 20 mmCR (×16.5)

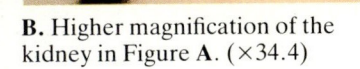

B. Higher magnification of the kidney in Figure A. (×34.4)

A and B. Metanephric kidney in the early embryo viewed from the left. Leg bud removed.

1. back
2. genital tubercle
3. gonad
4. intestine
5. mesonephric kidney
6. metanephric kidney
7. pancreas
8. stomach
9. suprarenal (adrenal) gland
10. umbilical cord

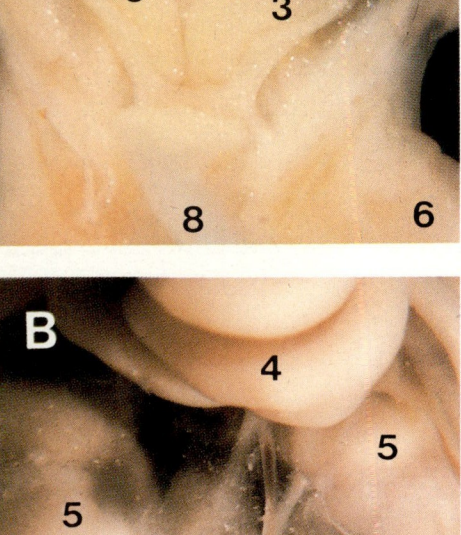

A. Week 8. 40 mmCR ♀ (×8.3)

A–F. Relative positions of the developing kidney viewed from the front.

1. bladder
2. external genitals
3. gonads
4. intestine
5. kidney
6. leg
7. suprarenal (adrenal) gland
8. umbilical cord

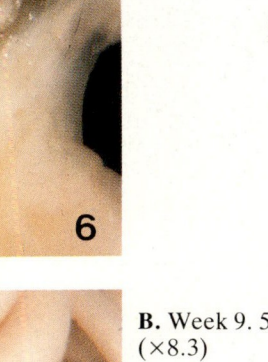

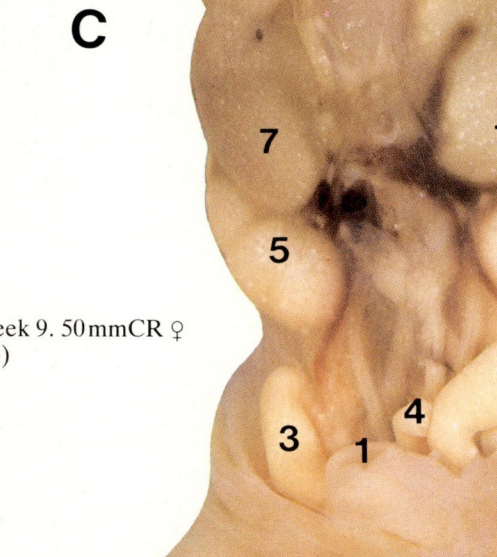

C. Week 9. 50 mmCR ♀ (×5.9)

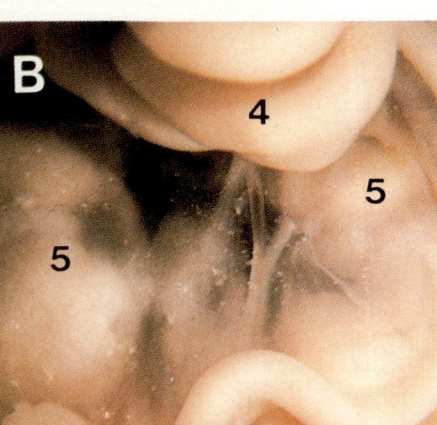

B. Week 9. 50 mmCR ♀ (×8.3)

1. bladder
2. external genitals
3. gonads
4. intestine
5. kidney
6. leg
7. suprarenal (adrenal) gland
8. umbilical cord
9. ureter

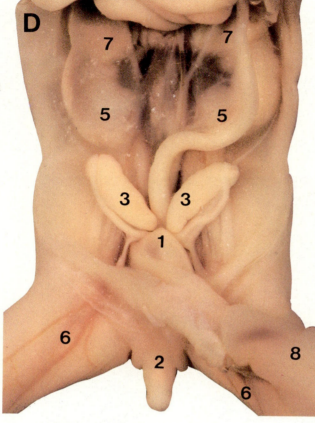

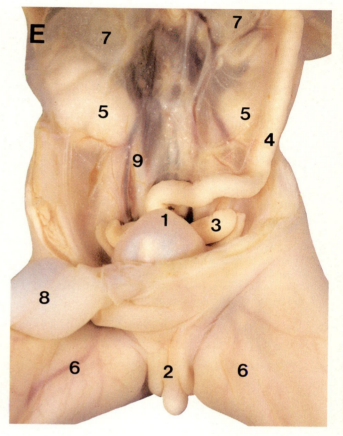

D. Week 9. 57 mmCR ♂
(×4.3)

E. Week 13. 92 mmCR ♀
(×3.5)

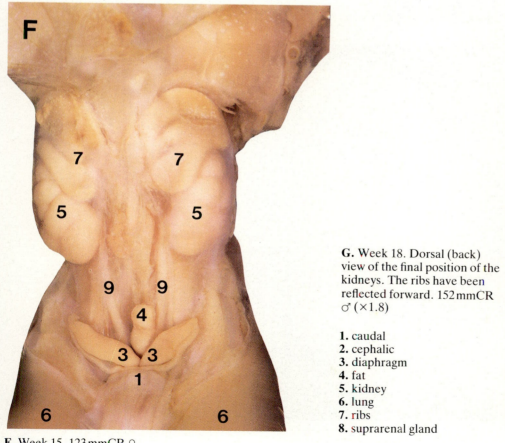

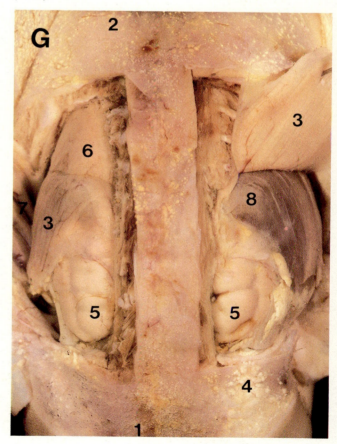

G. Week 18. Dorsal (back)
view of the final position of the
kidneys. The ribs have been
reflected forward. 152 mmCR
♂ (×1.8)

1. caudal
2. cephalic
3. diaphragm
4. fat
5. kidney
6. lung
7. ribs
8. suprarenal gland

F. Week 15. 123 mmCR ♀
(×2.6)

Suprarenal (adrenal) glands

The suprarenal has a dual origin: the medulla from neuroectoderm and the cortex from mesoderm. The fetal cortex appears in Week 6 when cells from the coelomic epithelium aggregate on each side between the developing gonad and the dorsal mesentery. The medullary cells migrate from adjacent sympathetic ganglia (neuroectoderm) and form a mass on the medial surface of the fetal cortex. Gradually the medullary mass, which forms the chromaffin cells, is surrounded by the fetal cortex. A second layer of investing mesoderm forms the adult cortex. Between Week 8 and 9 the cortex produces corticosteroids. The cortex also produces androgens and estriol precursors.
The medulla produces insignificant quantities of epinephrine (adrenalin).

- The neonatal gland is twenty times the relative size of the gland in the adult.
- The zona glomerulosa and the zona fasciculata are present in the neonatal suprarenal.
- The fetal cortex disappears by the first year of age and the suprarenal rapidly becomes absolutely smaller.
- The zona reticularis forms by the end of the third year.

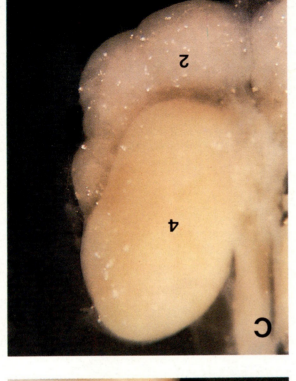

C. Higher magnification of the suprarenal gland in Figure **B.** (×18.9)

B. Week 8. View from the ventral surface. 40 mmCR (×9.5)

1. gonad
2. kidney (metanephric)
3. mesonephric kidney
4. suprarenal gland

A–G. Development of the suprarenal (adrenal) gland. (Also see Kidney.)

A. Horizon XIX (Day 38–40). Early suprarenal gland viewed from the right side. The liver has been removed. 20 mmCR (×39.4)

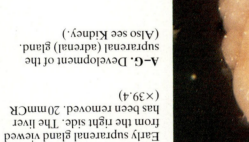

D. Week 10. View of the
ventral surface. 56 mm CR
(×9.9)

1. kidney
2. pelvis of kidney
3. suprarenal gland

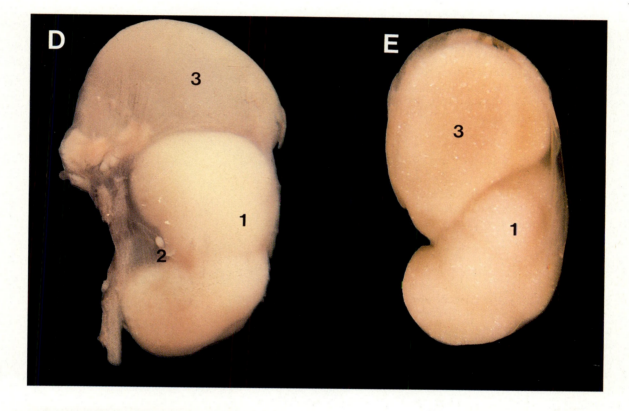

E. Week 10. View of the
ventral surface. 60 mm CR ♀
(×9.9)

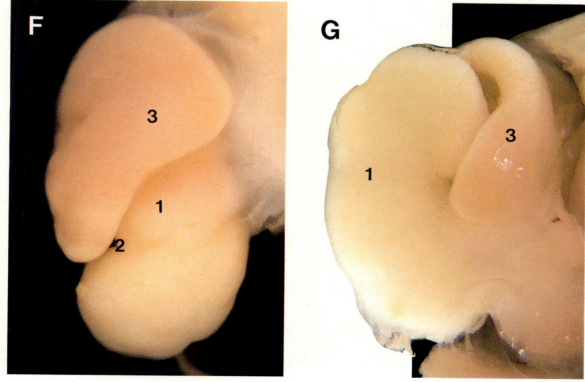

F. Week 11. View from the ventral
surface. 65 mm CR ♂ (×9.9)

G. Dorsal view of the specimen
in Figure **F**. (×9.9)

Bladder

The urorectal septum divides the cloaca into the urogenital sinus and the rectum and anal canal. The allantois is continuous with and ends in the urogenital sinus. The mesonephric ducts also end in the urogenital sinus. The bladder forms from the cranial part of the urogenital sinus. As the bladder enlarges the mesonephric ducts (the vasa deferentia in the male) and ureter are incorporated into the dorsal wall so that they enter the bladder separately. The mesonephric ducts contribute to the trigone of the bladder, but their mesodermal epithelium is soon replaced by urogenital sinus endodermal epithelium. In the female the caudal ends of the mesonephric ducts subsequently degenerate. The surrounding splanchnic mesoderm forms the other layers of the bladder.

As the bladder grows, the allantois forms the tubular urachus which then becomes a fibrous cord passing from the apex of the bladder to the umbilicus. This cord is the median umbilical ligament.

Female urethra

The epithelium is derived from the endodermal urogenital sinus. Adjacent splanchnic mesoderm forms the connective tissue and smooth muscle.

Male urethra

The epithelium is derived from the urogenital sinus (except the glandular part of the penile urethra). The connective tissue and smooth muscle are from adjacent splanchnic mesoderm. The epithelium of the cranial prostatic part is originally mesodermal, but is replaced by endodermal epithelium.

The glandular penile urethra forms by an ectodermal ingrowth at the tip of the penis splitting to form a urathral groove. This later closes.

- There is no true fundus in the neonatal bladder.

- The bladder contains a small amount of urine at birth.

- The fully distended bladder in the young infant is almost entirely abdominal and may extend up to the umbilicus.

- Hypospadius in the male is failure or incomplete fusion of the urogenital folds and results in an incomplete penile urethra.

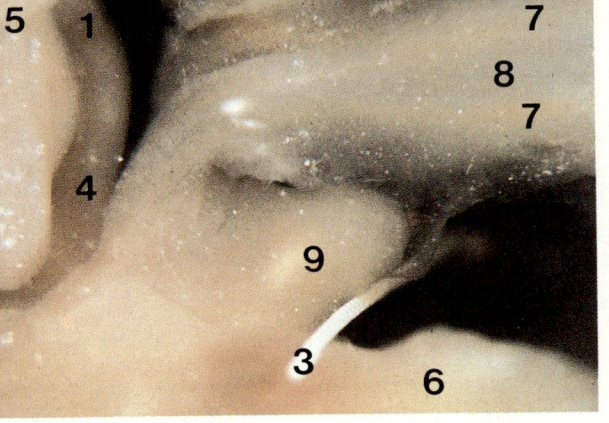

A–F. The bladder.

1. allantois
2. buttocks
3. cactus needle
4. early bladder
5. intestine
6. leg
7. umbilical arteries
8. umbilical cord
9. external genitals

A. Horizon XIX (Day 38–40). View from the right. 20 mmCR (×35.6)

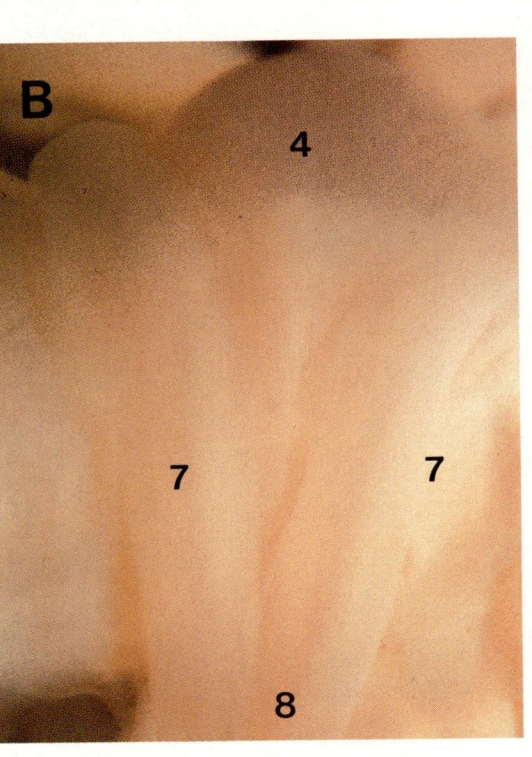

B. Week 9. The umbilical cord has been pulled taut. View from the front of the rostral surface. 48 mmCR (×18)

C. Week 10. The caudal surface of the bladder viewed from below. The legs have been removed. 56 mmCR (×9)

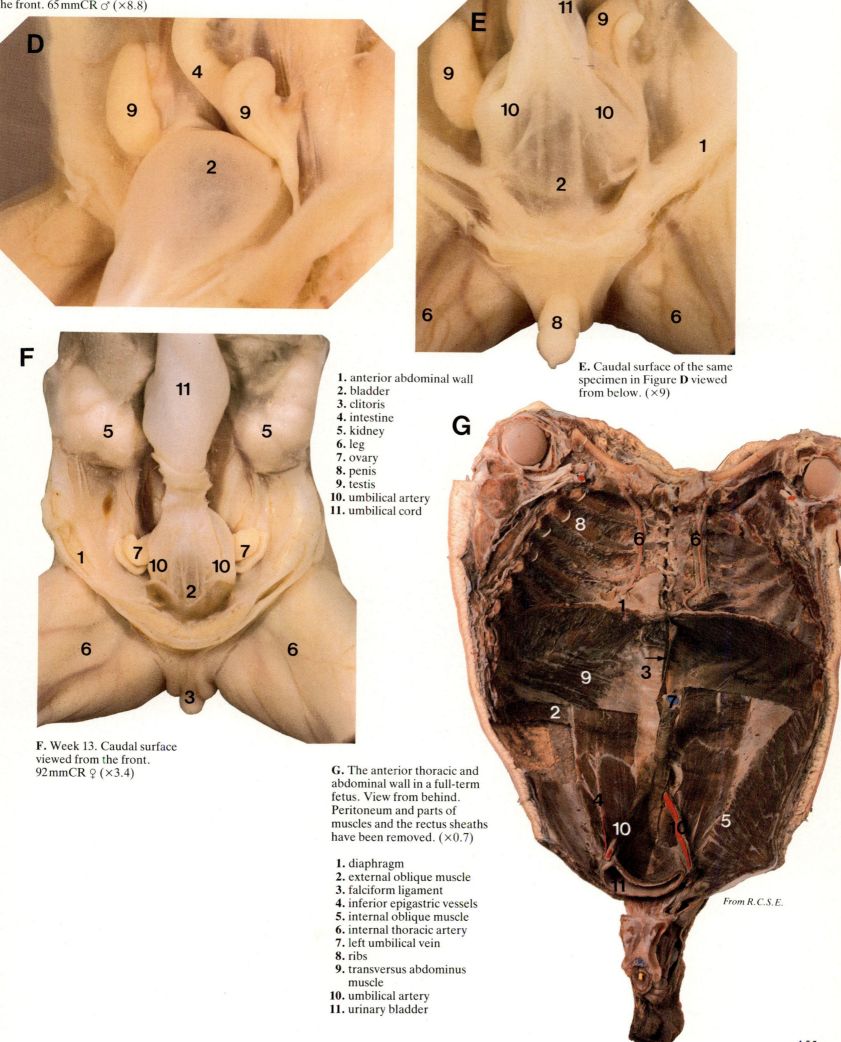

D. Week 11. Rostral surface viewed from the front. 65 mmCR ♂ (×8.8)

E. Caudal surface of the same specimen in Figure **D** viewed from below. (×9)

1. anterior abdominal wall
2. bladder
3. clitoris
4. intestine
5. kidney
6. leg
7. ovary
8. penis
9. testis
10. umbilical artery
11. umbilical cord

F. Week 13. Caudal surface viewed from the front. 92 mmCR ♀ (×3.4)

G. The anterior thoracic and abdominal wall in a full-term fetus. View from behind. Peritoneum and parts of muscles and the rectus sheaths have been removed. (×0.7)

1. diaphragm
2. external oblique muscle
3. falciform ligament
4. inferior epigastric vessels
5. internal oblique muscle
6. internal thoracic artery
7. left umbilical vein
8. ribs
9. transversus abdominus muscle
10. umbilical artery
11. urinary bladder

From R.C.S.E.

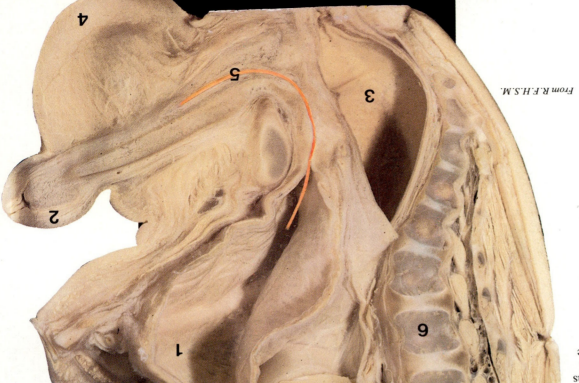

From R.F.H.S.M.

B. Full-term fetus. Sagittal section through the bladder and urethra. A red bristle has been inserted in the urethra. Note the fetal position of the bladder. (×2.1)

1. bladder
2. femur
3. labioscrotal swelling
4. phallus
5. rectum
6. spinal cord
7. urethra
8. vertebral body

A. Week 9. Transverse section through the bladder and urethra. 49mmCR (×7.3)

From C.C.H.M.S.

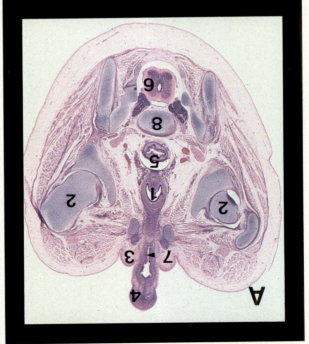

1. bladder
2. penis
3. rectum
4. scrotum
5. urethra
6. vertebral column

A. The developing bladder viewed in sagittal section. (×2)

A–E. Development of the genital tubercle viewed from the right side.

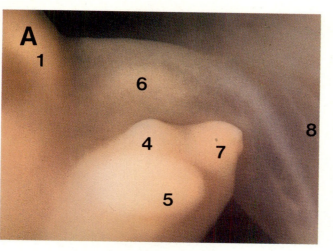

A. Horizon XVII (Day 34–36). 12mmCR (×15.9)

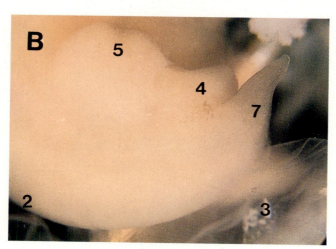

B. Horizon XVII (Day 34–36). 12mmCR (×15.9)

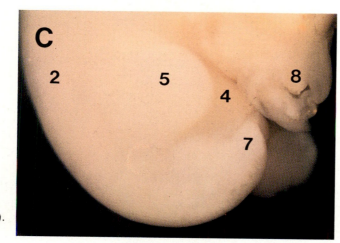

C. Horizon XVIII (Day 36–38). 14mmCR (×15.9)

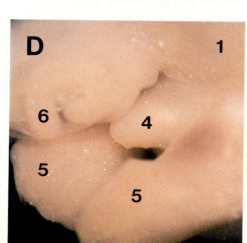

D. Horizon XIX (Day 38–40). 20mmCR (×15.9)

Genitals: external

Indifferent stage

Until Week 9 the external genitalia of the two sexes are similar in appearance.

Initially a midline genital tubercle is present cephalic to the proctodeal depression (Week 4). This tubercle will form the penis or clitoris. At the caudal surface of the genital tubercle are two labioscrotal swellings enclosing two urogenital folds which enclose the cloacal membrane. The genital tubercle elongates to form a phallus* and is as big in the female as in the male. As the tubercle elongates it carries a projection from the urogenital sinus (urethral groove). At Week 6 the urorectal septum fuses with the cloacal membrane dividing it into a ventral urogenital membrane and a dorsal anal membrane. Shortly after Week 6 the urogenital membrane breaks down and the urethral groove and urogenital orifice are continuous.

*The term 'phallus' is used to denote the indifferent stage of development.

1. abdomen
2. back
3. early membranes
4. genital tubercle
5. leg bud
6. midgut herniation in the umbilical cord
7. tail
8. umbilical cord

E. Horizon XIX (Day 38–40). 20mmCR (×15.9)

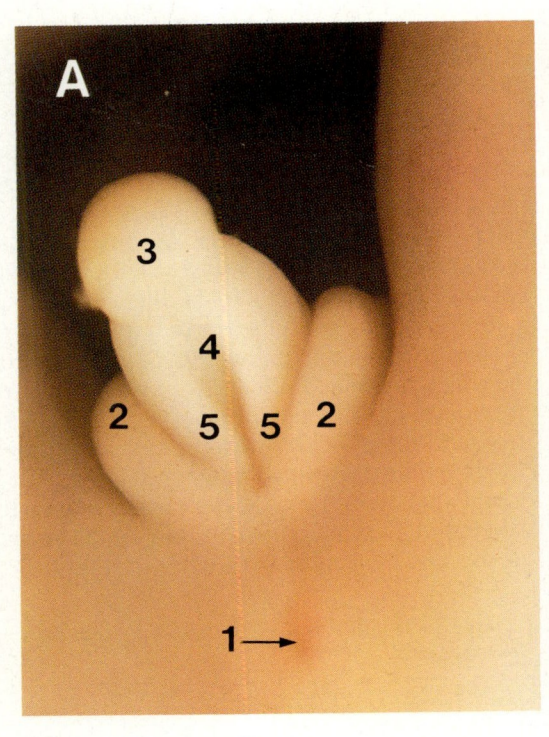

A. Unfused urogenital folds.

B. Urethral groove continuous
with the urogenital sinus
viewed by transmitted light.

A and B. Week 9. Formation of
the phallus viewed from below.
48mmCR (×18)

1. anus
2. labioscrotal swelling
3. phallus
4. urethral groove continuous
   with the urogenital sinus
5. urogenital folds

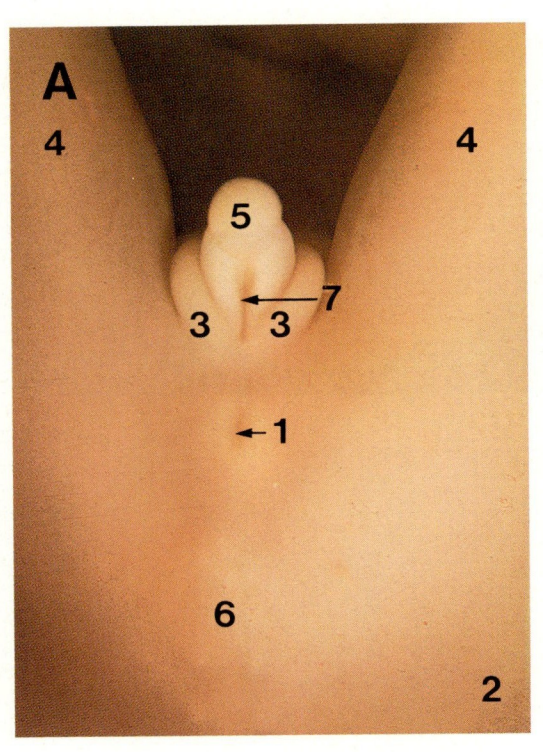

A. Week 9. Relationship
between the anus, genitals and
tail. 48mmCR (×9)

1. anus
2. back (dorsal) surface
3. labioscrotal swelling
4. leg
5. phallus
6. tail
7. urethral groove continuous
   with the urogenital sinus

A–G. Male external genitalia.
View from below.

1. anus
2. labioscrotal swelling
3. leg
4. penis (glans)
5. scrotal raphe
6. scrotum
7. urethral groove
8. urogenital folds

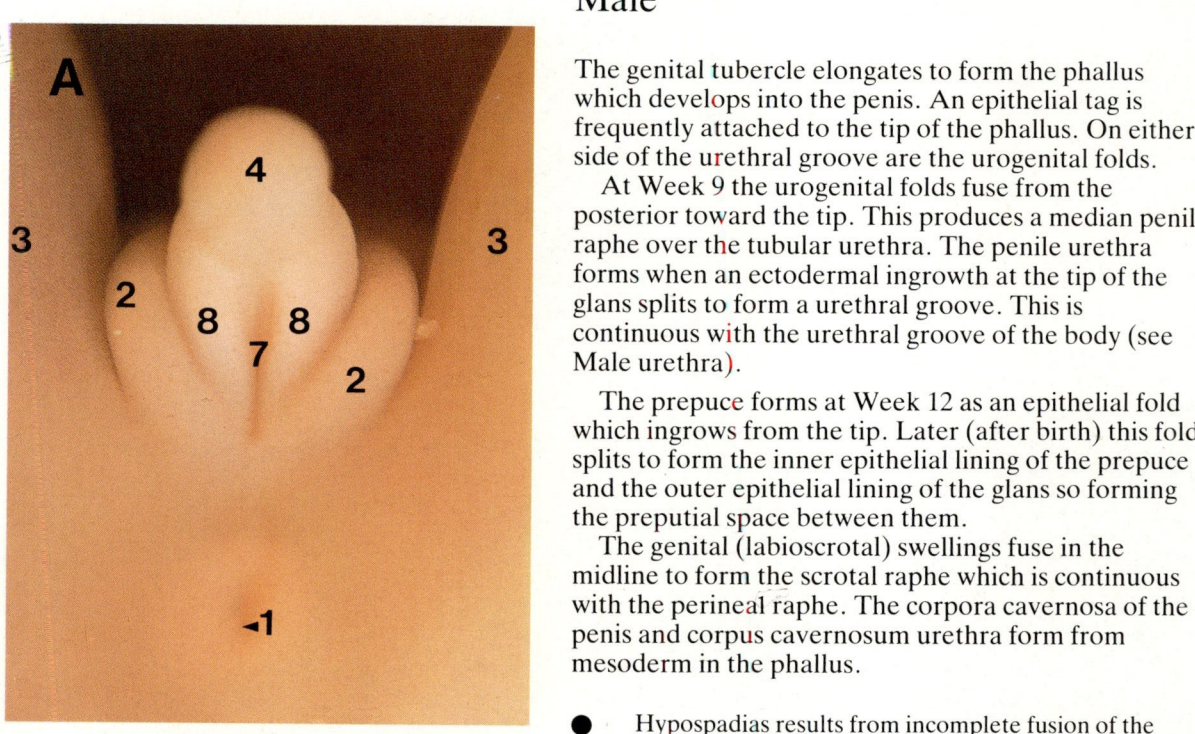

A. Week 9. The urogenital folds have started to fuse. 48 mmCR (×18)

Male

The genital tubercle elongates to form the phallus which develops into the penis. An epithelial tag is frequently attached to the tip of the phallus. On either side of the urethral groove are the urogenital folds.

At Week 9 the urogenital folds fuse from the posterior toward the tip. This produces a median penile raphe over the tubular urethra. The penile urethra forms when an ectodermal ingrowth at the tip of the glans splits to form a urethral groove. This is continuous with the urethral groove of the body (see Male urethra).

The prepuce forms at Week 12 as an epithelial fold which ingrows from the tip. Later (after birth) this fold splits to form the inner epithelial lining of the prepuce and the outer epithelial lining of the glans so forming the preputial space between them.

The genital (labioscrotal) swellings fuse in the midline to form the scrotal raphe which is continuous with the perineal raphe. The corpora cavernosa of the penis and corpus cavernosum urethra form from mesoderm in the phallus.

● Hypospadias results from incomplete fusion of the urogenital folds.

● The neonatal prepuce and glans may not be completely separated.

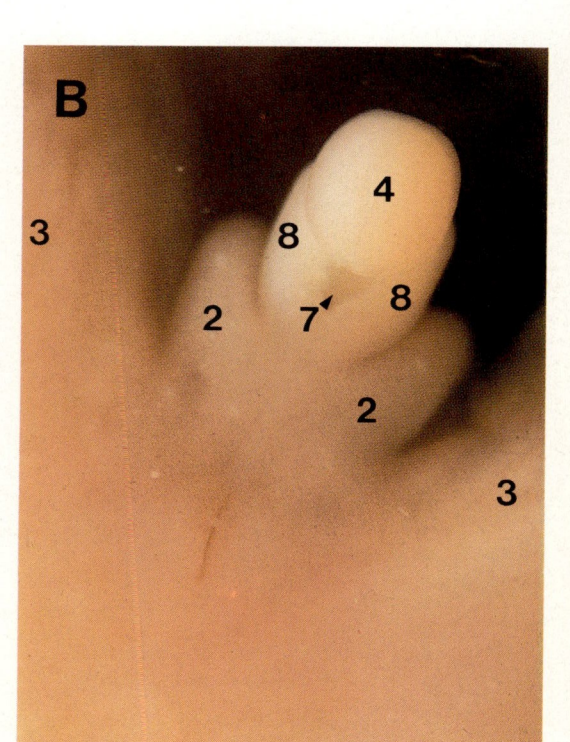

B. Week 9. The urogenital folds have fused except near the tip. 48 mmCR (×18)

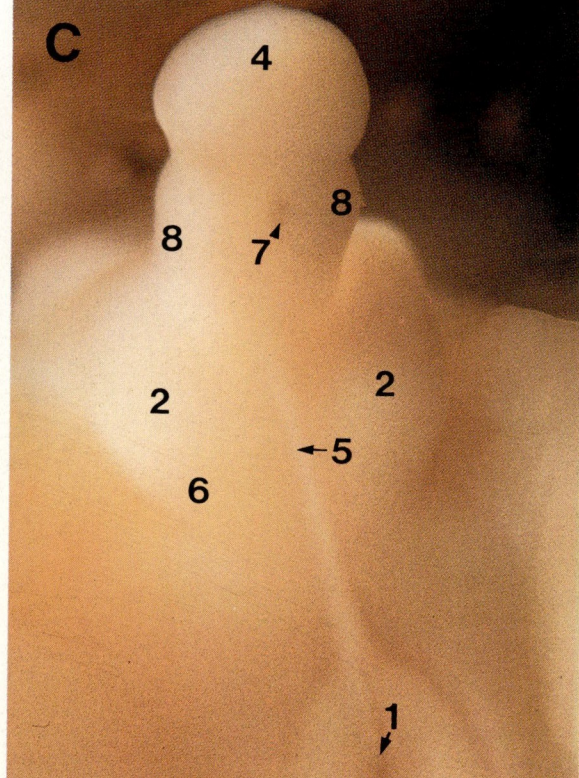

C. Week 10. The urogenital folds have almost completely fused. 56 mmCR (×19.8)

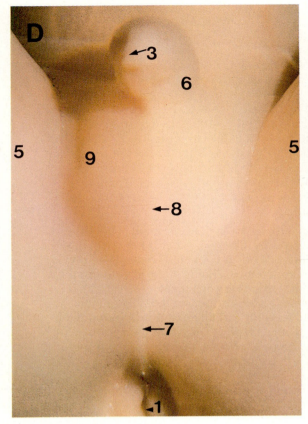

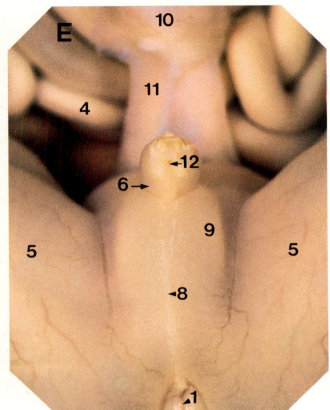

D. Week 12. The urogenital folds have fused. Note the epithelial tag. 85 mm CR (×10)

E. Week 13. The urethra is present at the top. 97 mm CR (×6.6)

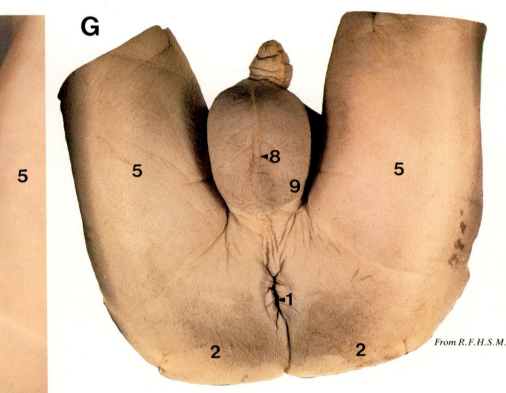

From R.F.H.S.M.

F. Week 18. The testes are not present in the scrotum. 152 mm CR (×3)

G. Full-term fetus. The testes are present in the scrotum. (×1.3)

Female

The genital tubercle forms the phallus which develops into the clitoris (Week 9). The urogenital folds do not fuse (except immediately in front of the anus) and form the labia minora. The labioscrotal swellings do not fuse (except cephalically to form the mons pubis and caudally to form the posterior labial commissure) and form the labia majora (Week 9–12). The labia majora are homologous with the male scrotum.

A primitive urethral groove forms but regresses. The female urethra is homologous to the upper portion of the prostatic part of the male urethra (see Male urethra).

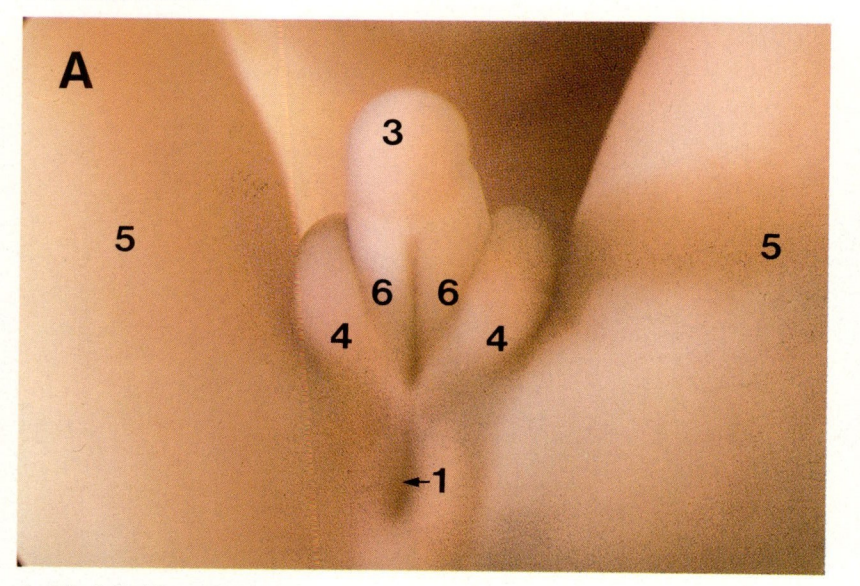

A. Clitoris of a female fetus. Note the epithelial tag. View from the side. 43 mmCR (×18.6)

1. clitoris
2. epithelial tag
3. leg

A and B. Development of the female external genitalia. View from below.

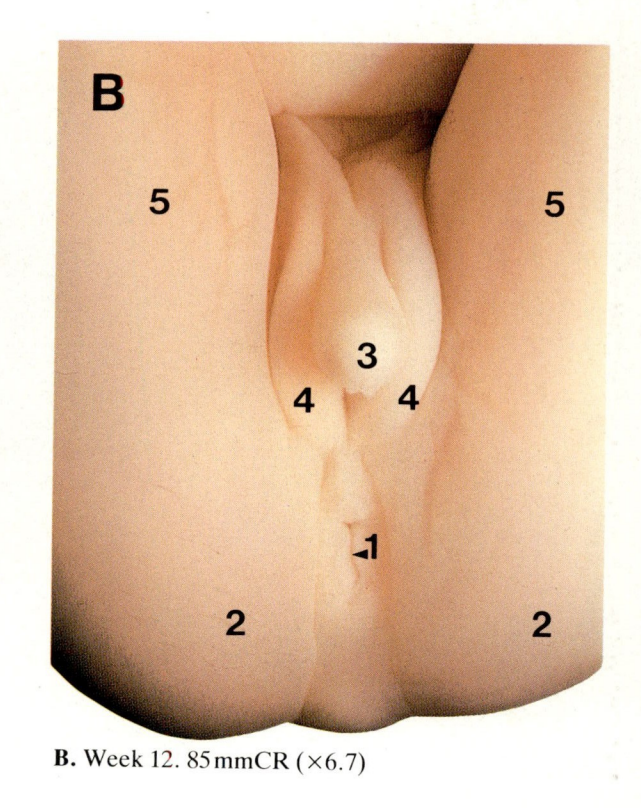

A. Week 9. 46 mmCR (×21)

1. anus
2. buttock
3. clitoris
4. labioscrotal swelling (labia majora)
5. leg
6. urogenital fold (labia minora)

B. Week 12. 85 mmCR (×6.7)

A–E. Development of the female external genitalia. View from below.

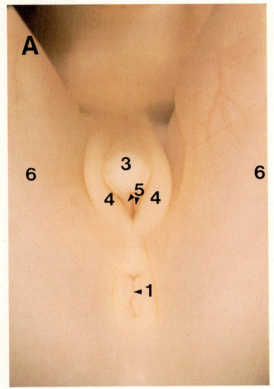

A. Week 13. 92 mmCR (×5.7)

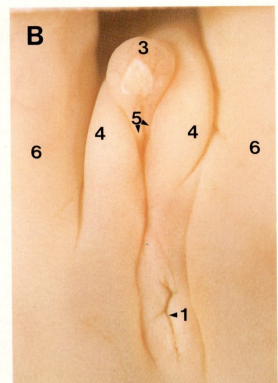

B. Week 13. 101 mmCR (×7.3)

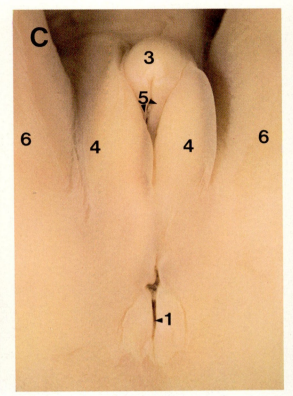

C. Week 17. 150 mmCR (×5.4)

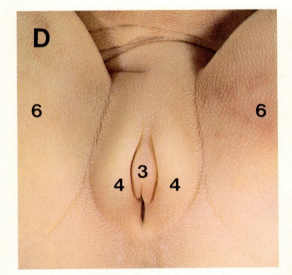

D. Week 20. 185 mmCR (×2.6)

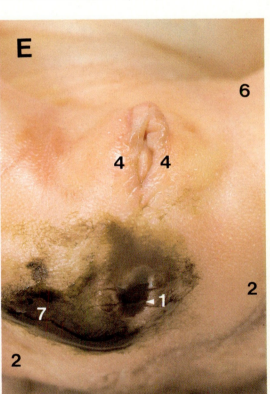

E. Week 35. (×2.6)

1. anus
2. buttock
3. clitoris
4. labia majora
5. labia minora
6. leg
7. meconium

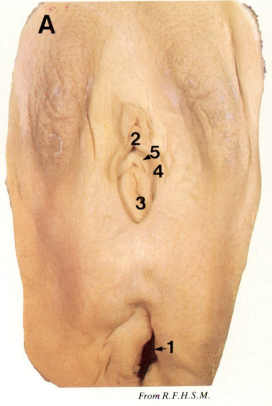

A. Neonatal external genitalia. A complete hymen is present. Note the small development of the labia minora. (×1.1)

1. anus
2. clitoris
3. hymen
4. labia majora
5. labia minora

From R.F.H.S.M.

Gonads: internal

Indifferent stage

Until Week 7 both sexes appear similar even though their sex is determined at fertilization. The early period is the 'indifferent' stage of development.

Early in Week 4 primordial germ cells from the yolk sac migrate to the gonadal ridges which have developed on the medial side of the mesonephros. Coelomic epithelial cords (primary sex cords) grow into the mesoderm of the gonadal ridge to produce an outer cortex and inner medulla. In the male the cords are very prominent but in the female they break up into cell clusters.

During Week 6 the germ cells become incorporated into the gonad. In the female the medulla regresses whilst in the male the cortex regresses and the medulla forms the testis.

Ducts. Two pairs of ducts form in both sexes; these are the mesonephric ducts (see Kidney) and the paramesonephric (Müllerian) ducts. The latter form from coelomic epithelium and lie lateral and generally parallel to the mesonephric ducts. Their cranial ends open into the coelomic cavity and the caudal ends cross ventral to the mesonephric ducts and fuse in the midline to form a 'Y' shaped uterovaginal primordium in the female which projects into the urogenital sinus. In the male, development of the paramesonephric duct is suppressed and the duct forms the appendix of the testis. The Müllerian tubercle is produced where the primordium enters the sinus. The mesonephric ducts enter the sinus on either side of this tubercle.

A. Horizon XV (Day 31–32). Transverse paraffin wax section of the gonadal ridge. 8mmCR (×75)

1. body wall
2. dorsal aorta
3. dorsal mesentery
4. gonadal ridge
5. common iliac artery
6. mesonephric glomeruli
7. notochord

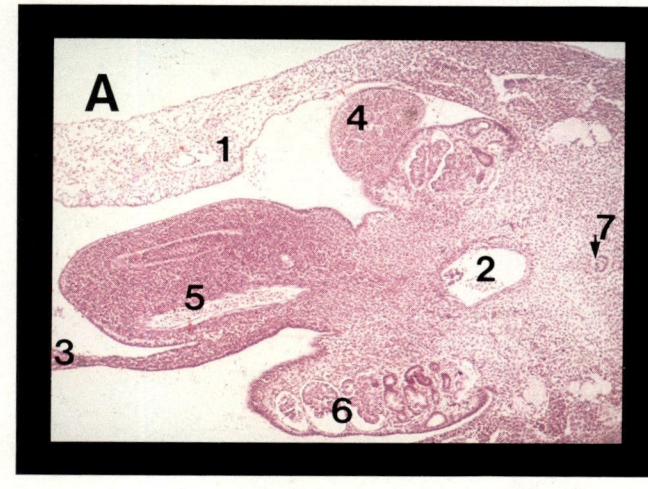

From L.H.S.M.

A–C. Horizon XVIII (Day 36–38). The gonadal ridge.

1. esophagus
2. gonadal ridge
3. mesonephric duct
4. mesonephric kidney
5. mesonephric tubules
6. midgut herniation (the umbilical cord has been removed)
7. paramesonephric duct
8. stomach

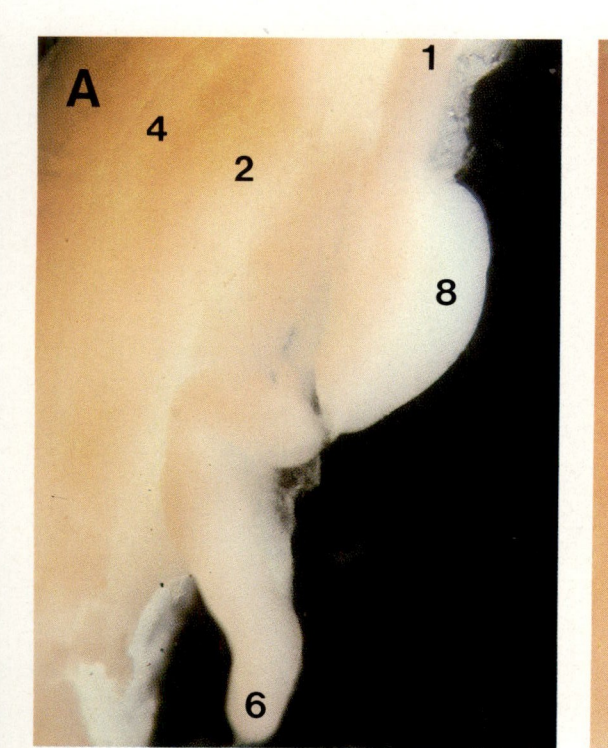

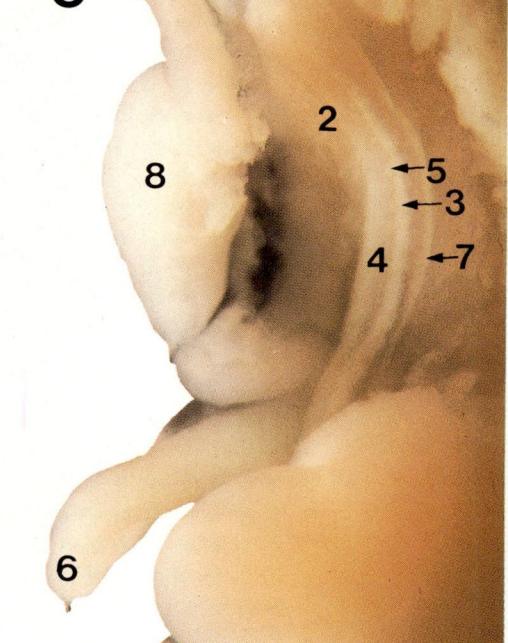

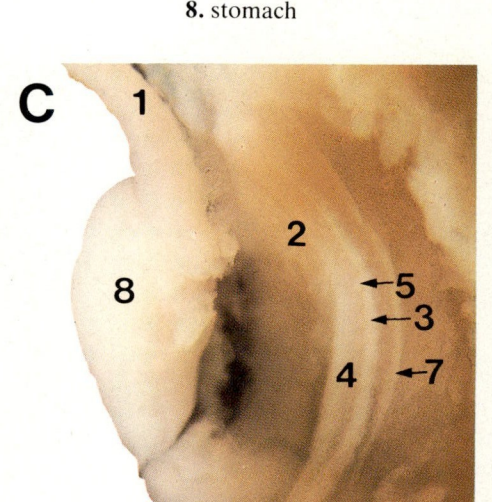

A. View from the right side. The liver has been removed. 14mmCR (×16.7)

B. Higher magnification of the ridge in Figure A. (×39)

C. View from the left side. (×18.6)

Male

Testis. In the male, the primary sex cords extend into the medulla where they branch, hollow out and their ends then anastomose to form the rete testis. The sex cords (seminiferous or testicular cords) lose their connection with the germinal epithelium as the connective tissue coat (tunica albuginea) forms. As the mesonephros regresses caudally the testis separates and is suspended by its own mesentery, the mesorchium.

The seminiferous cords form the seminiferous tubules, rete testis and tubuli recti. The walls of the seminiferous tubules are composed of two types of cells: supporting Sertoli cells derived from germinal epithelium and spermatogonia derived from primordial germ cells. The seminiferous tubules become separated by Leydig cells (mesoderm).

The cephalic end of the mesonephric duct forms the appendix of the epididymis. The mesonephric duct also forms the duct of the epididymis, the vas deferens and the ejaculatory duct. Where it enters the urogenital sinus the ampulla of the vas deferens forms and a diverticulum from the ampulla forms the seminal vesicles. The caudal tubules of the mesonephros form the paradidymis.

The paramesonephric duct disappears except from the cranial tip which forms the appendix of the testis and the caudal end which forms the utriculus masculinus.

A–C. Development of the testis. View from the ventral surface.

1. anterior abdominal wall
2. bladder
3. buttock
4. leg
5. rectum
6. scrotum
7. testis
8. umbilical arteries
9. umbilical cord

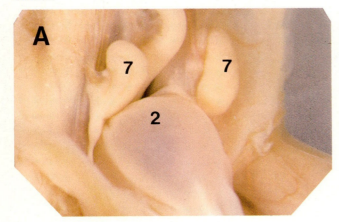

A. Week 11. 65 mmCR (×69)

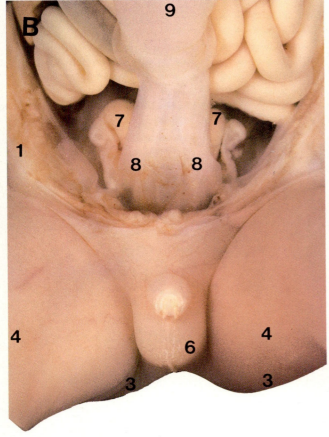

B. Week 13. 97 mmCR (×4.7)

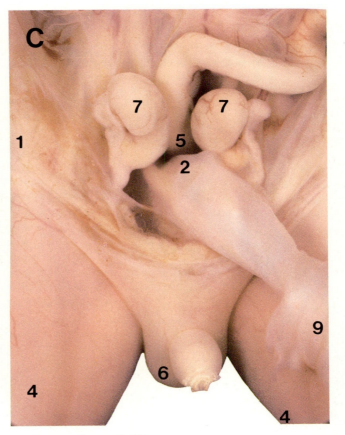

C. The same fetus as in Figure A. The bladder and urachus have been lowered. (×5.6)

Descent of the testis. As the mesonephros degenerates the gubernaculum forms on the lower side of the testis, passes obliquely through the abdominal wall and attaches to the scrotal swelling. The processus vaginalis, a sac of peritoneum carrying layers of the abdominal wall, forms ventral to the gubernaculum. These layers form the walls of the inguinal canal and the coverings of the spermatic cord and testis.

A–C. Descent of the testis into the scrotum

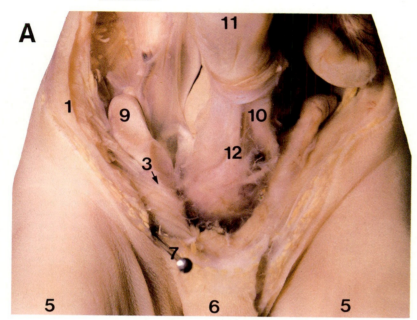

A. Week 18. Testis in the abdominal cavity viewed from the ventral surface. 152 mmCR (×2.4)

By Week 28 the testis, originally on the dorsal abdominal wall, has moved to the deep inguinal ring. The fetal body then elongates whilst the gubernaculum grows at a slower rate so that the testis descends into the scrotum (Week 32).

Prostate gland. The prostate has a dual origin; the glandular epithelium forms from the numerous outgrowths of the prostatic urethral endoderm and the stroma and smooth muscle form from surrounding mesoderm.

Bulbourethral gland. These glands have a dual origin: one part is an endodermal outgrowth of the membranous urethra and another part is stroma and smooth muscle from the surrounding mesoderm.

● Sometimes the testes are undescended at birth but descend into the scrotum during the first three months thereafter.

1. anterior abdominal wall
2. fat
3. inguinal canal
4. intestine
5. leg
6. penis
7. pin
8. scrotum
9. testis
10. umbilical artery
11. umbilical cord
12. urachus

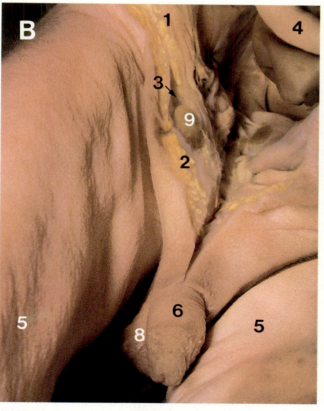

*B and C are in reverse order because B is less mature than C.

B.* Week 24. Testis in the inguinal canal. View from the ventral surface. 228 mmCR (×2.2)

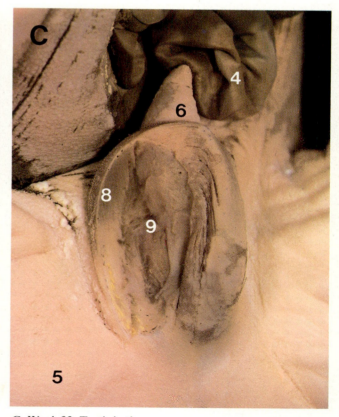

C. Week 23. Testis in the scrotum. View from below. 220 mmCR (×2.1)

165

Female

Ovary. The formation of the early ovary is similar to the testis, though the sex cords become broken up into isolated follicles and the tunica albuginea and rete are poorly developed.

Descent of the ovary. During Week 12 the ovary descends to a point below the pelvic brim. The middle part of the gubernaculum fuses with the body of the uterus dividing the gubernaculum into two parts: the upper part becomes the ovarian ligament and the lower part the round ligament of the uterus. The round ligament passes through the inguinal canal to end in the labium majus. A vaginal process forms but disappears before birth. Estrogen secretion by the fetal ovaries is insignificant.

Uterus and vagina. The fused paramesonephric ducts form the uterovaginal primordium. This forms the epithelium and glands of the body and cervix of the uterus and can be distinguished in Week 10. The cervix is longer than the body. The myometrium and endometrial stroma form from adjacent mesoderm. The unfused parts of the paramesonephric ducts form the uterine (Fallopian) tubes whose open ends develop fimbria. The gubernaculum forms from mesoderm of the inguinal folds.

The uterovaginal region of the fused paramesonephric ducts expands to form the vaginal walls and canalization forms the vaginal lumen. Dilatation of the cephalic end produces the fornices. The caudal end expands and increases the area of contact with the urogenital sinus. The vaginal plate forms from the sinovaginal bulbs and forms the hymen which is placed superficially at birth.

- In the first weeks after birth the uterus is no longer influenced by maternal hormones and involutes markedly.

- After birth, the ovaries assume their adult position on the posterior surface of the broad ligament.

1. bladder
2. kidney
3. ovary
4. rectum
5. round ligament of the uterus
6. suprarenal (adrenal) gland
7. uterine tube
8. uterovaginal primordium

A and B. Week 8. Urogenital organs of a female fetus dissected out. 40 mm CR

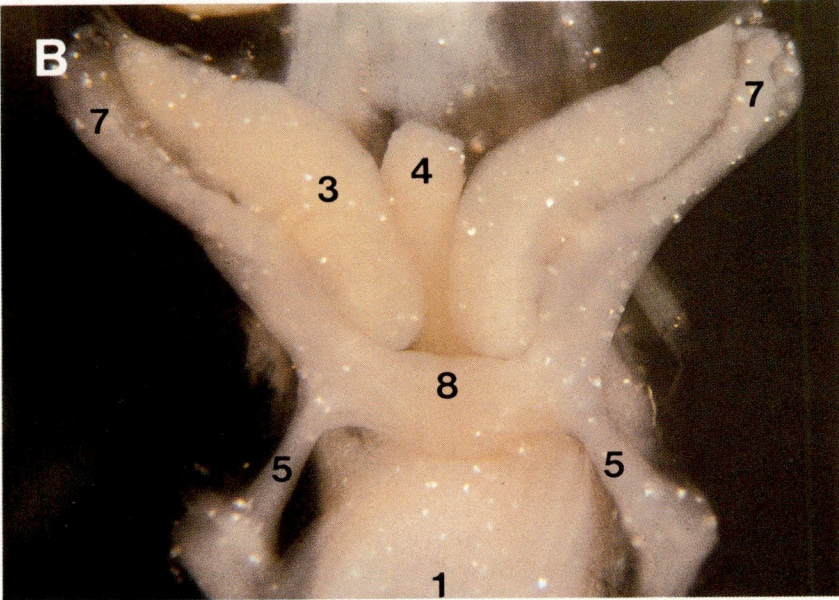

A. View from the ventral side. (×10)

B. Higher magnification of the organs in Figure **A**. (×20.4)

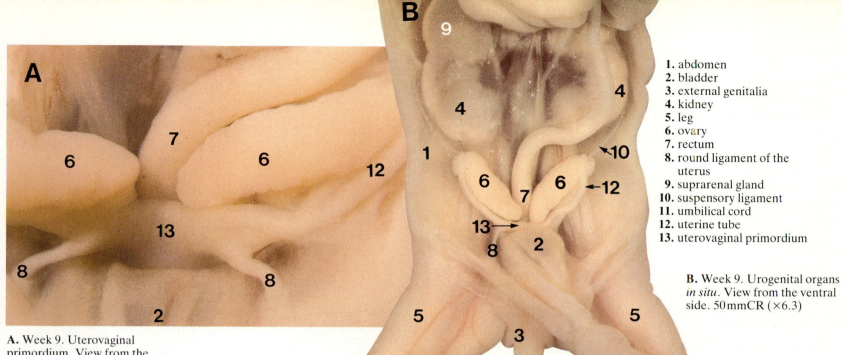

A. Week 9. Uterovaginal primordium. View from the ventral side. 48 mmCR (×20.4)

1. abdomen
2. bladder
3. external genitalia
4. kidney
5. leg
6. ovary
7. rectum
8. round ligament of the uterus
9. suprarenal gland
10. suspensory ligament
11. umbilical cord
12. uterine tube
13. uterovaginal primordium

B. Week 9. Urogenital organs *in situ*. View from the ventral side. 50 mmCR (×6.3)

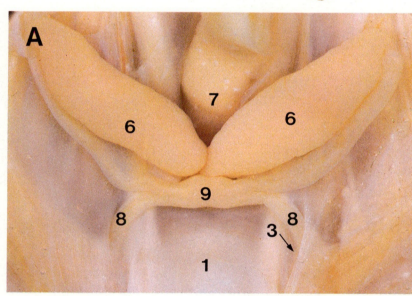

A. 123 mmCR (×7.2)

A and B. Week 15. Course of the round ligament of the uterus viewed from the ventral surface.

1. bladder
2. clitoris
3. vaginal process
4. labia majora
5. leg
6. ovary
7. rectum
8. round ligament of the uterus
9. uterovaginal primordium

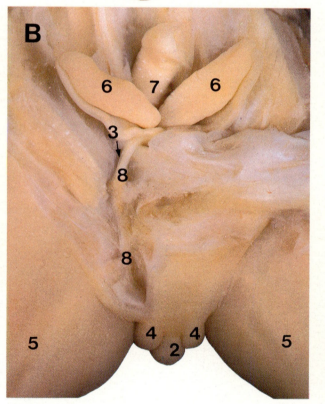

B. Same fetus as in Figure **A**. (×4.3)

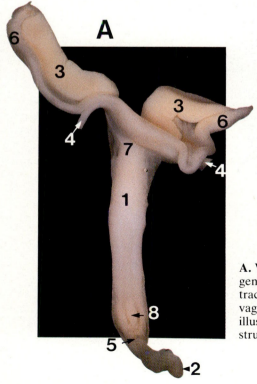

A. Week 13. Female internal genitalia dissected as a single tract. The lower uterus and vagina have been opened to illustrate the internal structure. 101 mmCR (×4.6)

1. body of the uterus
2. clitoris
3. ovary
4. round ligament of the uterus
5. solid epithelial plug where the vagina meets the urogenital sinus
6. uterine tube
7. uterus
8. vagina

Tail Formation

The human tail develops from the posterior body fold or tail fold. It normally reaches a maximum length of one tenth that of the embryo during Week 5 and then disappears during the next 3 or 4 weeks by regression, cell death, and by the rapid increase in size of the buttock region. At term, the coccyx represents the tail remnant.

● Abnormally a tail may be present at birth. It is usually 'soft' and is removed surgically.

1. anus
2. buttocks
3. genitals
4. head
5. heart
6. leg bud
7. liver
8. tail
9. umbilical cord

A-G. Regression and disappearance of the tail.

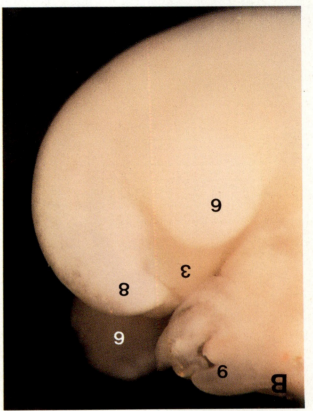

B. Horizon XVIII (Day 36–38). View from the right side. 14mmCR (×20).

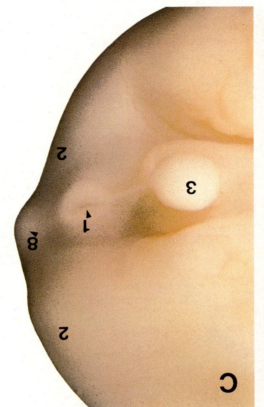

C. Week 10. View from below. 56mmCR ♂ (×11.1).

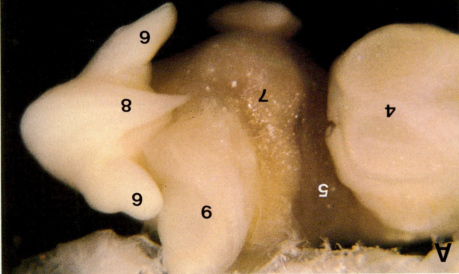

A. Horizon XVII (Day 34–36). View from the ventral surface. 12mmCR (×11.4).

D. Week 10. View from the right side. 57 mmCR ♂ (×11.1)

1. anus
2. buttocks
3. genitals
4. leg
5. tail

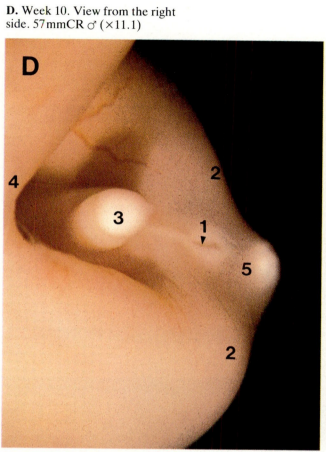

E. Week 10. View from below. 60 mmCR ♀ (×11.1)

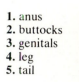

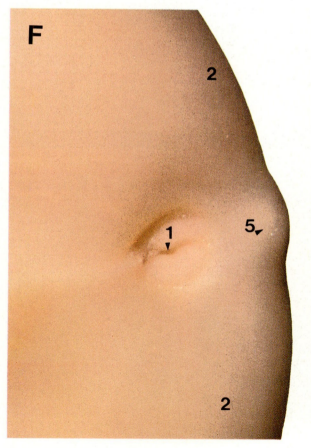

F. Week 12. View from below. 85 mmCR ♂ (×11.1)

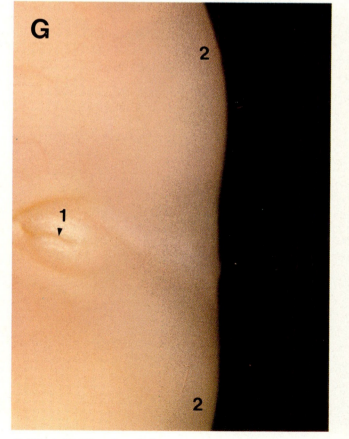

G. Week 13. View from below. 97 mmCR ♂ (×11.1)

Limbs

The upper and lower limbs develop from buds of mesoderm covered by a layer of ectoderm. The upper limb first appears late in Week 4 followed by the lower limb. This cephalo-caudal maturity gradient is retained throughout development.

Arm development and rotation

The upper limb bud projects 90° from the body. The cranial border is called the preaxial border and the caudal border the postaxial. An apical ectodermal ridge influences growth of the limb. As the arm, forearm and hand regions form (Week 5) the hand faces the trunk. At Week 7–9 the elbow is moved 90° dorsally.

Hand and foot development

In Week 6 the upper limb bud develops a plate (paddle) distally which is composed of radial ridges (digits) separated by grooves. In Week 7 the lower limb bud plate has radial ridges. Soon tissue in the radial grooves breaks down and fingers or toes are produced.

Fingernails and toenails

During Week 10 the fingernails appear followed by the toenails. The ectoderm covering the dorsal aspect of the tip of the digit thickens to form a nail field. As the nail field grows it moves onto the dorsal surface, but because of its slow growth rate it becomes depressed with the surrounding epidermis overlapping the proximal and lateral parts of the nail field. The proximal part of the nail field becomes the formative zone whose cells grow over the nail field, keratinize and form the nail.

At first a thin layer of epidermis, the eponychium, covers the developing nail; later this degenerates except for the cuticle.

The nails reach the fingertips by Week 32 and toetips by Week 36.

Nerve supply

Spinal nerves enter the brachial plexus from the cervical enlargement of the spinal cord. The plexus divides into anterior and posterior divisions which supply the flexor compartment and extensor compartment respectively.

● Infants are often born with faces scratched by their fingernails. It may be necessary to clip the nails at birth to prevent damage to the skin and eyes.

1. apical ectodermal ridge
2. arm bud
3. cervical and thoracic spinal nerves
4. postaxial border
5. preaxial border

A-1. Development and rotation of the arm.

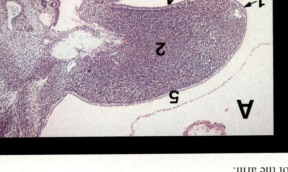

A. Horizons XIV-XV (Day 28-32). Coronal section of the early arm bud. 7mmCR (×75). From L.H.S.M.

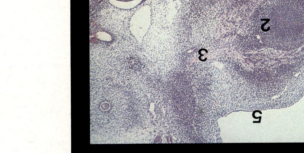

B. Horizon XVI (Day 32-34). Arm bud sectioned coronally. 10mmCR (×75).

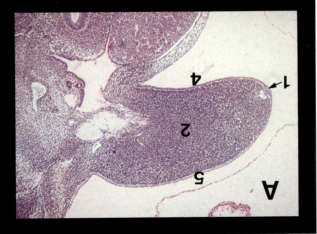

C. Horizon XVIII (Day 36-38). Arm bud. 14mmCR (×8).

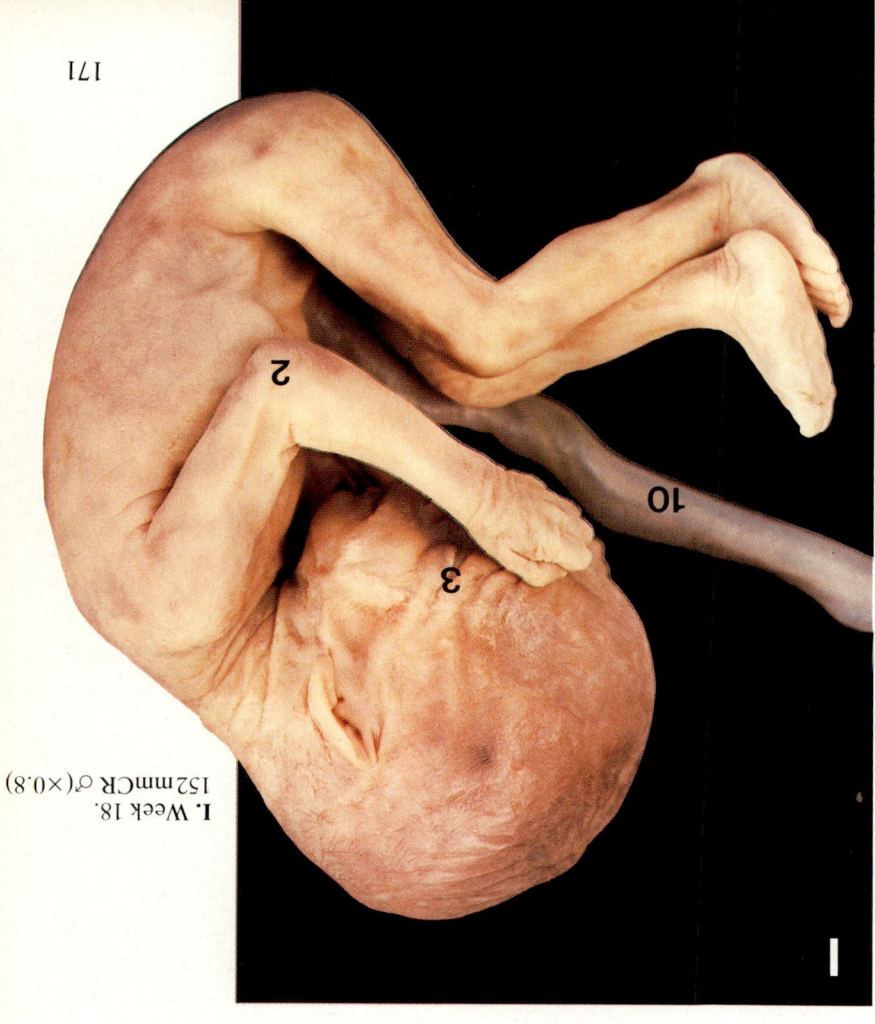

I. Week 18. 152 mmCR ♂ (×0.8)

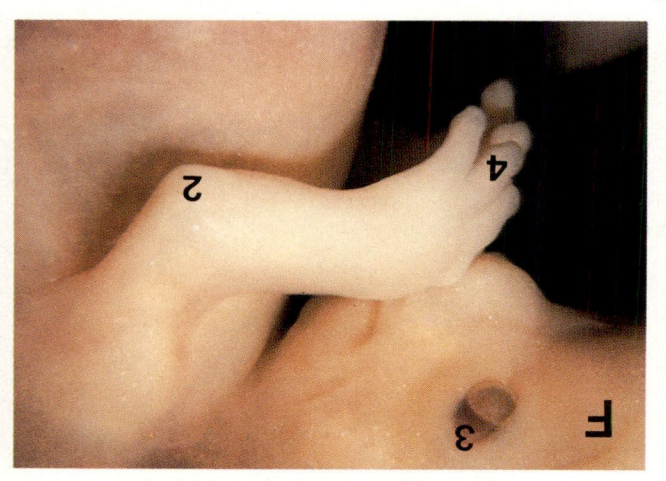

H. Week 13. 97 mmCR ♂ (×1.3)

F. Horizon XXII (Day 44–46). The arm has bent at the elbow which points caudally. The arms move *in utero* from Week 7–8. 27 mmCR (×7.8)

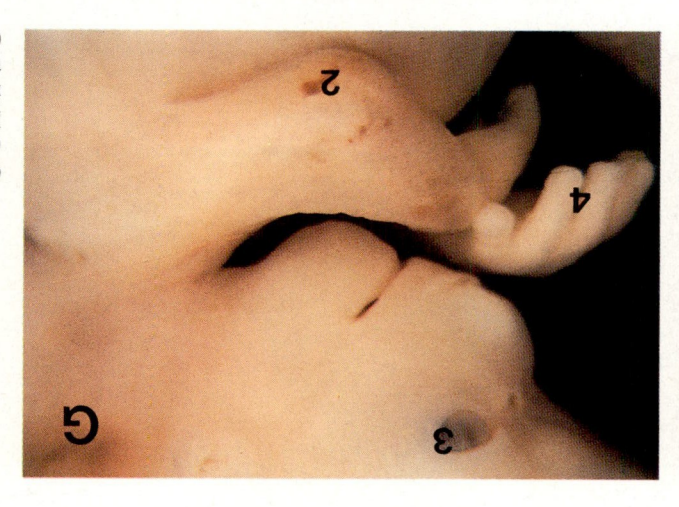

G. Horizon XXII (Day 44–46). The hands meet and cross in the midline over the thorax. 27 mmCR (×7.8)

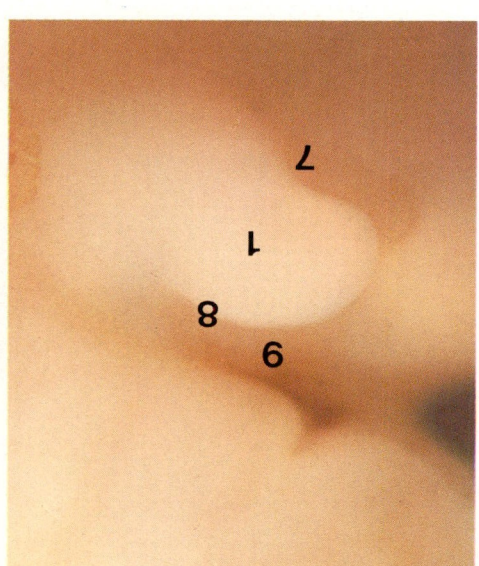

F.

E. Horizon XVII (Day 34–36). The hand paddle is present.* 12 mmCR (×15.6)

*The younger specimen is more mature than the embryo in Figure D.

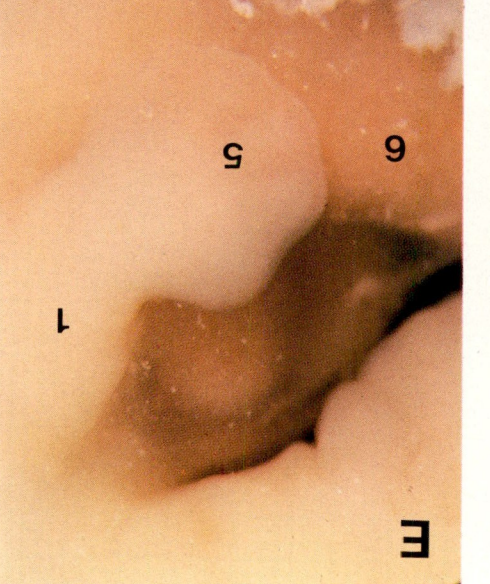

D. Horizon XVIII (Day 36–38). The arm bud has turned medially. 14 mmCR (×15.6)

1. arm bud
2. elbow
3. eye
4. fingers
5. hand paddle
6. liver
7. postaxial border
8. preaxial border
9. thorax
10. umbilical cord

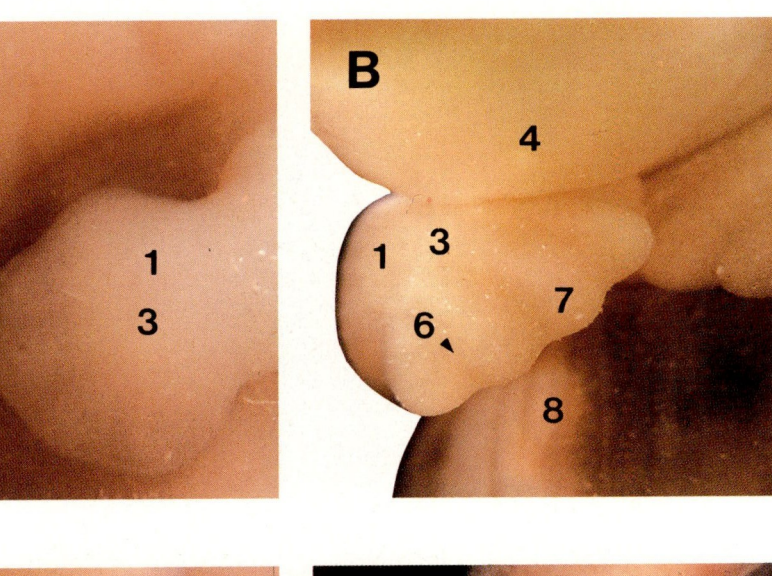

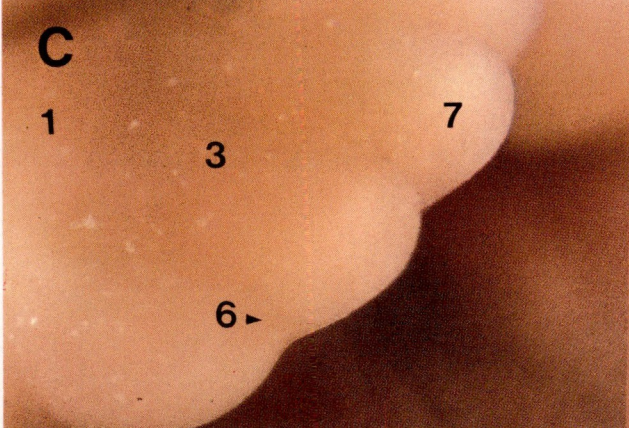

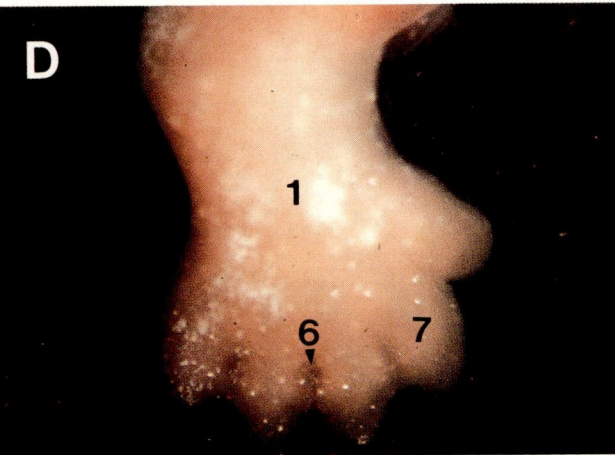

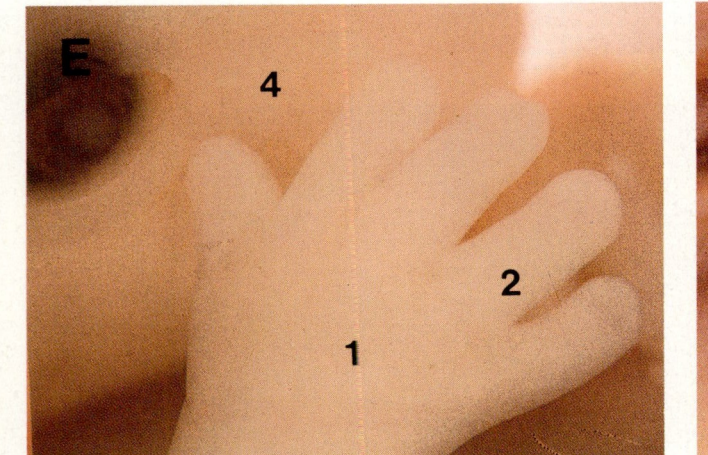

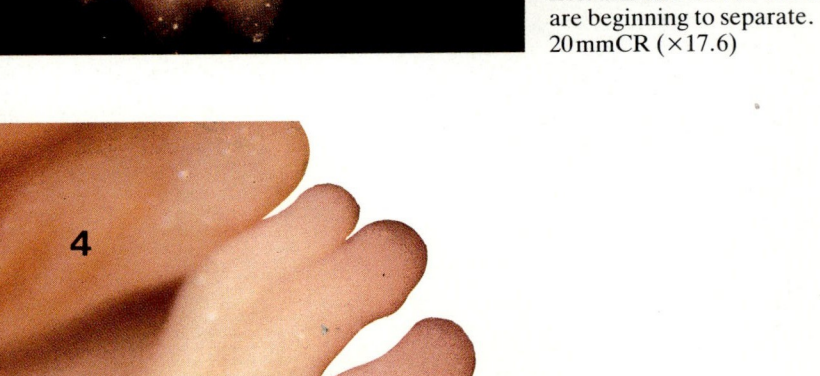

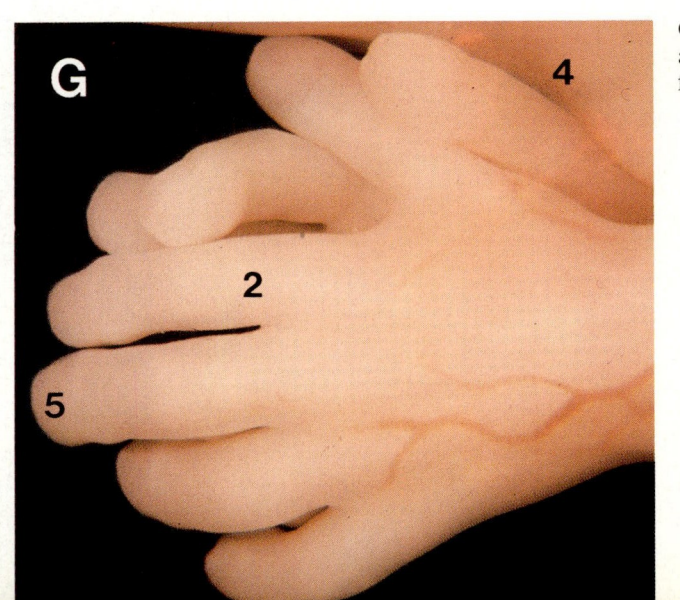

A–G. Hand and finger development.

1. dorsum of hand
2. finger
3. hand paddle (plate)
4. head
5. nail field
6. radial groove (digital groove)
7. radial ridge (digital ridge)
8. thorax

A. Horizon XVII (Day 34–36). Hand paddle viewed from the left side. 12 mmCR (×17.2)

B. Horizon XIX (Day 38–40). Radial ridges and grooves are present. View from the left. 20 mmCR (×17)

C. Higher magnification of Figure **B**. (×36)

D. Horizon XIX (Day 38–40). Left arm and elbow. The fingers are beginning to separate. 20 mmCR (×17.6)

E. Horizon XXII (Day 44–46). Fingers are separated. View from the right. 25 mmCR (×17.1)

F. Horizon XXII (Day 44–46). Fingertips are swollen where the touch pads are developing. 27 mmCR (×17.2)

G. Week 10. The hands are adducted. Fingernail fields are forming. 60 mmCR ♀ (×10.7)

172

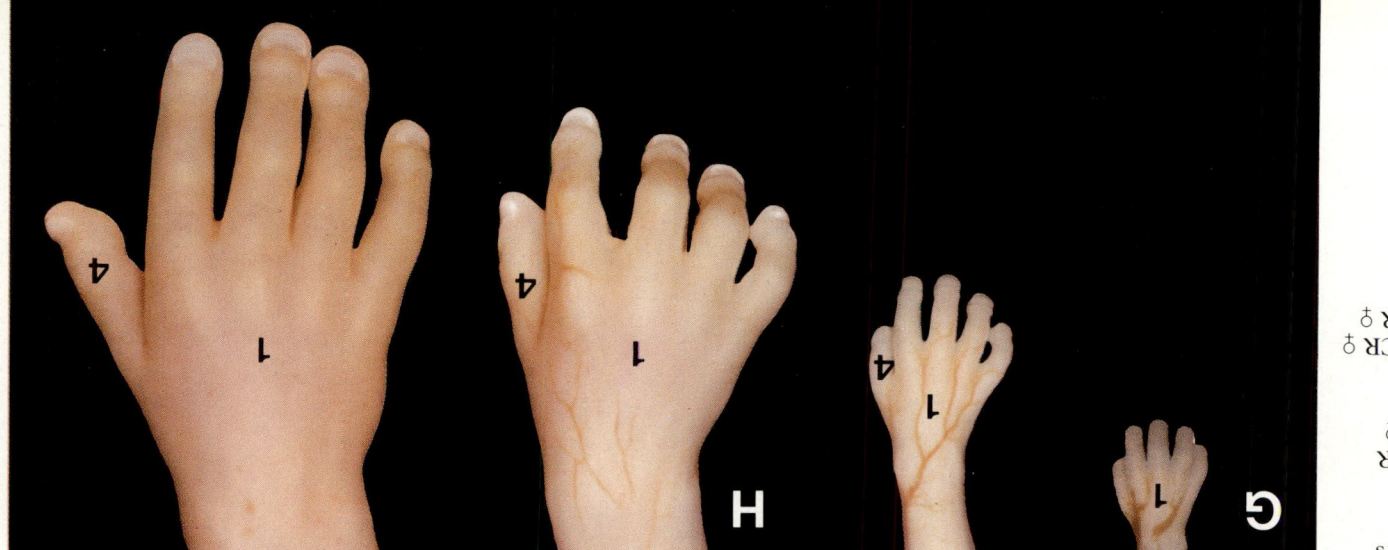

G and H. Developing fingers and nails. (×2.8)

G. Small: Week 8. 34 mmCR
Large: Week 9. 50 mmCR ♀

H. Small: Week 13. 92 mmCR ♀
Large: Week 15. 123 mmCR ♀

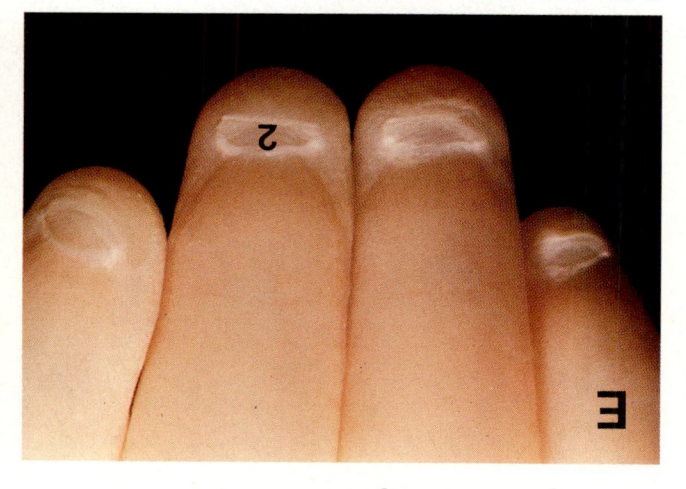

E. Week 15. 130 mmCR ♀ (×7.1)

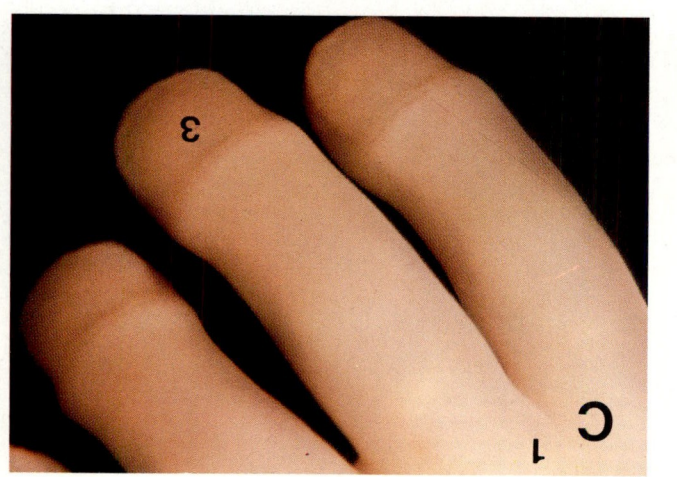

F. Week 23. Index finger. 220 mmCR ♂ (×17)

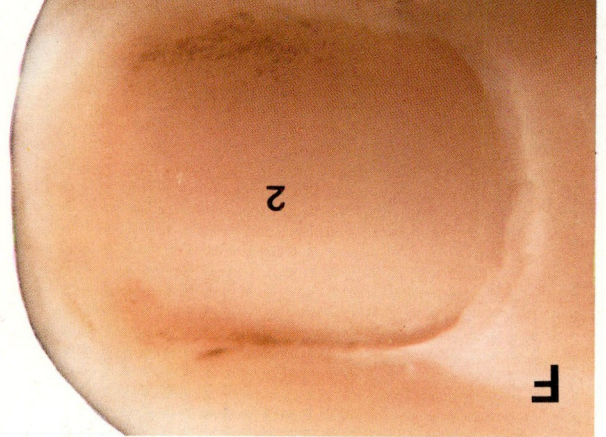

C. Same specimen as in Figure B.

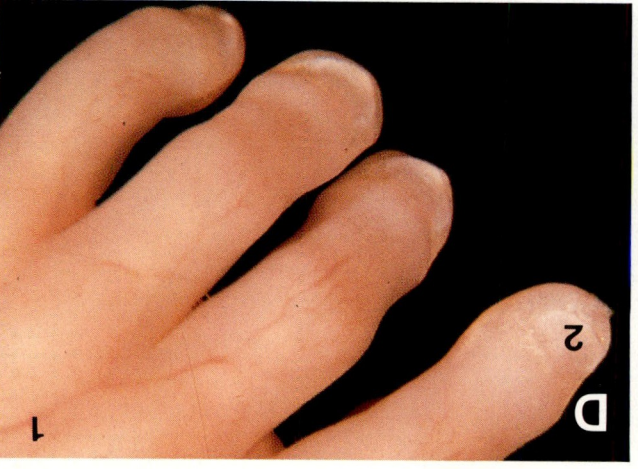

D. Week 13. 97 mmCR ♂ (×8.8)

1. dorsum of hand
2. fingernail
3. nail field
4. thumb

B–F. Development of the fingernails.

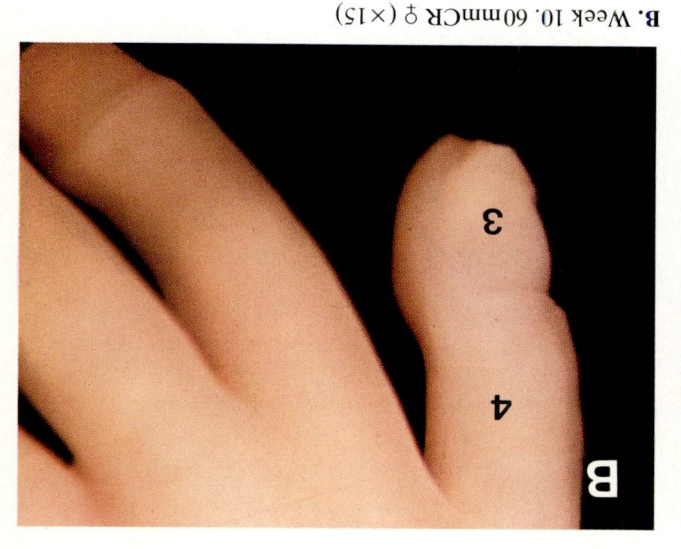

B. Week 10. 60 mmCR ♀ (×15)

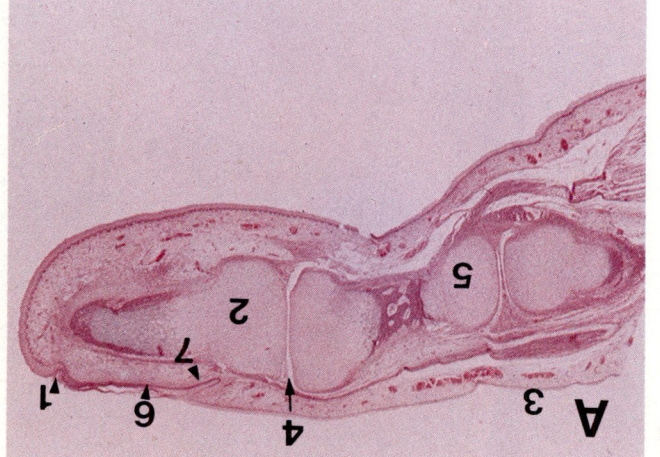

1. boundary furrow in epithelium
2. distal phalanx
3. dorsum of finger
4. joint cavity
5. middle phalanx
6. nail bed
7. nail fold

A. Horizon XXIII (Day 46–48). Longitudinal section of the index finger. 29 mmCR (×26)

Leg development and rotation

The lower limb projects 90° from the body (Week 4). The superior surface is called the preaxial border and the inferior surface the postaxial. As the thigh, leg and foot develop, the foot faces the trunk. The knee then rotates ventrally 90°.

Knee rotation occurs between Week 7 and 9.

At Week 17 epidermal ridges in the skin form on the plantar surface of the soles and toes.

- The neonatal lower limb tends to remain in its fetal position: the limb is flexed and abducted at the hip joint, the knee flexed, and the foot inverted in the talipes varus position.

- A thick plantar fibrous fat pad conceals the transverse and longitudinal arches of the neonatal sole.

- Congenital dislocation of the hip is not uncommon.

- Only during the second year of postnatal development are the leg and arm equal in length, an increase in leg length is a conspicuous feature of further development.

- Reduction of the limbs (phocomelia) or absence of the limbs (amelia) occurs very rarely naturally. Thalidomide can induce these abnormalities.

A–K. Development and rotation of the leg.

1. arm bud
2. genital tubercle
3. head
4. leg bud
5. midgut herniation
6. postaxial border
7. preaxial border
8. tail
9. umbilical cord

A. Horizon XVII (Day 34–36). 12 mm CR (×8)

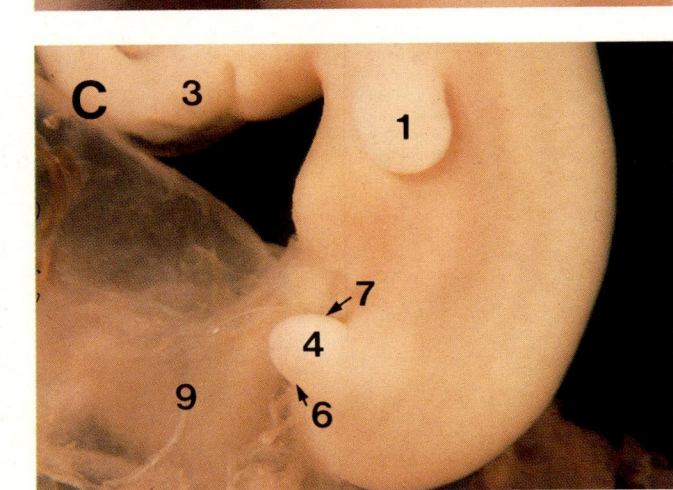

B. Higher magnification of Figure A. (×15.6)

C. Horizon XVIII (Day 36–38). 14 mm CR (×6.1)

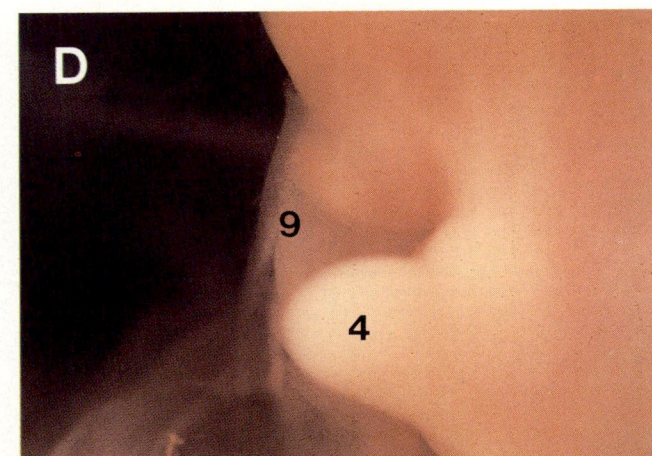

D. Higher magnification of Figure C. (×12)

C and D *from Dr E.C. Blenkinsopp*

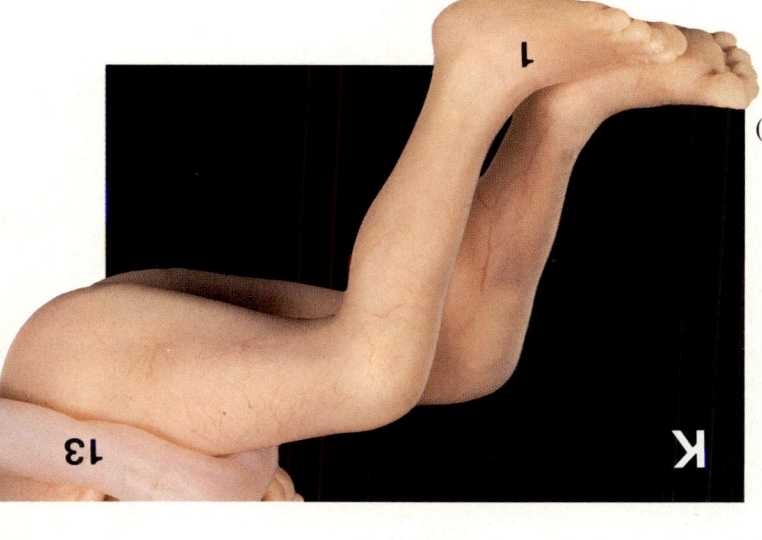

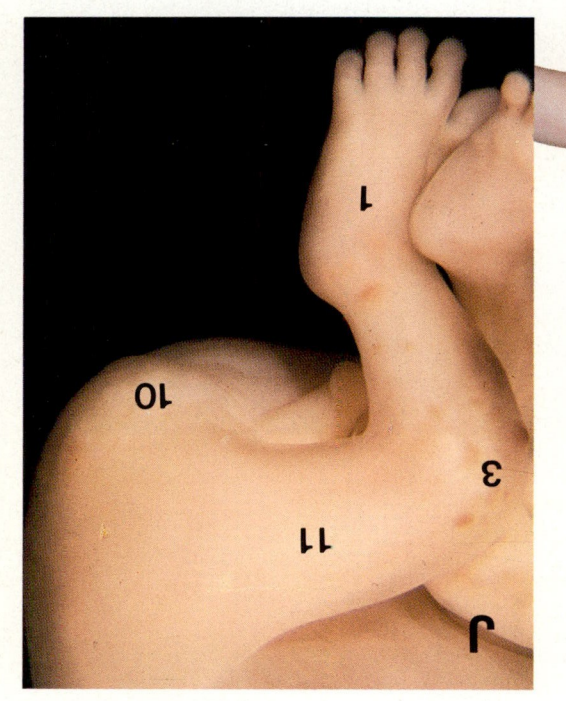

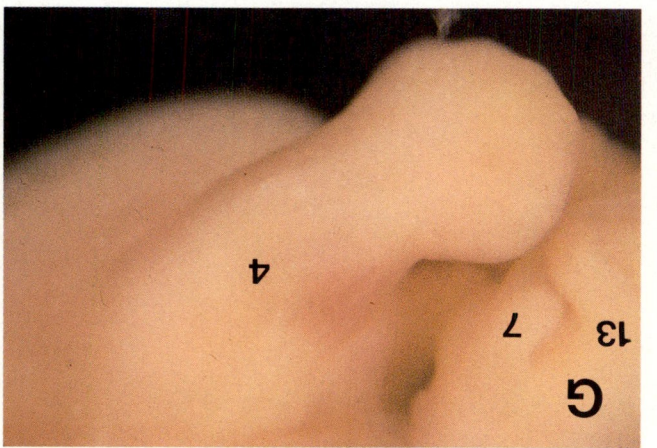

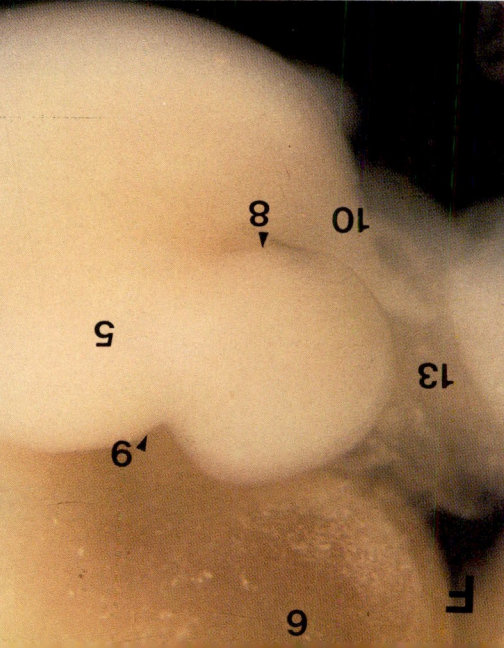

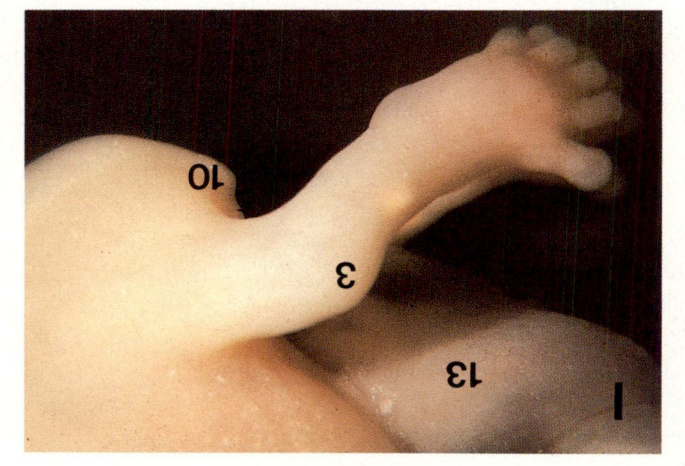

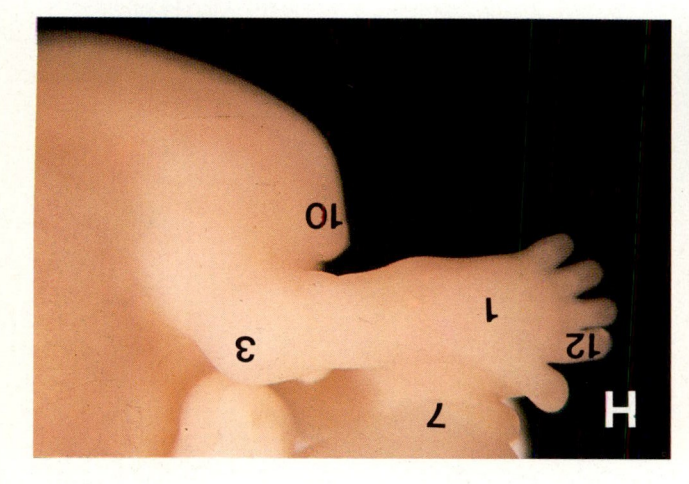

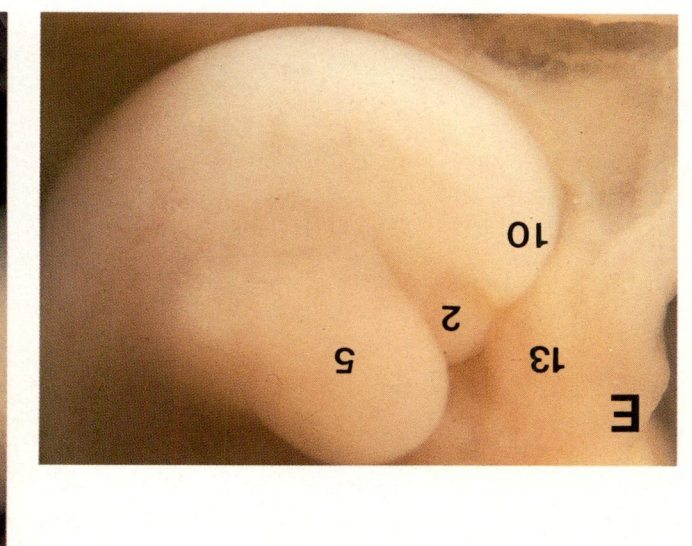

K. Week 13. 97 mmCR ♂ (×1.7)

J. Horizon XXII (Day 44–46). 27 mmCR (×8.9)

I. Horizon XXII (Day 44–46). The knee points cranially. 27 mmCR (×7.8)

H. Horizon XXII (Day 44–46). The soles of the feet face each other. 25 mmCR (×7.8)

G. Horizon XIX (Day 38–40). 20 mmCR (×15.9)

*This specimen is more mature than Figures C–E.

F. Horizon XVII (Day 34–36).* 12 mmCR (×15.8)

E. Horizon XVIII (Day 36–38). 14 mmCR (×15.6)

1. foot
2. genital tubercle
3. knee
4. leg
5. leg bud
6. liver
7. midgut herniation
8. postaxial border
9. preaxial border
10. tail
11. thigh
12. toes
13. umbilical cord

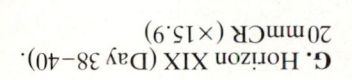

C. Week 24. 228 mmCR ♂ (×2.7)

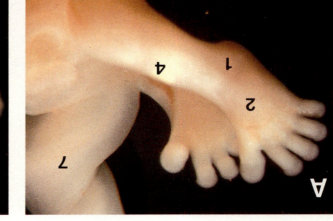

A. Week 8. No nail fields are present. 34 mmCR (×7.8)

B. Week 10. Nail fields are present on the toes. 60 mmCR ♀ (×7.8)

1. ankle
2. dorsum of foot
3. lateral border of foot
4. tibia
5. toe nail
6. toe nail field
7. umbilical cord

A–C. Development of the toenails.

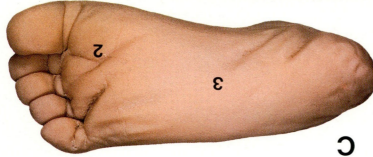

C. Week 23. Epidermal ridges are present on the sole of the foot. The arches are concealed by a fat pad. 220 mmCR ♂ (×1.7)

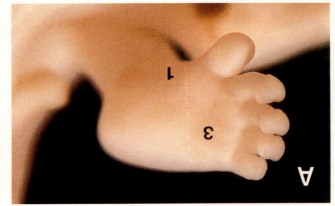

A. Horizon XXII (Day 44–46). The great toe is similar in appearance to the thumb. 27 mmCR (×16.8)

B. Week 9. The great toe has assumed its final position. 50 mmCR ♀ (×7.4)

1. ankle
2. epidermal ridges
3. plantar surface (sole)

A–C. Plantar surface (bottom) of the foot.

From L.H.S.M.

A. Horizon XIV (Day 28–30). Transverse section of the leg bud. 7 mmCR (×72)

B. Horizon XVII (Day 34–36). Note the ectodermal ridge on the leg bud. 12 mmCR (×16.5)

1. apical ectodermal ridge
2. leg bud
3. spinal cord
4. tail

A and B. Early development of the leg and foot.

Bones and Joints

Bones

Bone develops either by intracartilaginous (endochondral) or intramembranous ossification.

Endochondral ossification. Initially the mesoderm forms models of the bones in hyaline cartilage. Mesoderm adjacent to the cartilaginous model condenses to form a perichondrium and then periosteum of two layers: an outer fibrous and inner cellular layer. These cartilaginous models grow principally at the ends by the chondrocytes in the cartilage increasing in size and also by mitosis.

The long bones of the limbs are examples of intracartilaginous ossification. Ossification begins when chondrocytes in the shaft of the bone mature, phosphatase is produced and their matrix calcifies. The chondrocytes then die and their cavities remain. These cavities spread up and down the shaft.

The inner cellular layer of periosteum then ceases to form chondrocytes and forms osteoblasts instead. These osteoblasts invade the cavities in the shaft and, along with blood vessels, establish ossification centers. Osteoblasts positioned on the calcified cartilage deposit bone and ossification spreads up and down the shaft as the chondrocytes die.

The periosteum adds bone to the shaft surface by intramembranous ossification (see below). Bone in the center of the shaft is resorbed and replaced by hemopoietic mesoderm which forms the red marrow. Hemopoiesis begins at about Week 16 in the bone marrow. At Week 10 granulocytes enter the circulation from the bone marrow.

At each extremity of the marrow cavity is a zone of endochondral ossification which advances toward the end of the bone. At the same time cartilage is deposited at the ends of the bone.

At each end of the bone one (or more) ossification centers (epiphyses) form. Ossification continues until two types of areas remain: articular cartilage on the extreme ends of the bones and an epiphyseal disc of cartilage between the diaphyseal and epiphyseal centers.

Growth of the bone continues at this epiphyseal disc until the mature length is reached and the disc becomes bone.

The epiphyseal plate is divided into four regions (from the diaphyseal plate outwards towards the end of the bone): calcified cartilage with degenerating cells (chondrocytes), mature cells in columns, flat proliferating cells and resting cells. As the degenerating cells leave their lacunae they are replaced by osteoblasts which lay bone on the calcified cartilage.

Bones grow in length from the epiphyseal plates and in thickness from the periosteum.

Intramembranous ossification. Mesoderm cells (in flat bones of the skull) differentiate into osteoblasts and form an ossification center. They begin to secrete bone matrix (spicules) and trap the osteoblasts as osteocytes. Osteoblasts surrounding the matrix produce more osteocytes as the bony spicules grow and become more complex. Mesoderm at the periphery of the ossification center forms periosteum. Within the ossification center osteoblasts appear which resorb or destroy bone.

The growth and ultimate shape of a bone are the result of the combination of deposition of osteoblasts and destruction by osteoclasts. For example in the frontal bone new bone is added on to the external surface as older bone is destroyed on the internal surface.

●   Red marrow is present throughout the neonatal skeleton. After 5 years of age the red marrow in long bones is gradually replaced by yellow marrow.

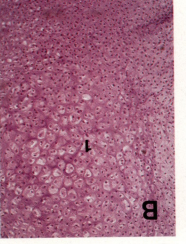

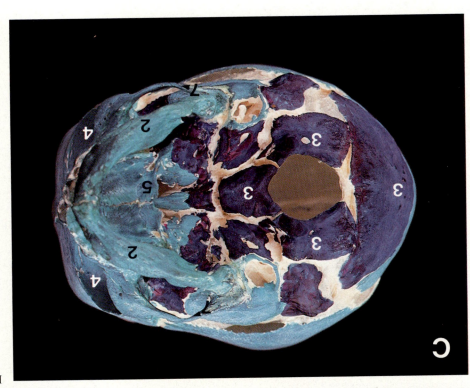

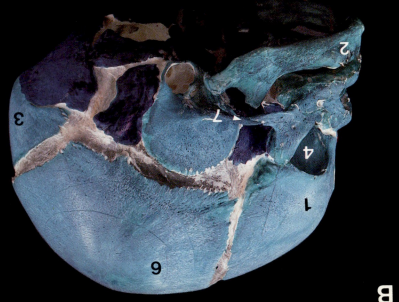

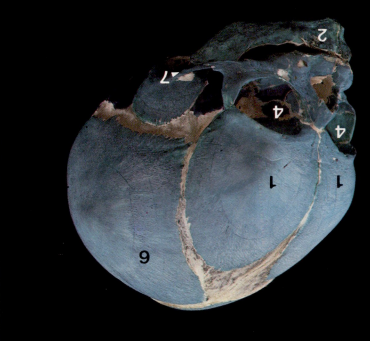

A and B. Week 11.
Developing vertebrae.
29 mmCR

1. cartilage beginning to hypertrophy in centrum
2. intervertebral disc

B. Higher magnification of Figure A. (×130)

A. (×82)

C. Base of the skull. (×1)

A–C. Neonatal skull painted to show intramembranous (turquoise) and cartilagenous (dark blue) origins of the bone.

1. frontal
2. mandible
3. occipital
4. orbit
5. palatine
6. parietal
7. zygomatic arch

A. Frontal and lateral view.
(×0.8)

B. Lateral view. (×1)

Skeleton

In Week 6 mesoderm in each limb condenses to form a skeleton which is continuous and has no joints. A cartilaginous center appears in the mesoderm of each bone and the cells differentiate to become cartilage. A cartilaginous model of each bone is formed while condensed mesoderm surrounding the models forms the perichondrium. The areas between the cartilaginous models are continuous with the perichondrium and will form the joints.

The perichondrium near the center of the shaft of a bone differentiates into a periosteum of two layers. The inner osteogenic layer contains osteoblasts which lay down bone matrix and fibers on the shaft. Calcium salts from the blood are then deposited and bone tissue is formed as a cylinder around the cartilaginous model.

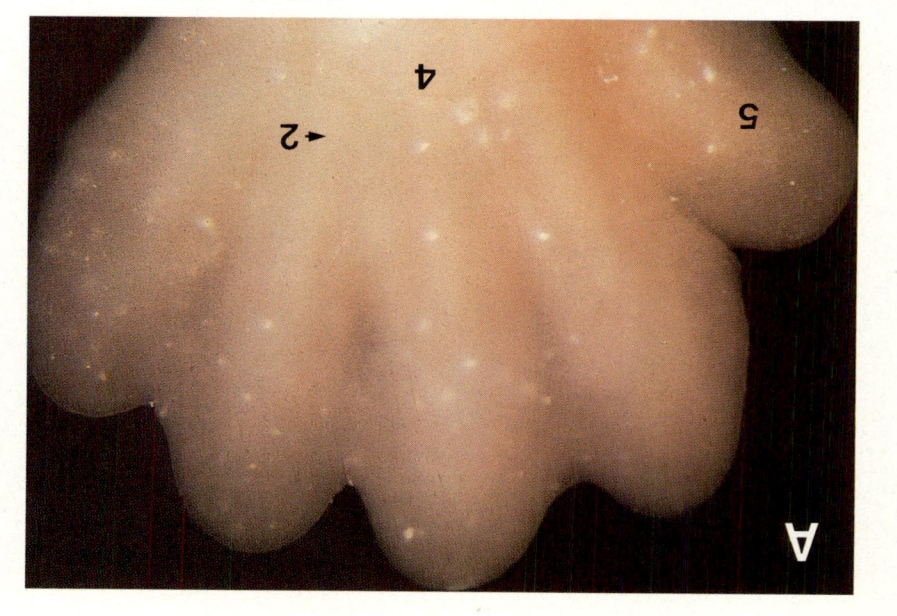

A. Horizon XIX (Day 38–40). 20mmCR (×41.8)

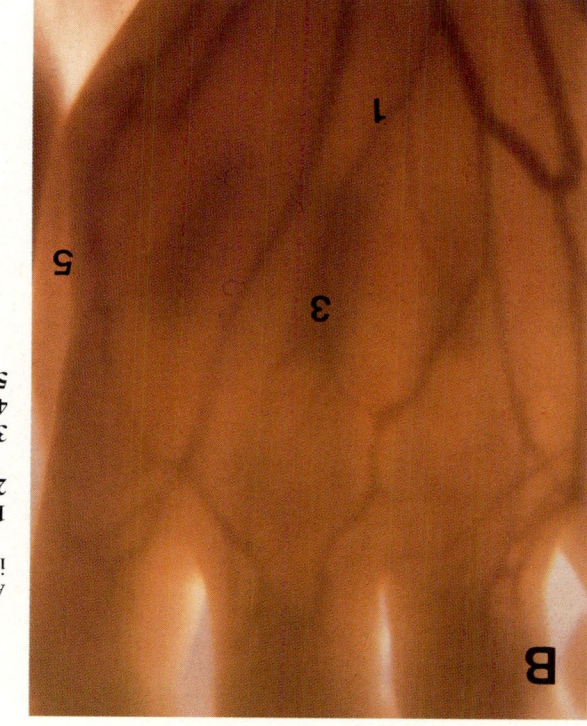

B

A and B. Developing skeleton in the hand.

1. dorsum of hand
2. mesodermal metacarpal primordia
3. metacarpals
4. palm of hand
5. thumb

A–C. Developing skeleton in the leg.

1. genital tubercle
2. greater saphenous vein
3. knee
4. leg bud
5. mesodermal metatarsal primordia
6. tibia

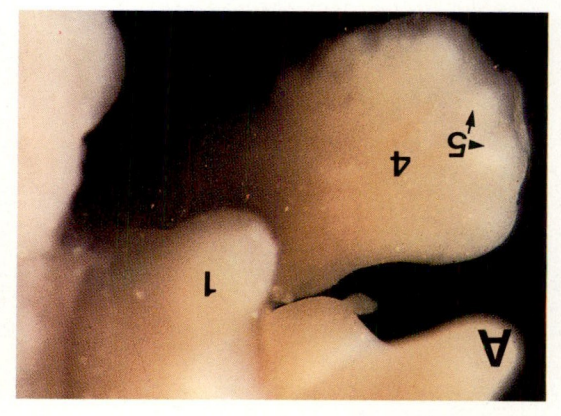

A. Horizon XIX (Day 38–40). 20mmCR (×15.9)

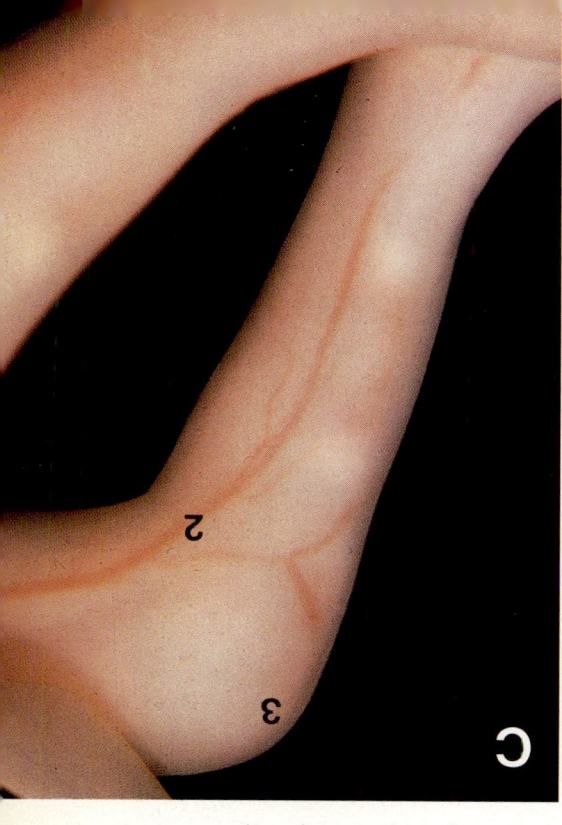

B. Week 13. 95mmCR (×10)

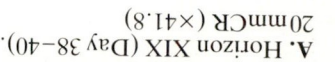

B. Week 8. 35mmCR (×10)

C. Week 9. 48mmCR ♀ (×9.7)

Joints

Synovial joints. Mesoderm surrounding the joint area condenses to form a capsule which is continuous with the shaft perichondrium and ligaments. Each bone end in the joint is covered by a layer of dense mesoderm which will form the articular cartilages and synovial membranes. Within the joint capsule fluid spaces appear in the loose mesoderm. These join to form the joint cavity.

Fibrocartilaginous joints. The mesoderm in the joint differentiates to form fibrocartilage (e.g. the symphysis pubis) or hyaline cartilage (e.g. the neurocentral joint).

Fibrous joints. The mesoderm in the joint differentiates to form dense fibrous connective tissue (e.g. the frontal or metopic suture of the skull).

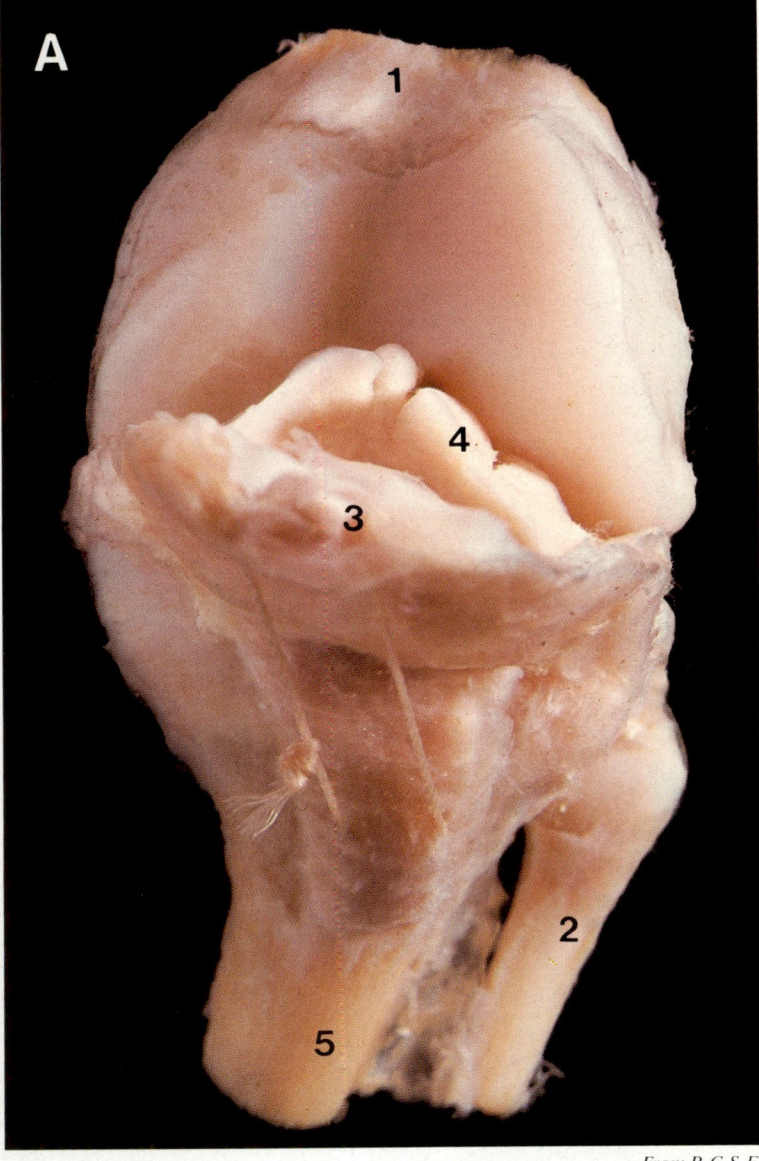

From R.C.S.E.

A. Left knee of a full-term fetus dissected and viewed from the front. The femur has been removed and the patella is reflected forward. (×3.3)

1. femur
2. fibula
3. patella
4. synovial folds
5. tibia

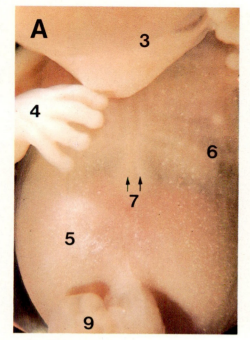

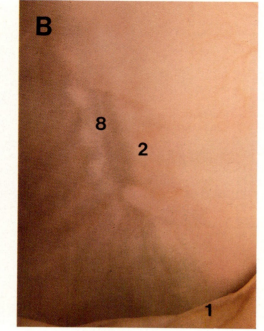

Sternum

Mesodermal condensations form two widely separated sternal bars in the thorax. During Week 9 the two sternal bars which are approximately parallel in the midline fuse to one another cephalo-caudally to form cartilaginous models of the manubrium, body and xiphoid process. These bars are connected to the ends of the costal cartilages.

Centers of ossification appear cephalo-caudally during Week 20 to 25 except in the xiphoid process.

- In the neonate the manubrium usually contains one main center of ossification, the upper segments of the body usually contain one main center and the lower segments paired centers. Ossification of the lowest segments begins shortly after birth and the xiphoid process during the third year of life.

- If fusion is incomplete a minor fissure or perforation may be present in the sternum.

A. Horizon XXII (Day 44–46). The two sternal bars. 27 mmCR (×7.6)

B. Week 10. 57 mmCR ♂ (×8.4)

A and B. Early sternum. View of the ventral surface.

1. arm
2. costal cartilages
3. face
4. hand
5. liver bulge
6. rib
7. sternal bars
8. sternum
9. umbilical cord

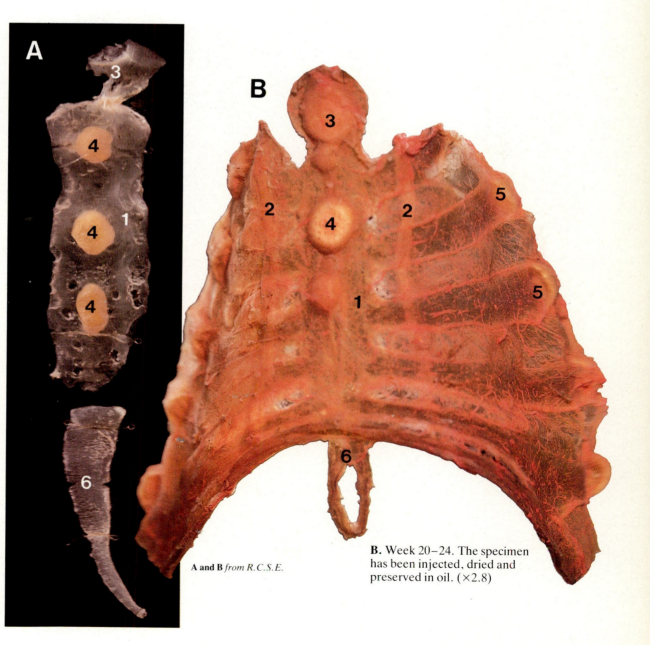

A and B. Centers of ossification in the sternum.

1. body of sternum
2. internal thoracic artery
3. manubrium sterni
4. ossification centers
5. rib
6. xiphoid process

A. Week 20–24. Four centers of ossification are present: one in the manubrium (removed) and three in the body. (×5)

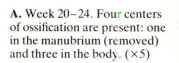

A and B *from R.C.S.E.*

B. Week 20–24. The specimen has been injected, dried and preserved in oil. (×2.8)

181

Ribs

The mesoderm models of the ribs form from the costal processes of the thoracic vertebrae. They become cartilagenous and during Week 13 and 14 a primary ossification center appears in the body of the rib.

- In the neonate the ribs are more horizontal and less curved than in the adult.

- Breathing in the neonate is primarily due to the musculature of the diaphragm and the abdominal wall.

- At puberty secondary centers of ossification appear for the head and tubercle of the rib.

A–E. Developing ribs.

1. arm bud and hand paddle
2. cactus needle and reflected skin
3. ear
4. elbow
5. eye
6. forebrain
7. hand
8. heart bulge
9. hindbrain
10. leg
11. leg bud
12. liver bulge
13. midgut herniation
14. precartilagenous rib
15. rib
16. umbilical cord

A. Horizon XVII (Day 34–36). Ribs are not present on the ventral surface at this stage. 12 mmCR (×8.6)

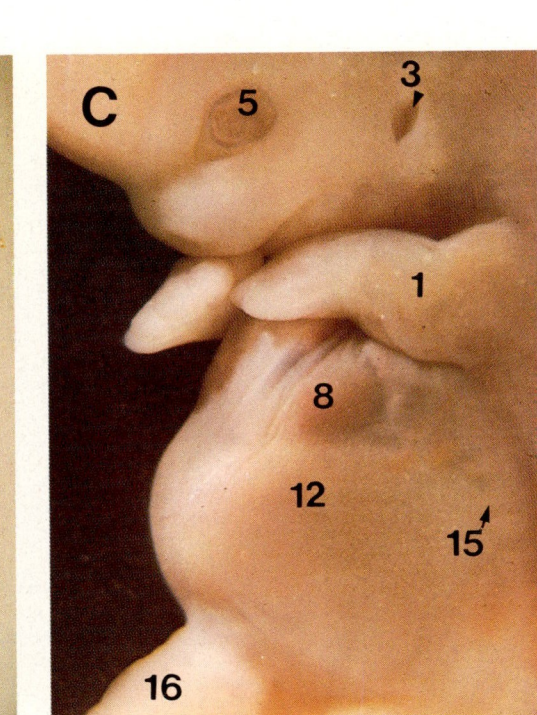

B. Horizon XVIII (Day 36–38). Precartilagenous ribs are present 14 mmCR (×17.1)

C. Horizon XIX (Day 38–40). The ribs have grown partly around the body wall. 20 mmCR (×8.6)

D. Horizon XXII (Day 44–46). 27 mmCR (×8.9)

E. Horizon XXII (Day 44–46). 27 mmCR (×8.6)

A. Week 8. Inner aspect of the ribs and costal cartilages. 40 mmCR ♀ (×8.6)

1. costal cartilages
2. rib
3. ventricle of heart

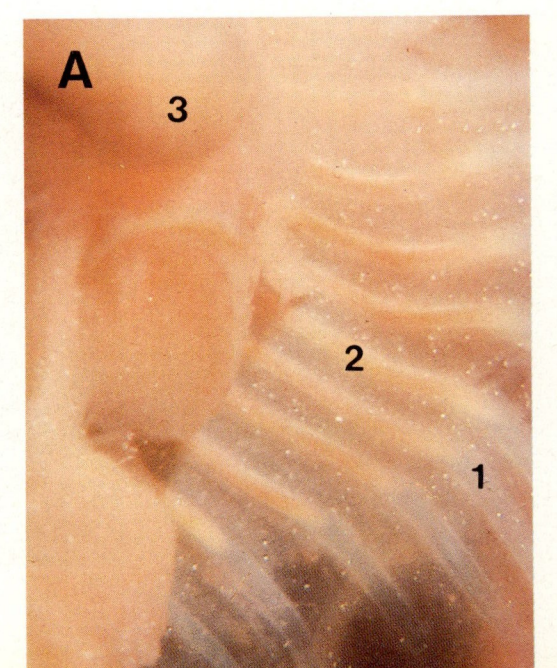

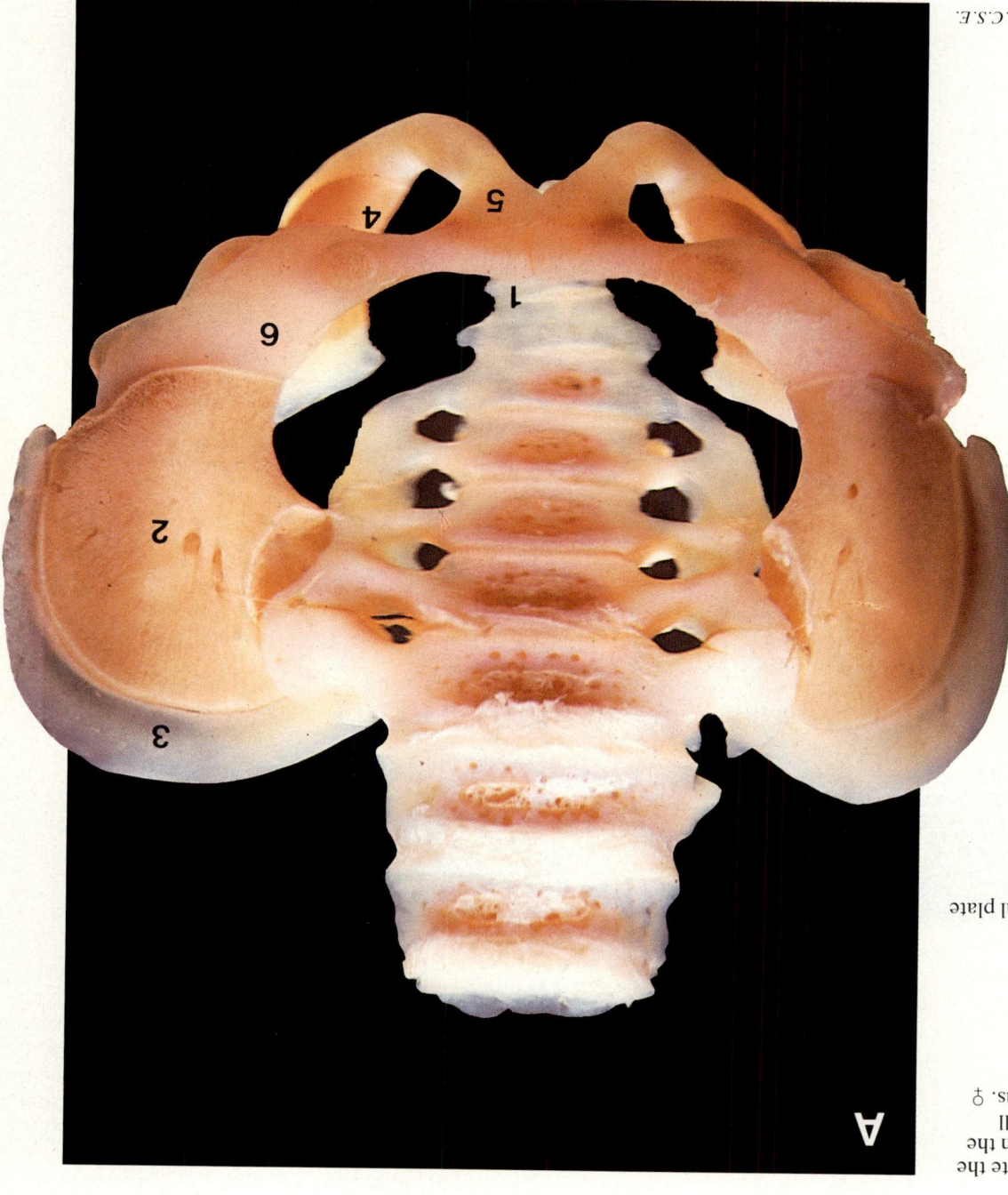

From R.C.S.E.

A. Full-term pelvis. Note the radiating ossific fibers in the ilium. The coccyx is still completely cartilaginous. ♀ (×2.1)

1. coccyx
2. ilium
3. iliac crest
4. ischium
5. pubis
6. 'Y' shaped epiphyseal plate

Pelvis

The neonatal pelvis is more vertical than in the adult and does not exhibit any sexual differences.
At birth the majority of the body of the ileum, the ramus of the ischium and the superior ramus of the pubis are ossified. They are separated by a 'Y' shaped cartilage forming the bulk of the acetabulum. The head of the femur is normally larger than the acetabulum and extends beyond its margins.

● When the infant walks (second year) the sacrum descends between the ilia.

183

Skull and arch derivatives

The skull consists of the neurocranium which protects the brain and the skeleton of the jaws. The basal part of skull is cartilaginous, i.e. the occipital bone, body of the sphenoid, lesser wings of the sphenoid, body of the ethmoid, otic capsules, nasal capsules and the petrous and mastoid parts of the temporals.

The flat bones of the skull are membranous, i.e. the frontals and parietals, the squamous parts of the temporals and occipitals, and the nasal and the lacrimal bones.

The skeleton of the jaws (or viscerocranium) is also formed by cartilaginous and membranous ossification. The cartilaginous parts form from the first and second branchial arches by mesoderm condensing to form a rod of cartilage. Some of the cartilage or its perichondrium is retained to form adult structures but most is later replaced by membranous bone.

The membranous parts of the viscerocranium include the maxillary process of the first branchial arch which forms the maxilla, the zygomatic and squamous parts of the temporal, the vomer and the palatine bone. The mandible forms around the ventral end of the first arch cartilage (Meckel's cartilage). Some cartilaginous ossification occurs at the mandibular condyle and the center of the chin.

As the brain grows the flat bones of the skull grow to accommodate it by the deposition of new bone on the external surface and the destruction of old bone on the internal surface.

In arches three to six cartilage bars only form at the ventral end of the arch. The dorsal end of arch one cartilage (Meckel's cartilage) forms the malleus and incus; dorsal end arch two cartilage (Reichert's cartilage) forms the stapes, styloid process; and the ventral end arch two cartilage forms the lesser cornu and upper body of the hyoid bone. Arch three cartilage (ventral end) forms the greater cornu and lower body of the hyoid. Arches four and six fuse to form the laryngeal cartilages with the exception of the epiglottis (from the hypobranchial eminence arches three and four).

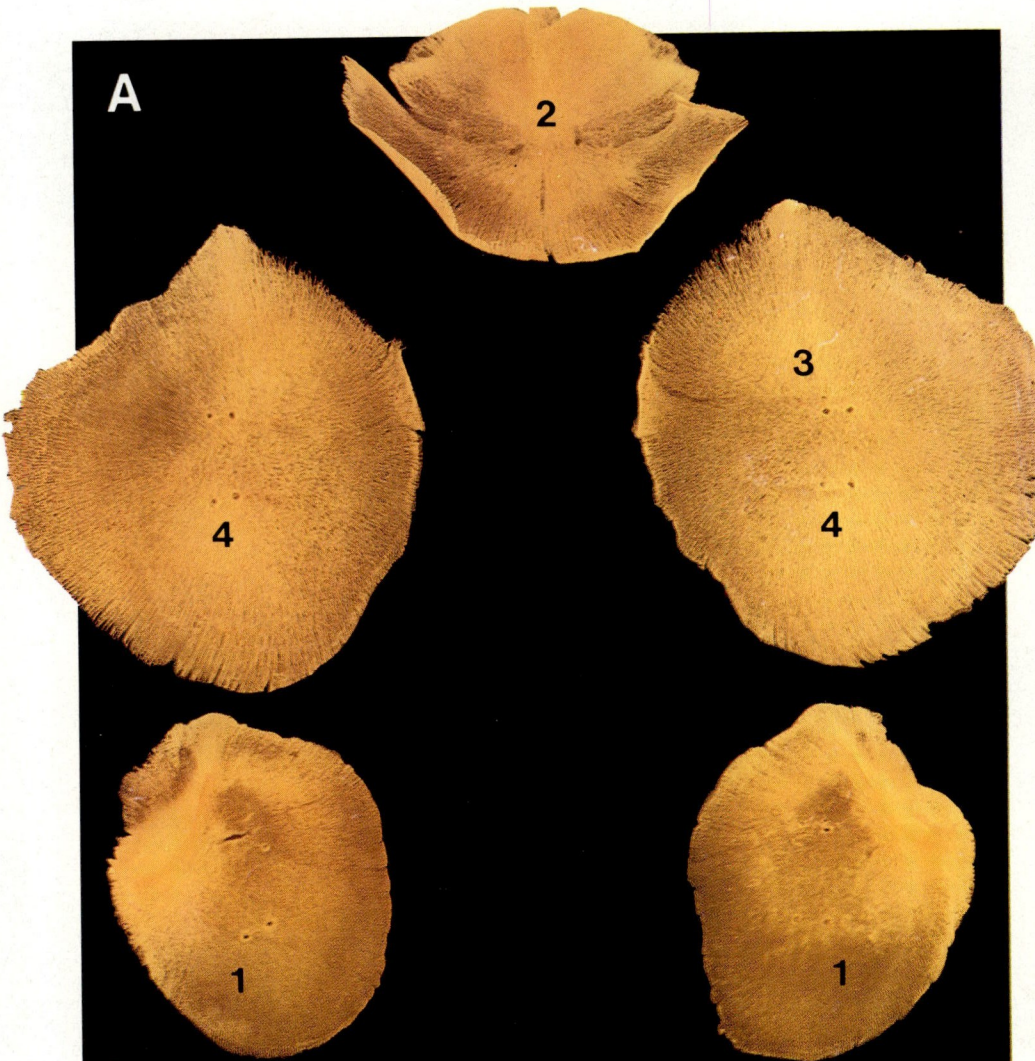

A. Week 20–24. Separated vault bones (inner aspect). Note the ossific fibers radiating from the ossification centers. (×1.2)

1. frontal
2. occipital
3. ossification center
4. parietal

From R.C.S.E.

Neonatal skull

The neonatal face is approximately one eighth of the total cranium. This will change in the adult to approximately one half. The small face in the neonate is due to the lack of erupted teeth and the small size of the nasal cavity and the maxillary sinuses.

The flat bones of the skull are separated by fibrous membranes along their sutures. Expansions in the sutures are called fontanelles. There are normally six fontanelles present at birth. The diamond-shaped anterior fontanelle is approximately 25 mm in diameter and the skin overlying it pulsates. This fontanelle is obliterated by the progressive ingrowing of the borders of the membranous bone. This process begins about 3 months after birth and the fontanelle is usually obliterated by the second year. The posterior fontanelle, two sphenoidal and two mastoidal fontanelles are obliterated between 6 months and 2 years after birth. Numerous accessory fontanelles may also be present. Palpation of the fontanelles allows clinical evaluation of hydration, intracranial pressure and bone growth.

Most of the bones of the skull are ossified at birth, but move relative to one another at the sutures because the bones are soft and loosely connected. This mobility is particularly important in childbirth since it allows the bones to overlap. The parietals overlap the frontals, though the frontals do not overlap each other as they are fixed at the root of the nose. The parietals also overlap the occipitals, and one parietal is driven under the other (see Childbirth).

The mastoid process does not develop until the second year and the facial nerve is relatively exposed and unprotected as it emerges from the stylomastoid foramen. In a difficult delivery forceps may damage the nerve.

- The neonate lacks superciliary arches.

- The skull continues to grow rapidly in the first 2 years after birth. New bone is added at the edges of the bones.

Mandible. The neonatal mandible is composed of two halves united by a midline suture (symphysis menti). The two halves fuse by the beginning of the second year.

The angle of the rami is broad (140°) and the mandibular notch is shallow.

Ten large alveolar fossae each containing a deciduous tooth are present.

- In the young adult the angle of the ramus is 120° or less, while in the elderly the angle becomes broader again due to resorption of bone.

Maxilla. The neonatal maxilla is low in height and its increase vertically in the child is due to an increase in the maxillary sinus and alveolar portion.

At birth the infraorbital foramina are large and the alveolar portion contains ten large alveoli with deciduous teeth.

Occipital bone. The occipital bone at birth is composed of four parts separated by cartilage: a squamous part, two lateral parts and a basilar part. All the parts are usually fused by the fourth year.

Sphenoid. The neonatal sphenoid is composed of three parts: a single middle portion and two lateral parts each consisting of part of the greater wing and the medial pterygoid plate which unite during the first year. The sphenoidal sinuses invade the sphenoid at 5 years of age.

Temporal bone. The newborn temporal bones are in three parts: squamous, petrous and tympanic. The mastoid process is absent and the styloid process is largely cartilaginous.

The tympanic part of the bone is an incomplete bony ring.

- The petrosquamous fissure separating the petrous and squamous temporal bone is a potential pathway for infection into the mastoid antrum of the middle ear.

Frontal bone. The two frontal bones fuse by 6 to 8 years and their suture is rarely present in the adult. The frontal sinuses are absent at birth and invade the bones at about 2 years of age.

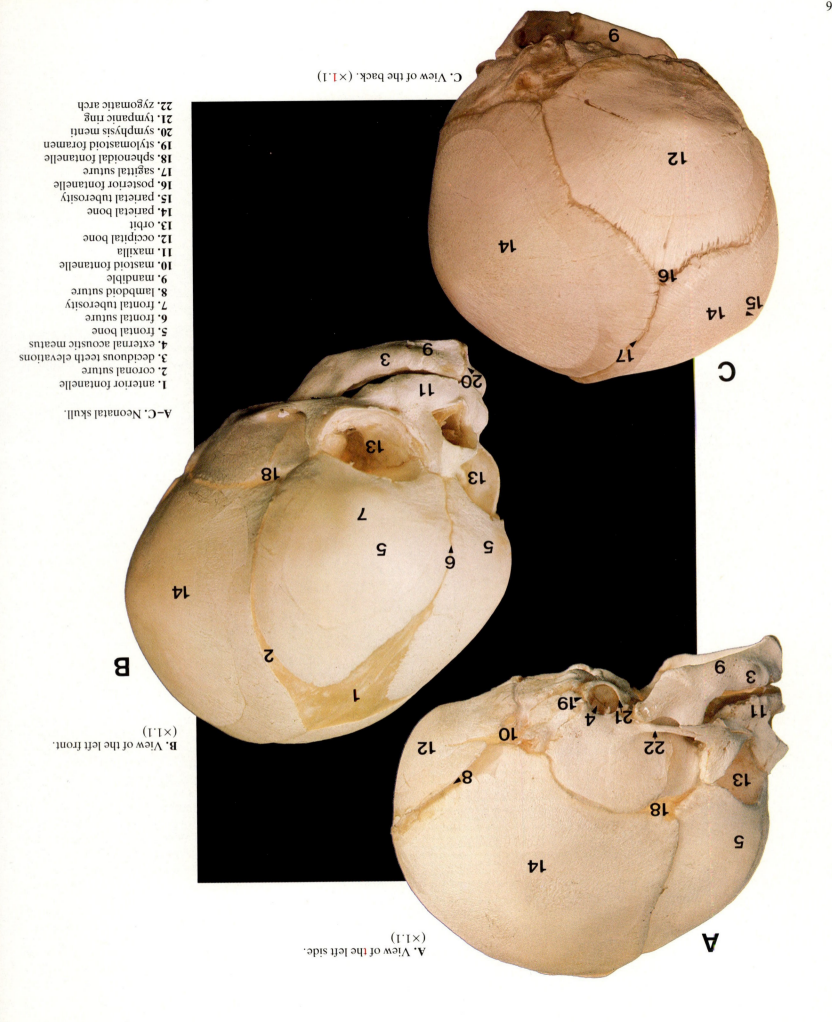

C. View of the back. (×1.1)

A–C. Neonatal skull.

1. anterior fontanelle
2. coronal suture
3. deciduous teeth elevations
4. external acoustic meatus
5. frontal bone
6. frontal suture
7. frontal tuberosity
8. lambdoid suture
9. mandible
10. mastoid fontanelle
11. maxilla
12. occipital bone
13. orbit
14. parietal bone
15. parietal tuberosity
16. posterior fontanelle
17. sagittal suture
18. sphenoidal fontanelle
19. stylomastoid foramen
20. symphysis menti
21. tympanic ring
22. zygomatic arch

B. View of the left front. (×1.1)

A. View of the left side. (×1.1)

Vertebral column

During Week 4 sclerotome cells from the somites surround the (1) ventromedial aspect of the notochord to form the centrum and intervertebral disc, (2) dorsal to the neural tube and (3) ventrolateral aspect of the body wall to form the costal processes. In the thorax these form ribs. Those cells ventromedial to the notochord arrange themselves in alternating bands of loose and densely packed cells. The centrum of a vertebra is formed when a region of packed cells fuses with a region of loose cells immediately caudal which has arisen from an adjacent sclerotome. Some densely packed cells from each region also migrate cranially opposite the myotome to form the intervertebral disc. The intersegmental nerves lie close to the discs, while the arteries lie close to the bodies.

The notochord persists as the nucleus pulposus of the intervertebral disc but disappears in the vertebral body.

Chondrification begins in Week 6. Ossification begins before birth and ends during the 25th year. At birth three primary centers are present: in the centrum and in each half of the vertebral arch.

- During the first year the two halves of the vertebral arch fuse.

- Joints between the arch and centrum allow the spinal cord to enlarge. When the arch fuses with the centrum between 3 and 6 years of age these joints disappear.

- The thoracic vertebral column gradually develops a relatively fixed curve after birth.

- The cervical curve appears when the infant begins to lift its head.

- The lumbar curve appears at the end of the first year when the infant begins to walk.

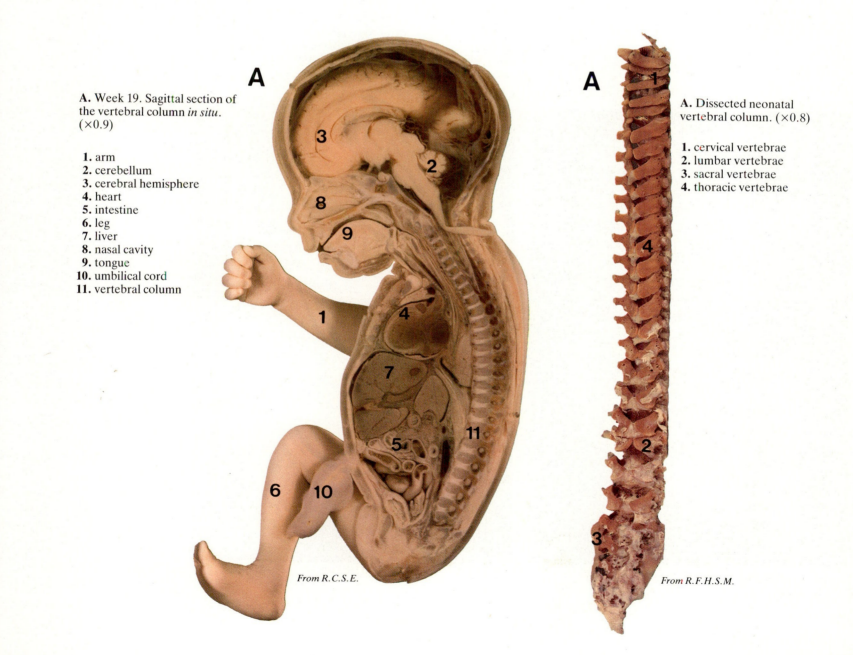

A. Week 19. Sagittal section of the vertebral column *in situ*. (×0.9)

1. arm
2. cerebellum
3. cerebral hemisphere
4. heart
5. intestine
6. leg
7. liver
8. nasal cavity
9. tongue
10. umbilical cord
11. vertebral column

From R.C.S.E.

A. Dissected neonatal vertebral column. (×0.8)

1. cervical vertebrae
2. lumbar vertebrae
3. sacral vertebrae
4. thoracic vertebrae

From R.F.H.S.M.

Developmental series (alizarin red stain)

The cartilaginous or membranous skeleton is ossified when discrete centers of ossification appear. The first center occurs in the clavicle at Week 6, in the jaws and palate at Week 7, and in the frontal bone at Week 8 to 9.

The skeleton of embryos and fetuses can be stained with alizarin red and the other body tissues cleared. Such preparations show the ossification centers and demonstrate the progress of ossification in the body.

- In the female the centers of ossification appear before those in the male and complete their ossification first.

- At birth all bones in the skeleton have red marrow (centers of hemopoiesis). In the adult hemopoiesis is limited to the red marrow of cancellous bone, i.e. the ribs, sternum, vertebral bodies, femur, humerus and diploë of the skull.

- The calcanial center of ossification (Week 16–20) is used medico-legally to establish maturity.

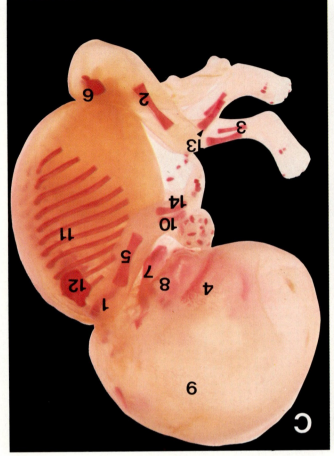

A. Horizon XVIII
(Day 36–38). (×5.9).

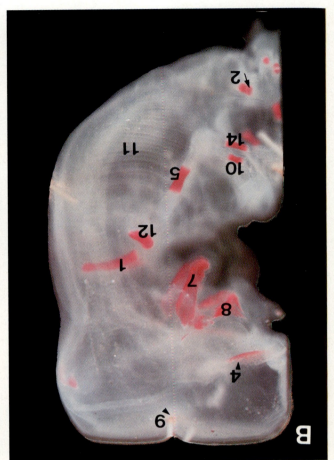

B. Horizon XXII
(Day 44–46). (×4.4).

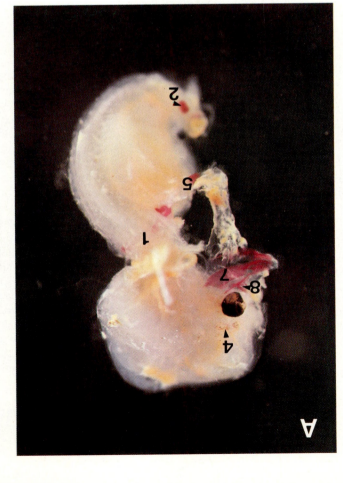

C. Week 8. (×3.1).

1. clavicle
2. femur
3. fibula
4. frontal
5. humerus
6. ilium
7. mandible
8. maxilla
9. parietal
10. radius
11. ribs
12. scapula
13. tibia
14. ulna

A–R. Primary ossification centers demonstrated by alizarin red staining and clearing.

A, B, C, E, H, K, M, N, O and P from
R.C.S.E.

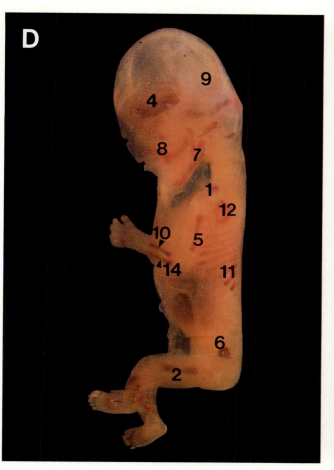

D. Week 11. The specimen has been stretched during mounting. (×1.7)

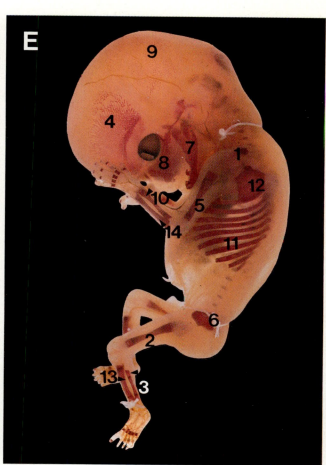

E. Week 11. (×1.9)

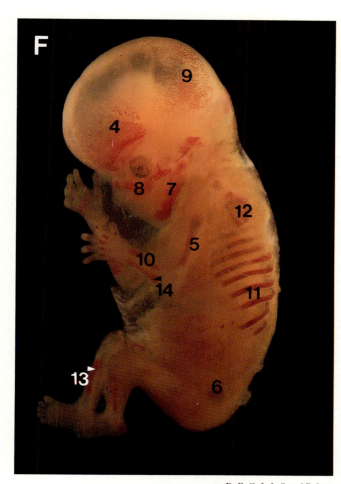

F. Week 11–12. (×1.8)

D, F, G, I, J, Q and R *from R.F.H.S.M.*

1. clavicle
2. femur
3. fibula
4. frontal
5. humerus
6. ilium
7. mandible
8. maxilla
9. parietal
10. radius
11. ribs
12. scapula
13. tibia
14. ulna

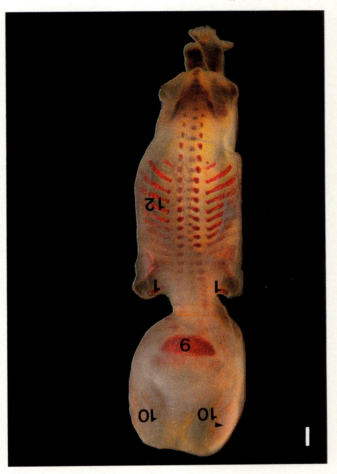

I. Week 13. (×1.4)

1. clavicle
2. femur
3. fibula
4. frontal
5. humerus
6. ilium
7. mandible
8. maxilla
9. occipital
10. parietal
11. radius
12. ribs
13. scapula
14. tibia
15. ulna

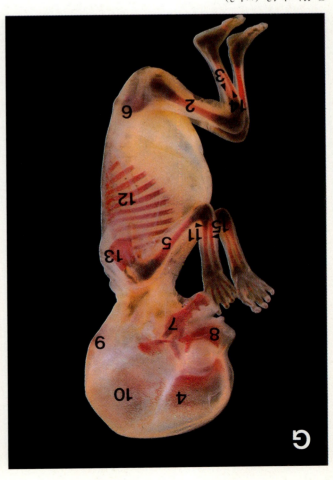

G. Week 13. (×1.3)

H. Week 13–14. This specimen has been damaged during preparation. (×1.6)

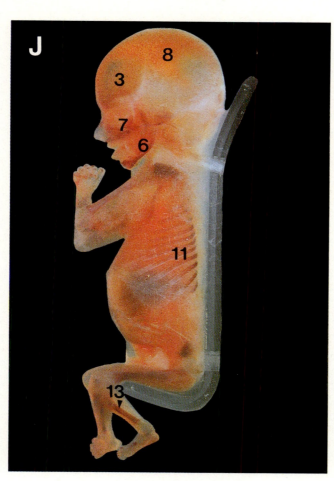

J. Week 14. This specimen has been stretched in preparation. (×1.1)

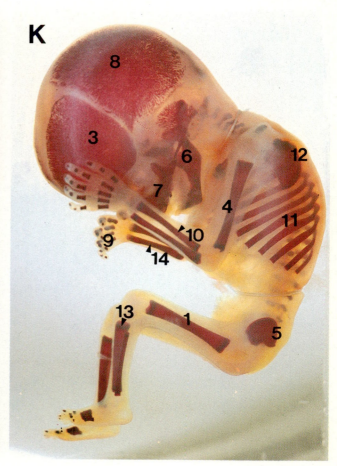

K. Week 14. (×1.5)

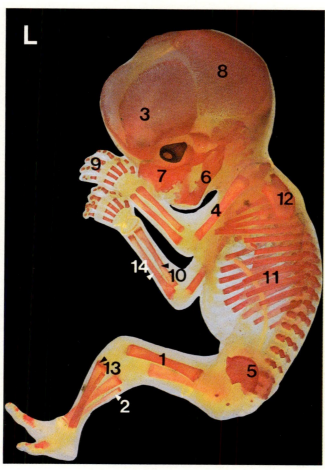

L. Week 15. (×1)

1. femur
2. fibula
3. frontal
4. humerus
5. ilium
6. mandible
7. maxilla
8. parietal
9. phalanges
10. radius
11. ribs
12. scapula
13. tibia
14. ulna

L *from Dr D. Dooley*

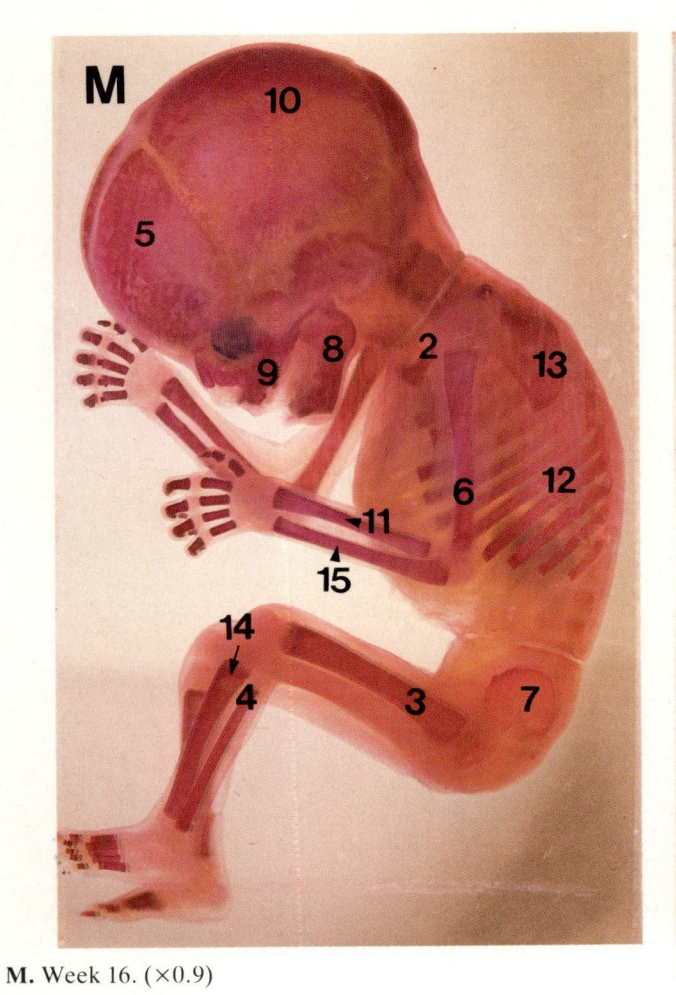

M. Week 16. (×0.9)

N. Week 16. (×0.9)

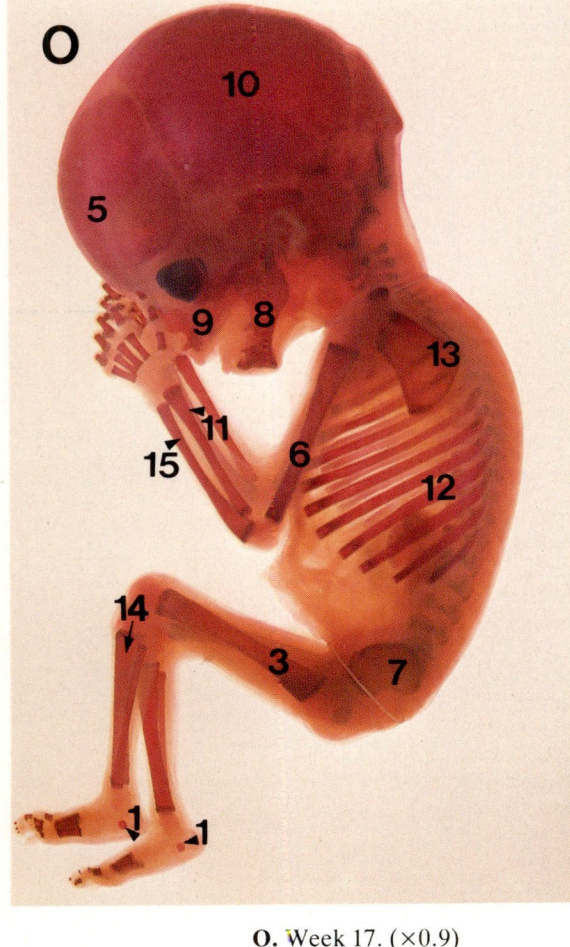

1. calcaneum
2. clavicle
3. femur
4. fibula
5. frontal
6. humerus
7. ilium
8. mandible
9. maxilla
10. parietal
11. radius
12. ribs
13. scapula
14. tibia
15. ulna

O. Week 17. (×0.9)

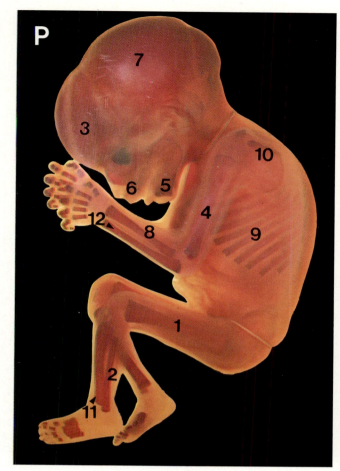

P. Week 18. (×1)

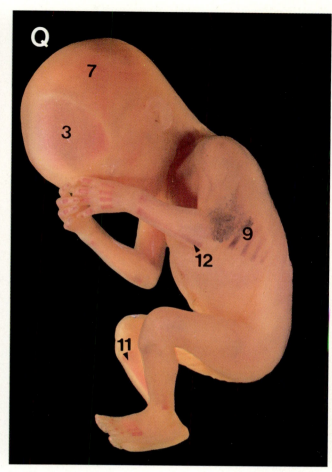

Q. Week 18. (×0.8)

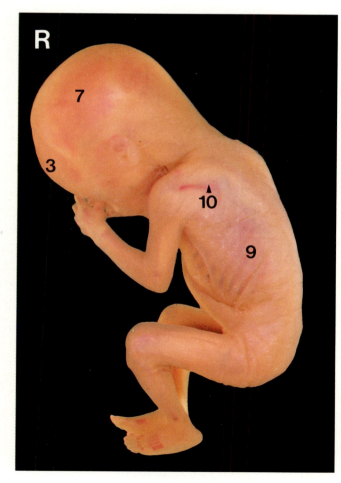

R. Same specimen as in Figure **Q**. After Week 18 the ossification centers are obscured by the muscles. (×0.8)

1. femur
2. fibula
3. frontal
4. humerus
5. mandible
6. maxilla
7. parietal
8. radius
9. ribs
10. scapula
11. tibia
12. ulna

Fetal skeleton

From R.F.H.S.M.

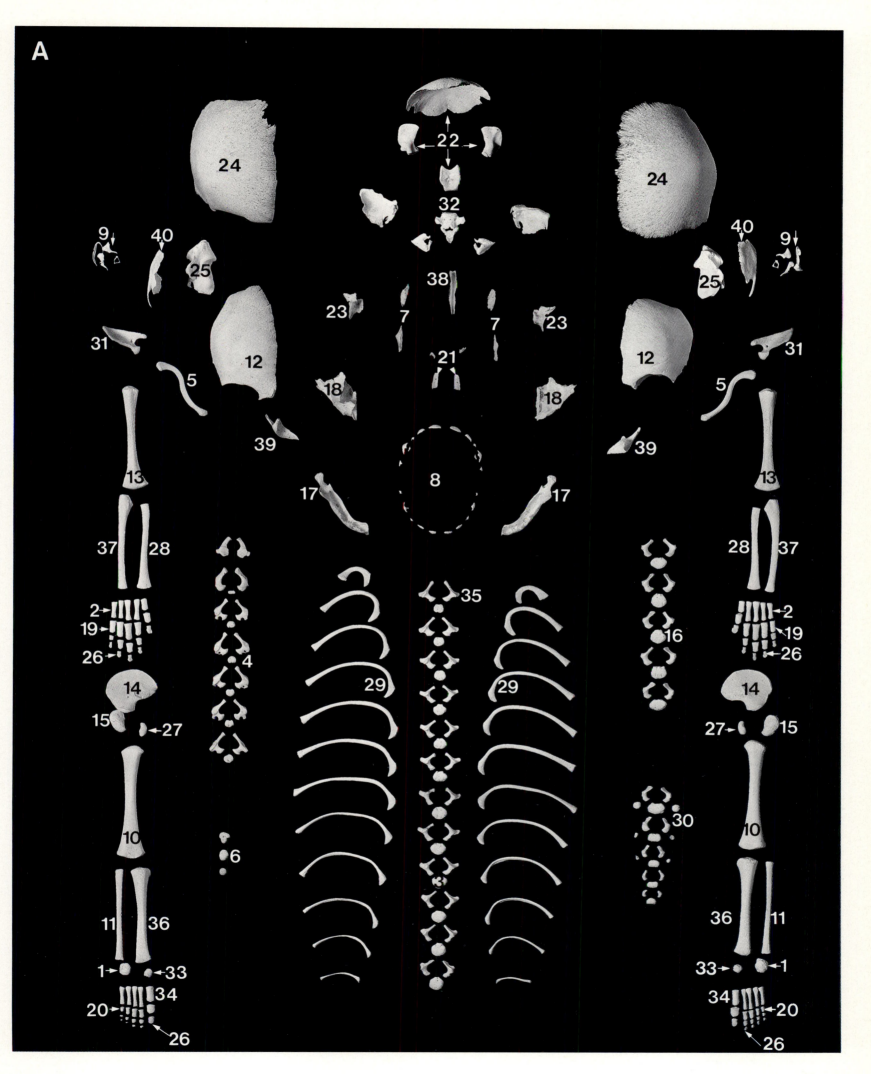

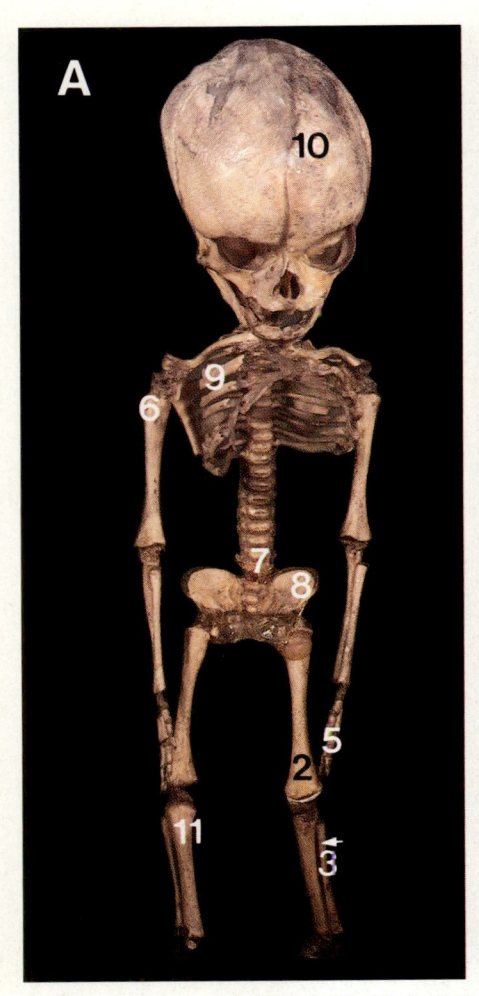

A. Week 13–16. (×0.9)

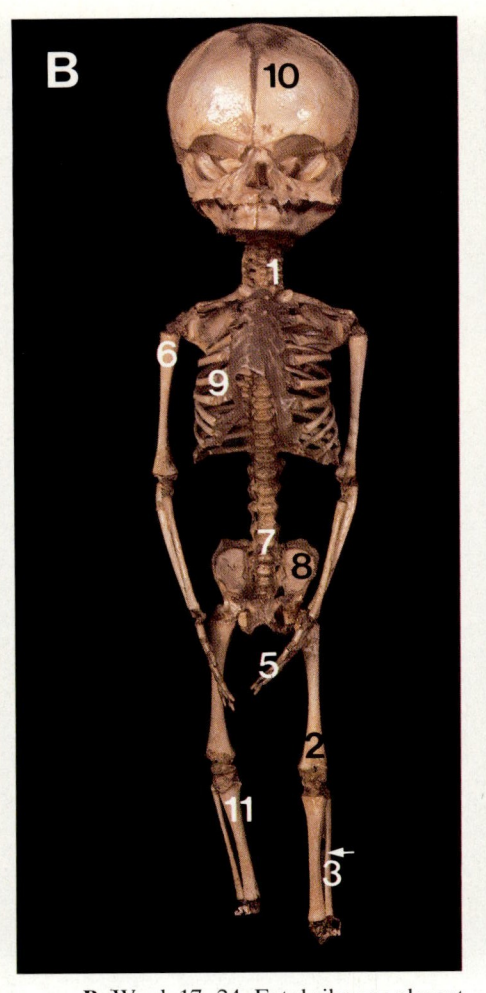

B. Week 17–24. Fetal ribs are almost horizontal. (×0.6)

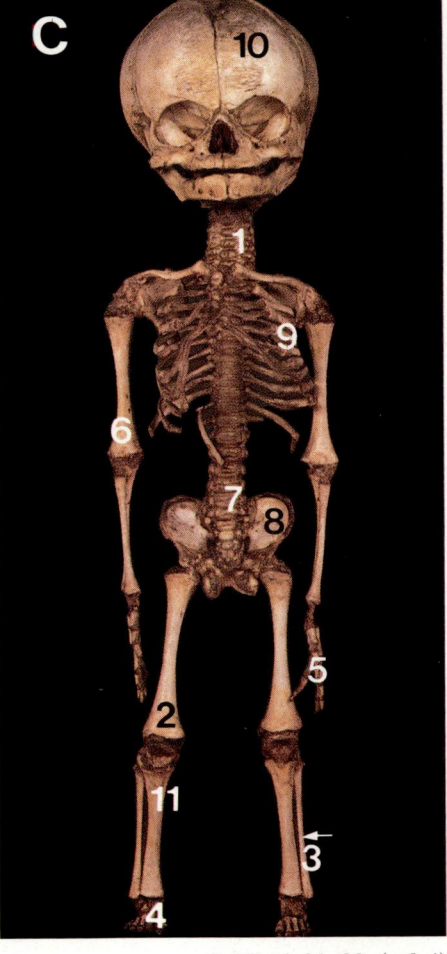

C. Week 21–28. (×0.4)

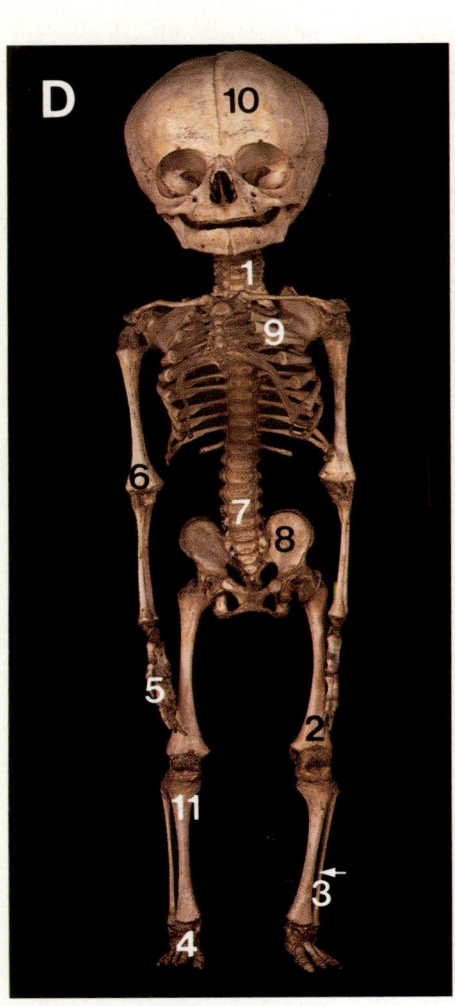

D. Week 25–32. The fetal skull is as wide as the pectoral girdle. (×0.3)

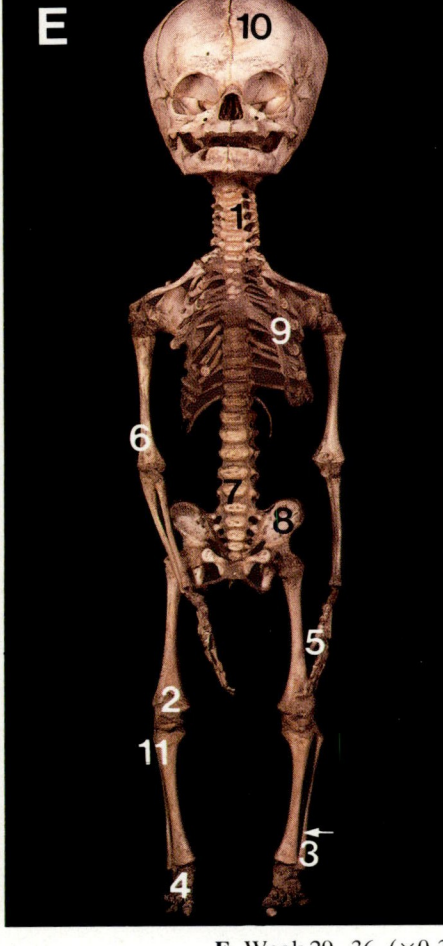

E. Week 29–36. (×0.3)

A–E. Articulated fetal skeleton to demonstrate relative size differences. The legs have been extended and adducted.

1. cervical vertebrae
2. femur
3. fibula
4. foot
5. hand
6. humerus
7. lumbar vertebrae
8. pelvis
9. ribs
10. skull
11. tibia

A–E *from R.F.H.S.M.*

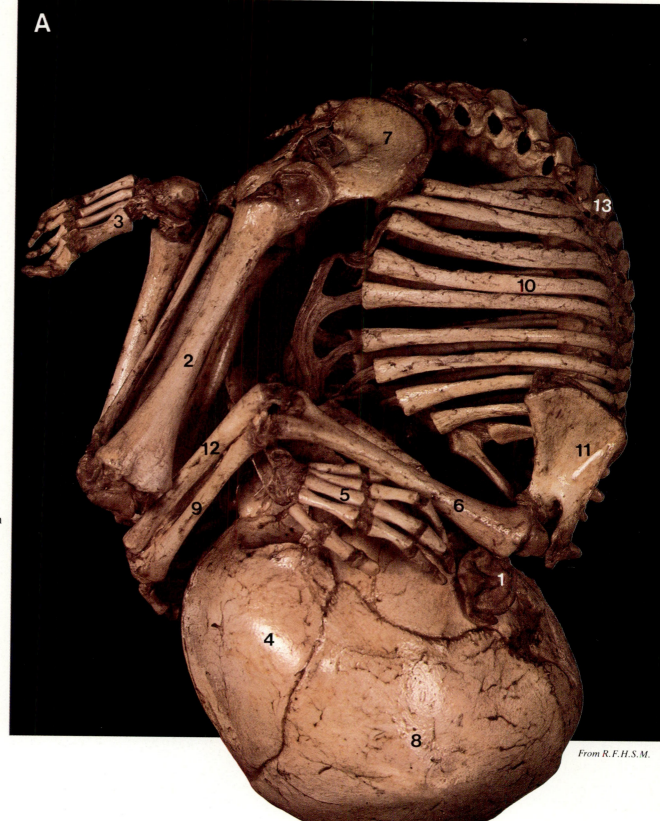

A. Full-term fetal skeleton in the normal position *in utero*. (×1.2)

1. ear
2. femur
3. foot
4. frontal
5. hand
6. humerus
7. ilium
8. parietal
9. radius
10. ribs
11. scapula
12. ulna
13. vertebral column

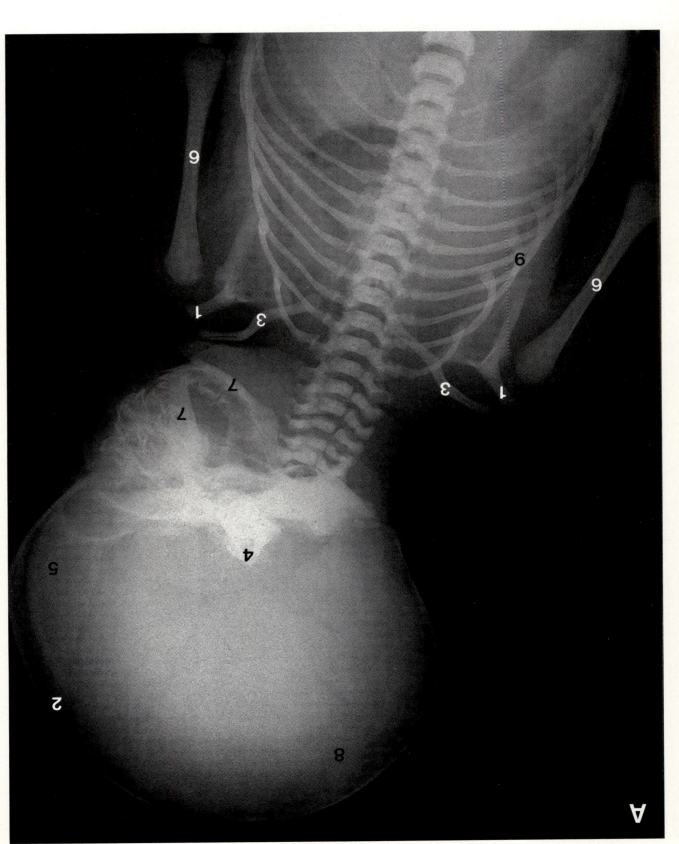

Fetal radiology

A. Week 35. Radiograph of
the head, neck and thorax.

1. acromion
2. anterior fontanelle
3. clavicle
4. external auditory meatus
5. frontal bone
6. humerus
7. mandible
8. parietal bone
9. rib

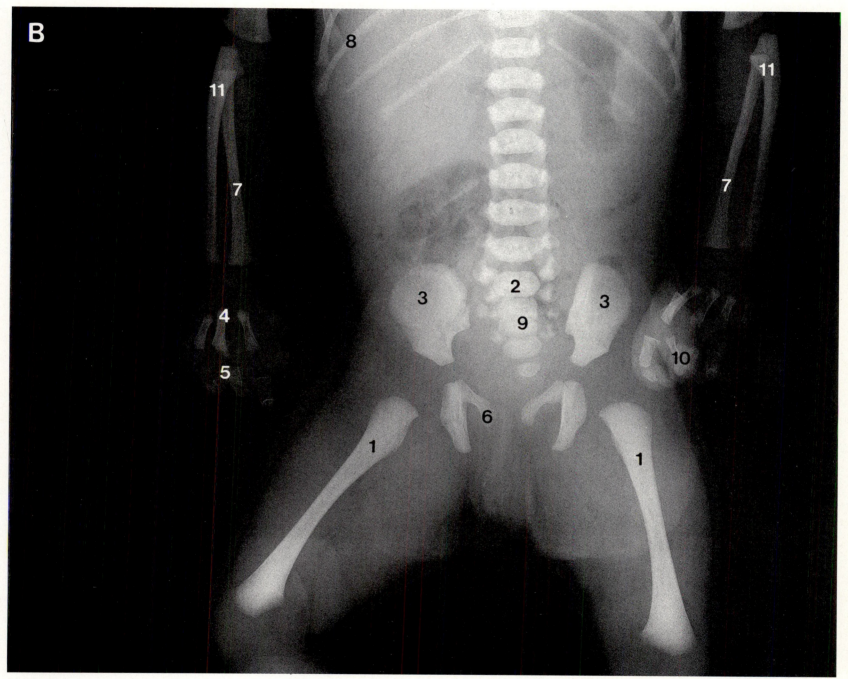

B. Antero-posterior radiograph of the abdomen and pelvis.

1. femur
2. fifth lumbar vertebra
3. ilium
4. metacarpals
5. proximal phalanges
6. pubis
7. radius
8. rib
9. sacral vertebra
10. thumb (pollex)
11. ulna

Muscles

Muscles form from myoblasts which have differentiated from mesoderm except for those of the iris which are derived from ectoderm.

Skeletal muscles form primarily from the myotome region of somites, but some head and neck muscles are formed from branchial arch myoblasts. Somatic mesoderm forms limb muscles *in situ*.

Each myotome divides into dorsal and ventral parts and as the spinal nerve develops it sends a branch to each part: the dorsal and ventral primary rami. The myoblasts then migrate to their final positions although some muscles remain segmentally arranged, e.g. the intercostals.

Most smooth muscles and cardiac muscles form from splanchnic mesoderm. The first heartbeats occur during Week 3 to 4.

At Week 7 some of the neck and trunk muscles begin to contract spontaneously. arm and leg movements then occur and are detectable by ultrasound methods, and by Week 12 the fetus can respond to skin stimulation and some postural reflexes are also present.

By Week 16–20 the fetal movements are felt by the mother, a phenomenon known as 'quickening'.

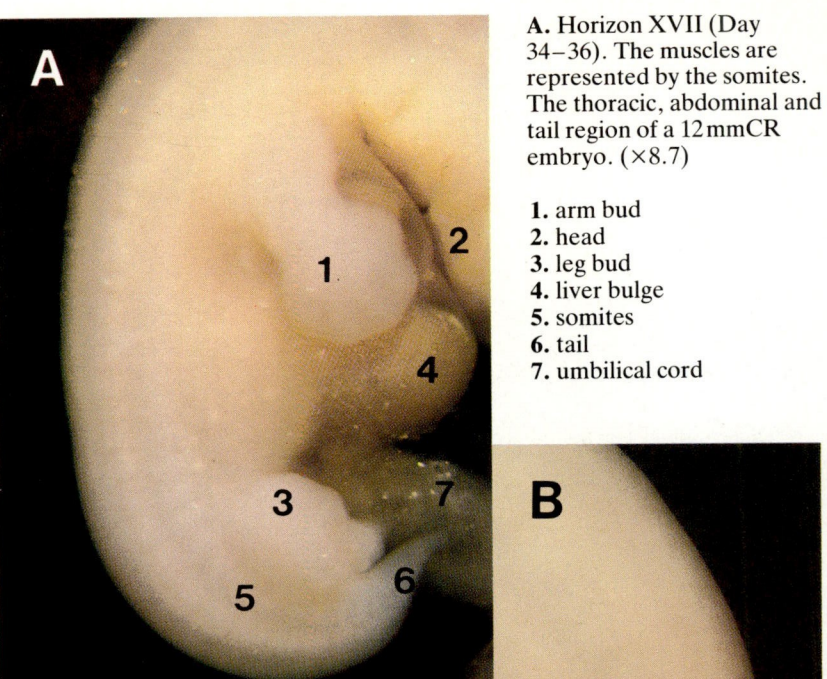

A. Horizon XVII (Day 34–36). The muscles are represented by the somites. The thoracic, abdominal and tail region of a 12 mmCR embryo. (×8.7)

1. arm bud
2. head
3. leg bud
4. liver bulge
5. somites
6. tail
7. umbilical cord

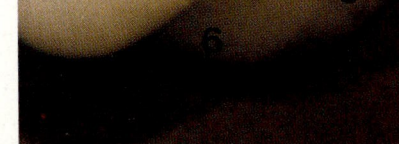

B. Horizon XVIII (Day 36–38). Somites in the lumbar region. 14 mmCR (×8.7)

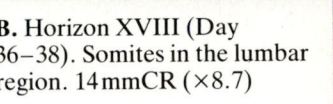

Swallowing reflexes

At Week 11 the fetus will open its mouth if the oral region is stimulated and suck a finger, at Week 12 the fetus regularly swallows amniotic fluid and near term it is swallowing approximately 750 ml daily. In addition to the fluid numerous other materials are swallowed, e.g. sloughed cells from the skin, oral cavity and respiratory tract, lanugo hairs and *vernix caseosa*.

A. Week 13. In addition to swallowing amniotic fluid a fetus may suck a finger from approximately Week 11. 92 mmCR ♀ (×3.4)

1. arm
2. ear
3. eye
4. superficial temporal artery

Integument

A–C. Development of the skin, samples taken from the arm above the elbow.

1. developing collagenous and elastic fibers (dermis)
2. epidermal ridge
3. intermediate layer
4. periderm
5. stratum corneum
6. stratum granulosum
7. stratum lucidum
8. stratum spinosum and germinativum

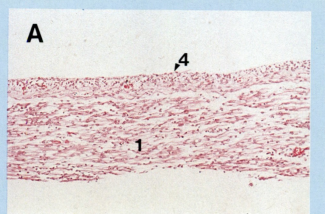

A. Week 10. 60 mmCR ♀ (×94)

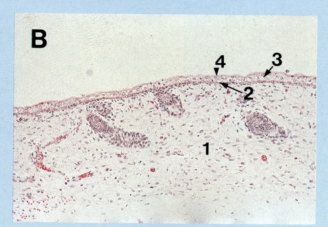

B. Week 13. 101 mmCR ♀ (×94)

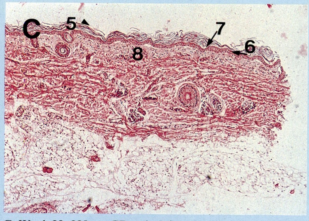

C. Week 23. 220 mmCR ♂ (×94)

Epidermis

The epidermis forms from ectoderm and the dermis forms from mesoderm associated with the ectoderm.

The epidermis is a simple epithelium at Week 4 but by Week 7 a superficial layer of periderm is present which keratinizes and desquamates. Cells are replaced by the basal layer, the stratum germinativum. At Week 11 an intermediate layer forms from cells of stratum germinativum. All of the adult layers are present at birth. Until approximately Week 17 the skin is very thin and the underlying blood vessels are visible.

The desquamated periderm cells together with sebum from sebaceous glands, lanugo hairs and amniotic cells form a white protective covering *(vernix caseosa)* for the fetal skin. This is primarily found on the back, on hair and in joint creases. It also fills the external auditory meatus at birth. From Week 21 the periderm cells gradually disappear and desquamated epidermal cells replace them in the *vernix caseosa*.

During Week 13–16 downgrowths of stratum germinativum penetrate into the dermis producing epidermal ridges which appear on the palmar surfaces of the hands and fingers and the plantar surfaces of the feet and toes. Each individual has a distinctive pattern.

Melanocytes

Around Week 8 melanoblasts migrate from the neural crest to the basal layer of the epidermis and form melanocytes. Melanin is produced before birth.

Dermis

The dermis originates from somatic mesoderm and the dermomyotome part of the somites. At Week 11 elastic and collagenous fibers are produced.

- Down's syndrome can be recognized by an abnormal epidermal ridge pattern, e.g. there is only one palmar crease rather than the normal two.

- Neonates of dark-skinned races are only slightly darker than those of white-skinned races. After birth their skin darkens due to increased melanin production in response to light. In the sacral region pigmented dermal melanocytes appear as a slate-blue or 'Mongolian' spot which disappears during the first year of life.

A. Week 13. The skin is very thin and the developing blood vessels are easily distinguished. Note the lack of *vernix caseosa*. 97 mmCR ♂ (×1.4)

1. arm
2. back
3. eye
4. hand
5. superficial temporal artery

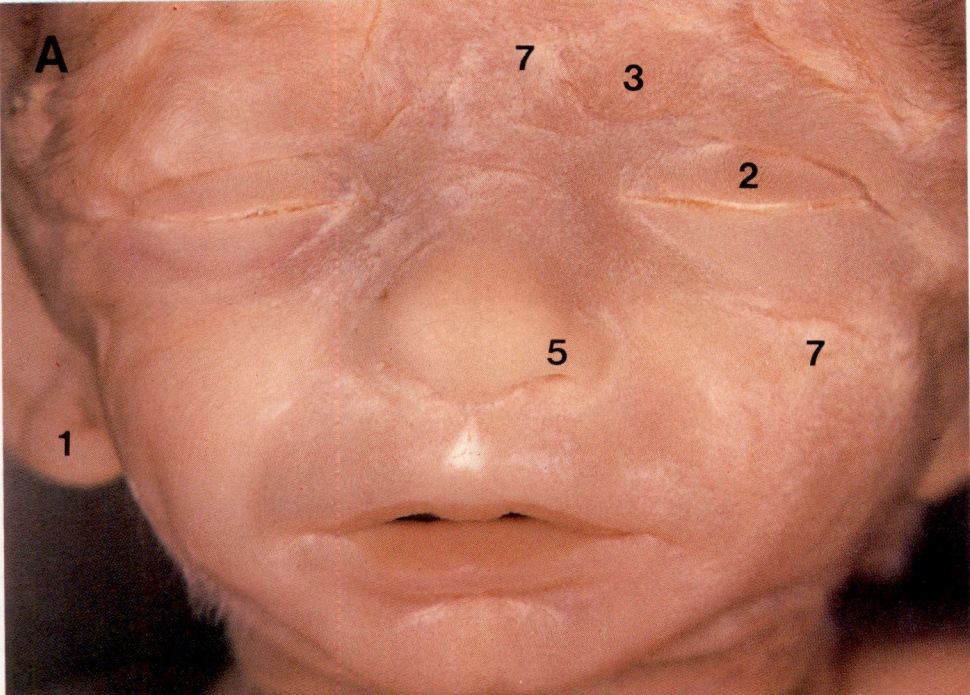

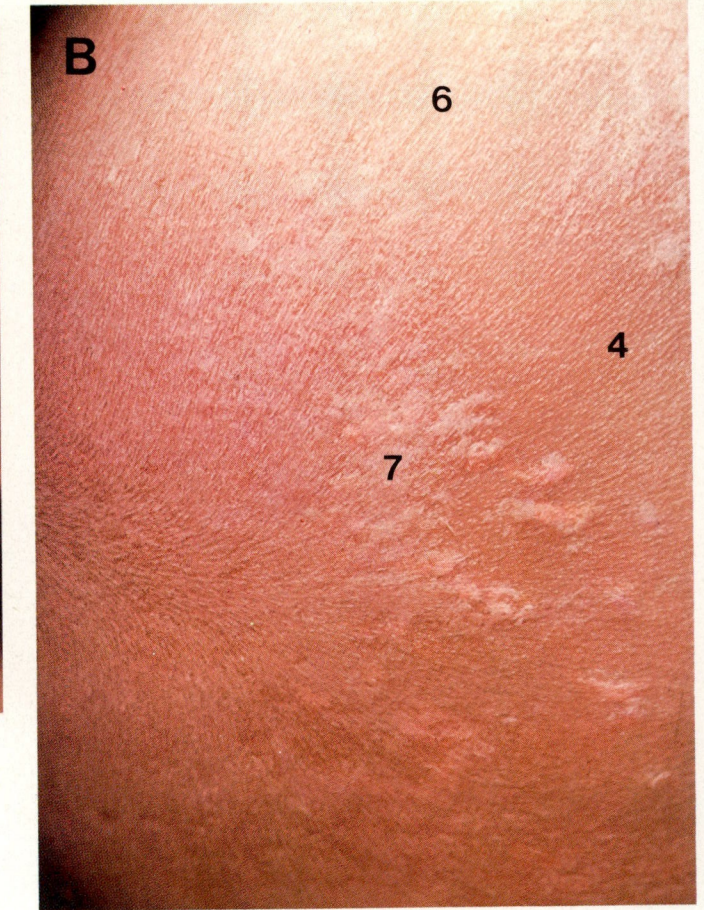

A and B. *Vernix caseosa* on the face and scalp.

1. ear
2. eye
3. eyebrow
4. lanugo
5. nose
6. scalp
7. *vernix caseosa*

A. Week 18. 152 mm CR ♂ (×2.6)

B. Week 18. *Vernix caseosa* on the back of the head. 160 mm CR ♀ (×3)

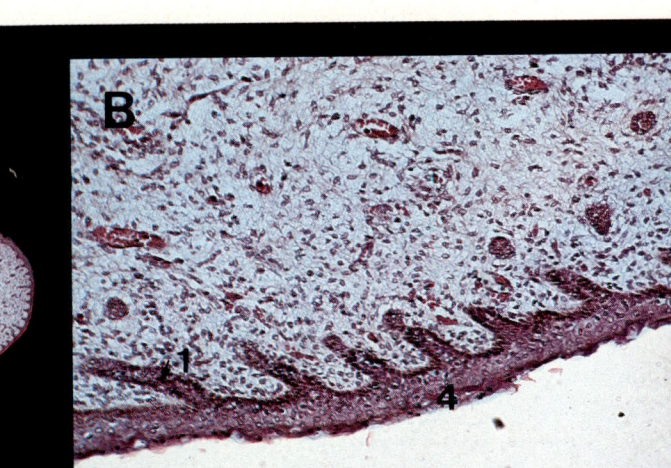

A and B. Week 13. Dermal ridges on the thumb.

1. dermal ridges
2. distal phalanx of thumb
3. fingernail
4. palmar surface

A. 101 mm CR ♀ (×24)

B. Higher magnification of the palmar surface of the thumb in Figure **A**. (×158)

A and B. **A and B.** Development of the
eyebrow viewed from the
front.

1. eyebrow
2. forehead
3. fused eyelid
4. lanugo

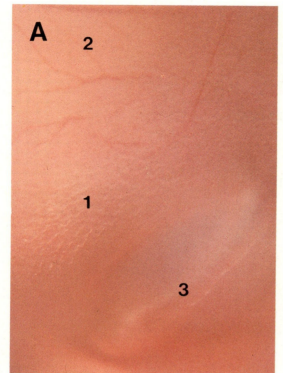

A. Week 13. 97mmCR ♂ (×10)

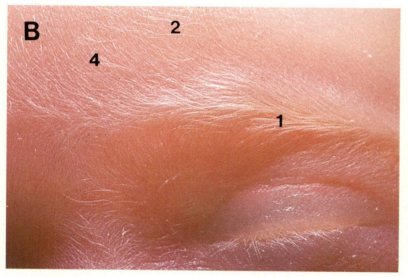

B. Week 15. 130mmCR ♀ (×5)

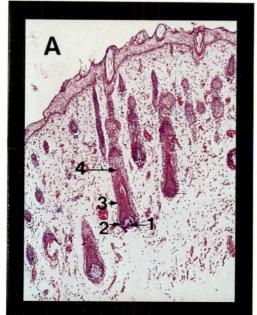

A. Week 13. Transverse
paraffin wax section of the
eyebrow. 101mmCR ♀ (×77)

1. blood vessels in hair papilla
2. bulb
3. dermal root sheath
4. hair shaft

Hair

Hair follicles form when downgrowths from the stratum germinativum penetrate into the dermis. The ends form hair bulbs containing the germinal matrices which produce the hairs. Melanocytes differentiate in the bulb from melanoblasts. Melanin is transferred from the melanocytes to the germinal matrix before birth. A hair papilla (mesoderm) invaginates the base of each hair bulb. The root sheath forms: the epithelial part from the hair follicle and the dermal portion from surrounding mesoderm.

The germinal matrix proliferates and the hair shaft cells are pushed up, keratinize, pierce the epidermis and protrude above the skin surface. Arrector pili muscles form from surrounding mesoderm.

Very fine hairs or lanugo first appear on the eyebrows and upper lip, and by Week 20 cover most of the body. Lanugo is replaced by secondary hairs (vellus) arising from new hair follicles. By Week 26–29 the secondary hair on the head is longer than the lanugo which is being shed. The new hair follicles cover almost all of the body.

● Lanugo is from the Latin *lana* meaning fine wool.

● Lanugo is shed before and shortly after birth, the last parts being shed from the eyelashes, eyebrows and scalp.

Sebaceous glands

Most of the sebaceous glands form as buds from a hair follicle root sheath except for those of the glans penis and the labia minora which bud from the epidermis. The sebaceous gland buds form several alveoli and ducts. The central alveolar cells break down to form oily sebum which is released into the hair follicle, onto the skin and so forms part of the *vernix caseosa*.

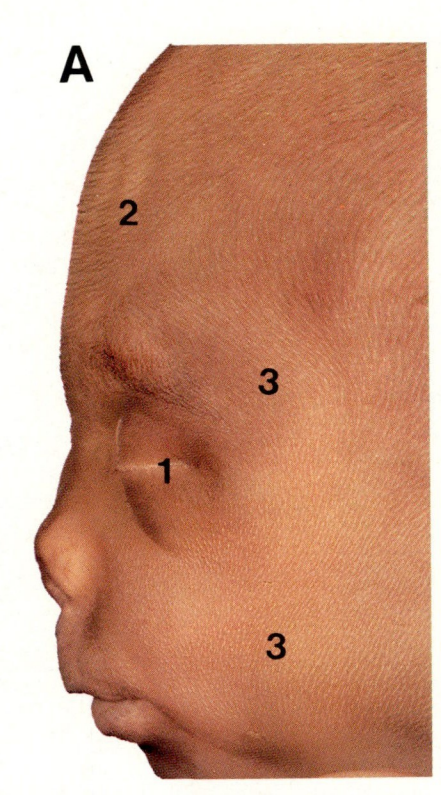

A. Week 17. Lanugo hairs on the face. 150 mmCR ♀ (×2)

1. eye
2. forehead
3. lanugo

A and B. Lanugo and vellus hairs.

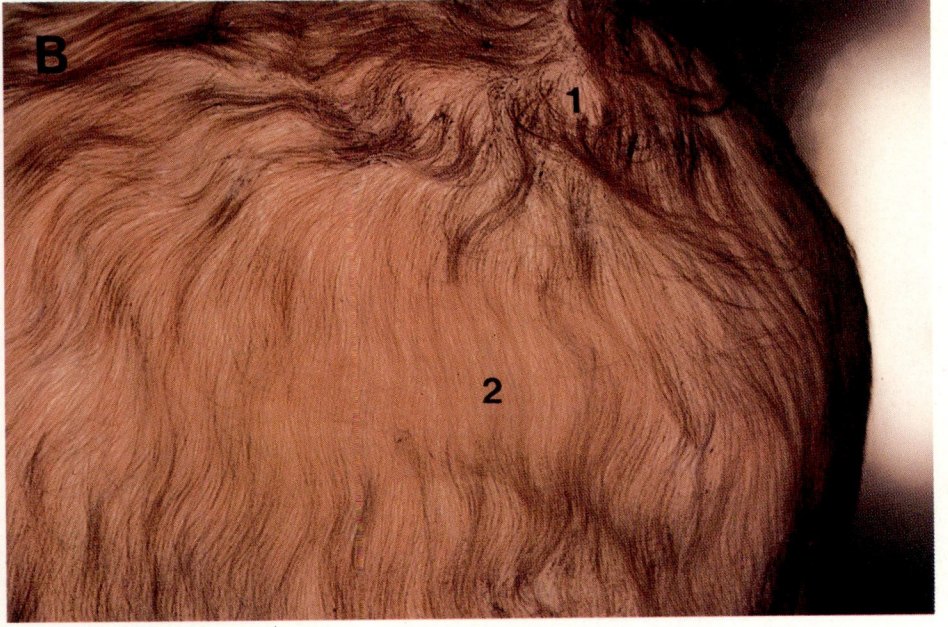

A. Week 20. Scalp showing both lanugo and scalp hairs. View from the right side. 185 mmCR ♀ (×7.5)

1. hair
2. head
3. lanugo

B. Week 23. Scalp covered with scalp hairs. View from behind. 220 mmCR ♂ (×1.5)

1. crown of head
2. hair

A and B. Developing mammary gland in transverse paraffin wax sections.

1. dermis
2. developing mammary gland
3. mammary pit
4. secondary bud

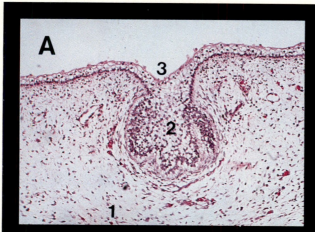

A. Week 18. 152 mmCR ♂ (×94)

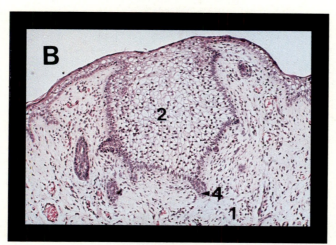

B. Week 18. 155 mmCR ♀ (×94)

A–C. Developing nipple.

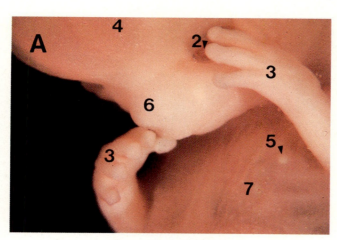

A. Horizon XXII (Day 44–46). 27 mmCR (×7.5)

1. arm
2. eye
3. hand
4. head
5. nipple (areola)
6. nose
7. thorax

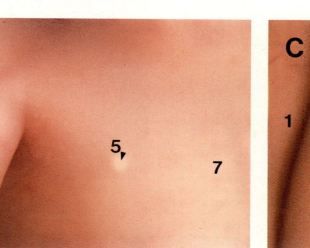

B. Week 9. 48 mmCR ♀ (×7.8)

Sweat glands

Merocrine sweat glands form as solid epidermal downgrowths into the dermis, the tip becoming a coiled gland and the stalk a duct. The lumen of the sweat gland forms by canalization; the peripheral cells form secretory and myoepithelial cells (smooth muscle).

Apocrine sweat glands bud from the epithelial downgrowths which will form the hair follicles.

Teeth – see Lips and teeth.

Fingernails and toenails – see Limbs.

Mammary gland

At the beginning of Week 4 a ridge of thickened ectoderm extends from the axilla to the inguinal region. During Week 6 it thickens and becomes depressed in the pectoral region. Numerous secondary epithelial cords then grow from it into the underlying mesoderm and at Week 32–36 the downgrowths and the cords become canalized.

- Either at full-term or in the neonatal period the nipple is formed when a proliferation of mesoderm beneath the downgrowth elevates it above the adjacent skin.

- At birth the mammary glands have the same appearance in either sex.

- As a result of maternal sex hormones crossing the placenta the breast in either sex may, for the first few days following birth, secrete a milky substance known as 'witches milk'.

- As the thorax grows in childhood the two nipples move further away from the midline.

- In the female at puberty estrogen stimulates further duct growth and the deposition of fat.

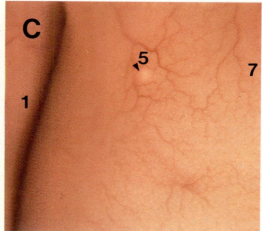

C. Week 13. 97 mmCR ♂ (×7.8)

Fat Deposition

Around Week 27 subcutaneous fat storage commences and the body becomes plump. Two colours of fat may be distinguished: white (yellow) and brown. Brown adipose tissue, which is important in metabolism and heat production, is present at the root of the neck, in the perirenal area, and behind the sternum.
around the organs in the thorax and on the posterior abdominal wall.

● A fetus born prematurely at Week 25 to 26 looks old and wizened due to the lack of subcutaneous fat and the fact that the skin grows faster than the underlying connective tissue.

● Fat also accumulates in the cheeks forming 'buccal fat pads' over the buccinator muscles which prevent the cheeks being drawn in during suckling.

● At birth the neonatal temperature is the same or slightly higher than the mother's but it then immediately drops below hers.

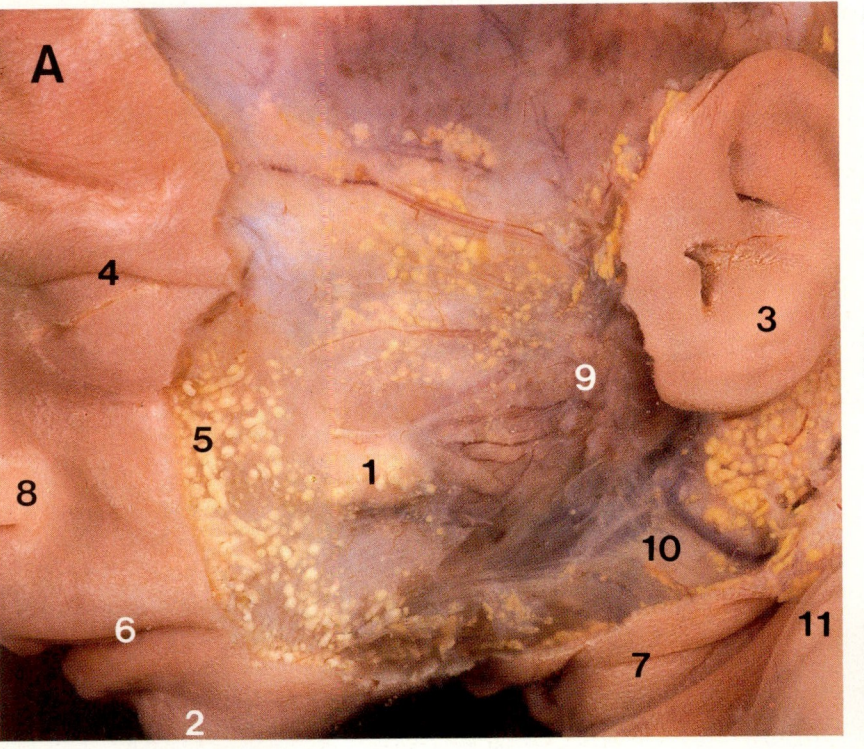

A. Week 18. Buccal fat pad.
152 mmCR ♂ (×2.6)

1. buccal fat pad
2. chin
3. ear
4. eye
5. fat
6. mouth
7. neck
8. nose
9. parotid gland
10. platysma muscle (cut)
11. shoulder

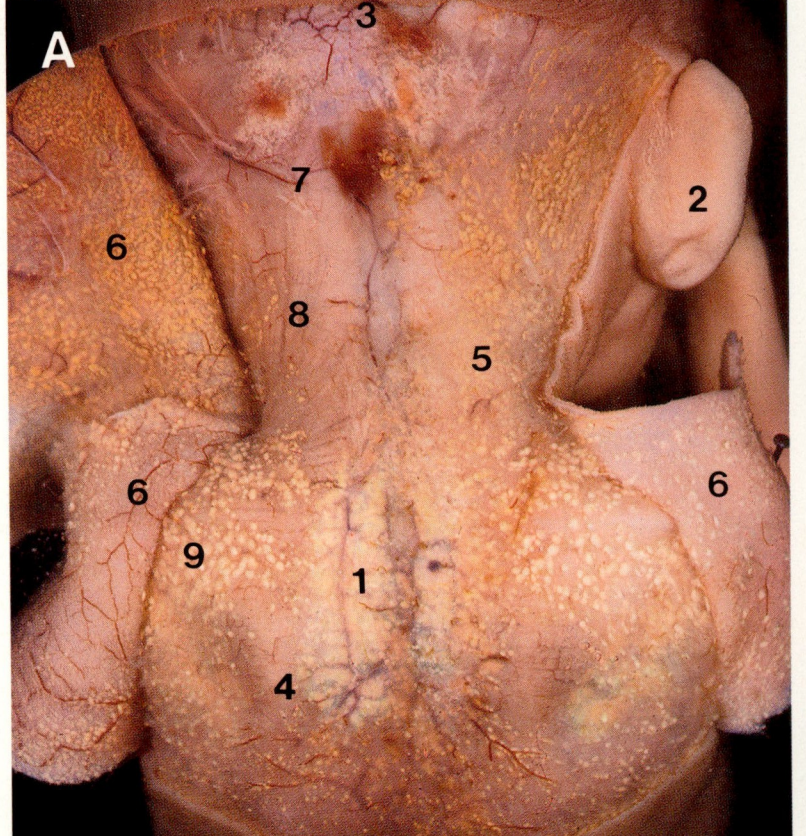

A. Week 18. Distribution of white (yellow) fat on the neck and shoulders.
152 mmCR ♂ (×1.4)

1. fat deposited in a pad
2. ear
3. head
4. medial border of the scapula
5. neck
6. reflected skin
7. superior nuchal line
8. trapezius muscle
9. white fat

Lymphatics

The lymphatic system develops at the end of Week 5. Two pairs of lymph sacs develop, the jugular sacs and the iliac sacs. Two single sacs also form: the retroperitoneal sac and the cisterna chyli. Lymphatic vessels grow out from these sacs and spread throughout the body.

Mesoderm surrounding the sacs invades them and forms the connective tissue framework and capsule of the lymph nodes. Lymphocytes invade from the thymus. Later, some lymphocytes form from the node mesoderm.

● Lymphoid nodules and germinal centers appear shortly after birth.

Tonsils

The lingual tonsils form from lymph nodules in the root of the tongue, the palatine tonsils from the second pharyngeal pouch, the pharyngotympanic tonsils from lymph nodules around the Eustachian tubes, and the pharyngeal tonsils (adenoids) from lymph nodules in the nasopharynx.

● The pharyngeal tonsil reaches its maximum size at the age of 6 years and usually involutes by puberty.

● The palatine tonsil atrophies between 5 years and puberty.

Spleen – see page 124.

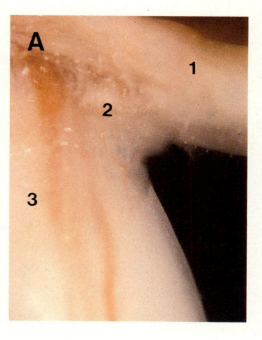

A. Week 9. Developing axillary lymph node. View of the ventral surface. 50 mmCR ♀ (×16)

1. arm
2. lymph node
3. thorax

A. Full-term fetus in utero.
(×1.1)

1. abdomen
2. arm
3. cervix (maternal)
4. head
5. leg
6. ovary (maternal)
7. uterus (maternal)

Growth of the Pregnant Uterus

The non-pregnant uterus lies within the pelvis.

During pregnancy the uterus expands due to hypertrophy of the existing muscle fibers and the addition of some new ones. In the first trimester the uterus reaches the level of the umbilicus and by Weeks 28–30 it is in the epigastric region.

Childbirth

There are three stages of labor, the first of which extends from the onset of labor until there is complete dilatation of the cervix. At the start of the first stage a blood stained mucous discharge occurs then the amnion and chorion form a wedge known as the 'bag of waters' which dilates the internal os. As the internal os dilates the cervix is shortened or 'taken up' into the lower uterine segment. Late in the first stage the wedge of amnion and chorion ruptures and the amniotic fluid lying in front of the advancing head escapes as the 'forewaters'. Regular contractions are then established less than 10 minutes apart and the cervix dilates completely. The first stage lasts about 10–12 hours in primigravidas or about 7 hours or less in multigravidas.

The second stage of labor begins when the cervix is completely dilated and ends with the delivery of the fetus. This stage lasts about 30–90 minutes in primigravidas and 20 minutes or less in multigravidas. As the amniotic fluid has escaped the uterine contractions can act directly on the fetus forcing it down the birth canal and through the vagina. If the head presents in a vertex presentation it undergoes the following movements: engagement when the head passes the pelvic brim, descent, flexion of the head on the body pressing the chin against the chest, internal rotation, a spiral movement which starts when the head reaches the pelvic floor and continues during its descent until complete rotation occurs with the occiput usually rotating forward, extension of the head occurs as it escapes from the birth canal, flexion of the head occurs after the face and chin pass the perineum and finally as the head is born the trunk descends into the pelvis, the shoulders are rotated into the anteroposterior diameter of the outlet and the birth of the trunk and legs follows quickly. The remaining liquor amnii then escapes.

The third stage of labor, which lasts 5–25 minutes, begins with the birth of the baby and ends with the delivery of the placenta and membranes. As the uterus continues to contract the placenta separates from the decidua, more of the umbilical cord appears and the placenta and membranes are delivered. The spiral arteries constrict with further myometrial contractions.

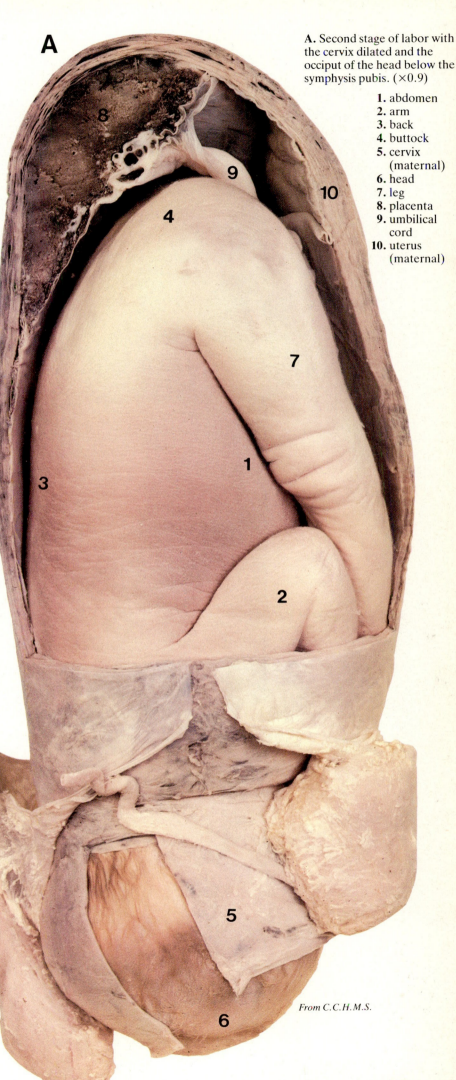

A. Second stage of labor with the cervix dilated and the occiput of the head below the symphysis pubis. (×0.9)

1. abdomen
2. arm
3. back
4. buttock
5. cervix (maternal)
6. head
7. leg
8. placenta
9. umbilical cord
10. uterus (maternal)

From C.C.H.M.S.

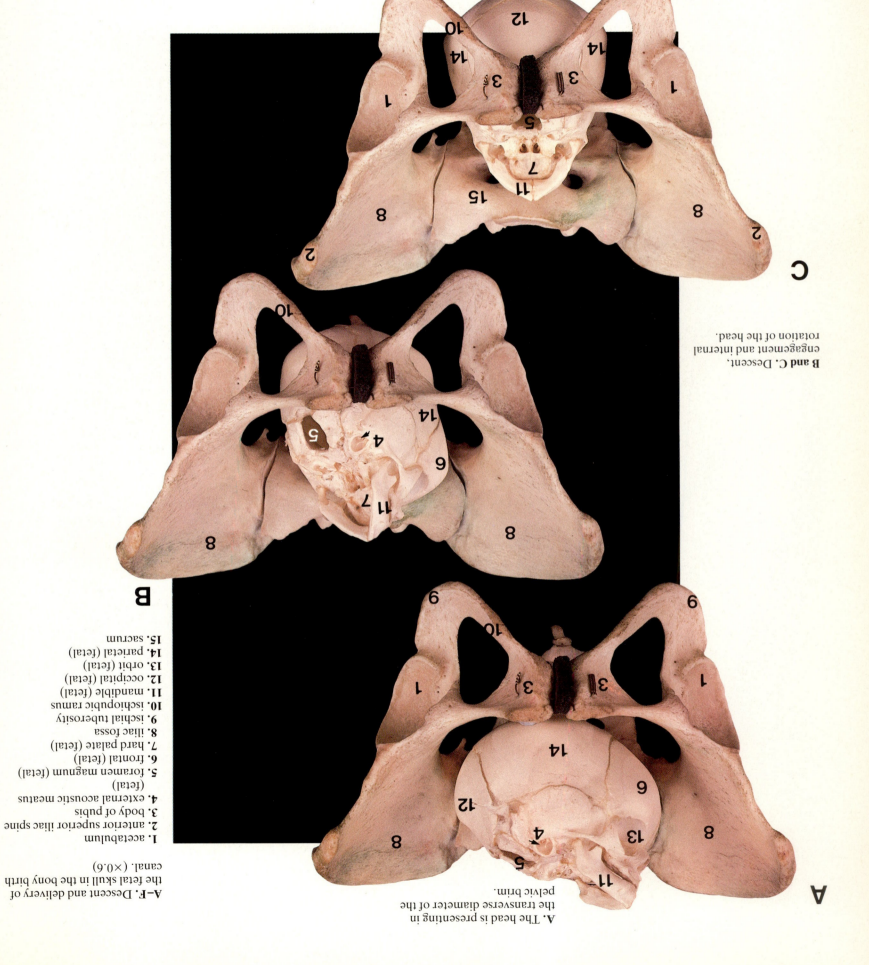

A-F. Descent and delivery of the fetal skull in the bony birth canal. (×0.6)

1. acetabulum
2. anterior superior iliac spine
3. body of pubis
4. external acoustic meatus (fetal)
5. foramen magnum (fetal)
6. frontal (fetal)
7. hard palate (fetal)
8. iliac fossa
9. ischial tuberosity
10. ischiopubic ramus
11. mandible (fetal)
12. occipital (fetal)
13. orbit (fetal)
14. parietal (fetal)
15. sacrum

A. The head is presenting in the transverse diameter of the pelvic brim.

B and C. Descent, engagement and internal rotation of the head.

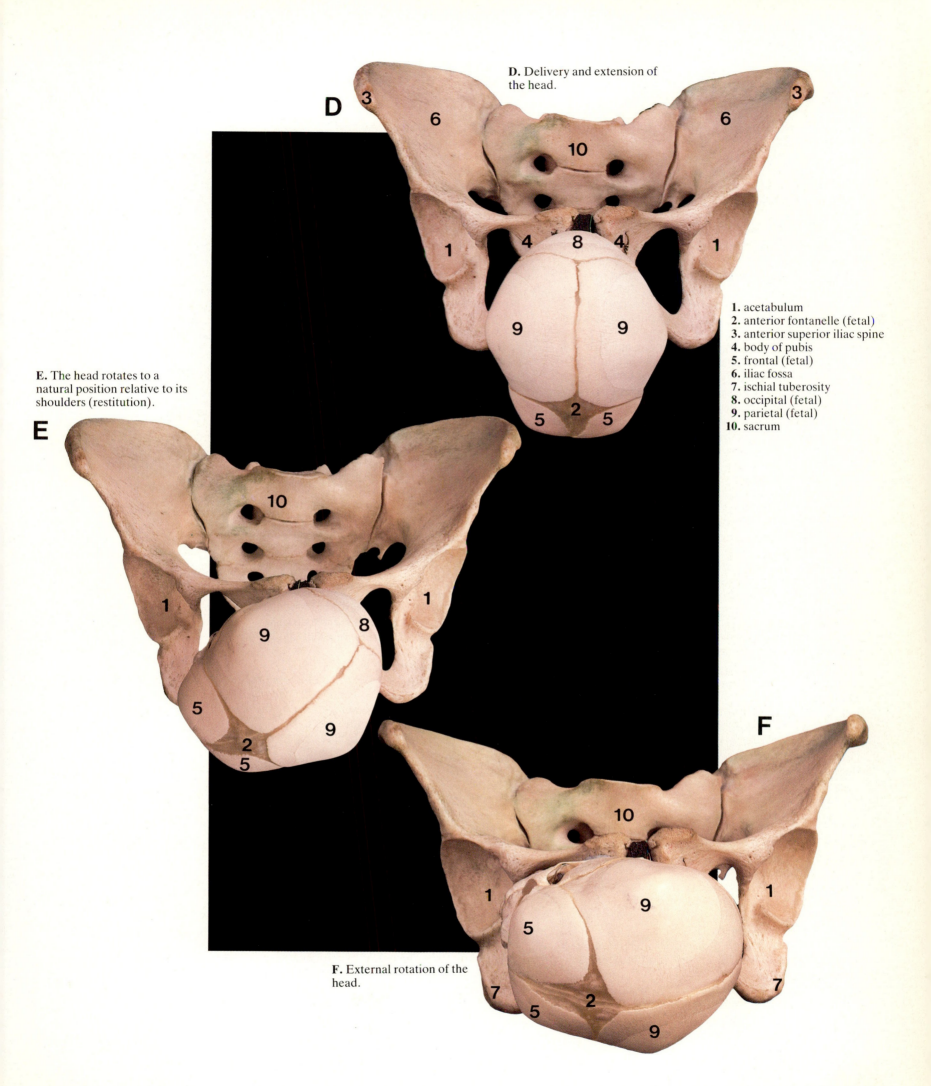

D. Delivery and extension of the head.

E. The head rotates to a natural position relative to its shoulders (restitution).

F. External rotation of the head.

1. acetabulum
2. anterior fontanelle (fetal)
3. anterior superior iliac spine
4. body of pubis
5. frontal (fetal)
6. iliac fossa
7. ischial tuberosity
8. occipital (fetal)
9. parietal (fetal)
10. sacrum

Glossary

Abduction   Movement away from the midline of the body.

Abortion   Pregnancy ending before viability (20 weeks). Spontaneous (naturally occurring) abortions usually occur in the first 12 weeks. Therapeutic abortions are those induced purposefully.

Adduction   Movement toward the midline of the body.

Afterbirth   At birth the umbilical cord, placenta, amnion and chorion are delivered after the fetus.

Alar plate   Dorsal portion of the neural tube.

Allantois   Endodermal diverticulum of the yolk sac.

Amnion   The innermost membrane surrounding the embryo/fetus. It also forms the epithelial covering of the umbilical cord.

Amniotic fluid   Fluid filling the amniotic cavity which cushions the embryo/fetus from external injuries to the mother and allows the fetus to move freely.

Anal membrane   A membrane formed from part of the cloacal membrane.

Anal pit   The external depression marking the site of the anal membrane. See also *Proctodeum*.

Anencephaly   Defective development of the brain and absence of the cranial vault.

Apical ectodermal ridge   Thickening of the ectoderm in the distal limb bud tip.

Arm bud   Primordium of the arm.

Auricular hillocks   Six swellings around the margin of the first branchial groove form the auricle of the ear.

Basal plate   Ventral portion of the neural tube.

Bilaminar embryo   The early embryo consisting of ectoderm and endoderm layers before the appearance of the mesoderm layer.

Bi-parietal diameter   A measurement of the distance between the two parietal bones.

Blastocyst   Early embryo consisting of a sphere of trophoblast and embryoblast cells.

Blood islands   Hemopoietic (blood-forming) areas on the yolk sac.

Body stalk   Stalk connecting the early embryo to the chorion (connecting or umbilical stalk).

Branchial arches   Arches in the walls of the neck region and floor of the pharynx.

Branchial grooves   Depressions in the ectoderm marking the boundaries of the branchial arches.

Buccopharyngeal membrane   The oral membrane which ruptures at about Day 24 linking the mouth and amniotic cavity.

Caudal   Towards the tail, inferior.

Caul   An unruptured amniotic sac surrounding the neonate at birth.

Cervical flexure   The second brain flexure to appear.

Cervix   The neck of the uterus.

Chorion   Trophoblast and associated underlying extra-embryonic mesoderm.

Chorionic plate   The chorion containing the main branches of the umbilical vessels on the fetal placental surface.

Chorionic sac   Contains the embryo and its amnion and yolk sac and is surrounded by the chorion.

Cloaca   The dilated terminal part of the hindgut caudal to the allantoic diverticulum.

Cloacal membrane. An area caudal to the primitive streak where the ectoderm and endoderm layers are in contact. Later (Week 6) this membrane is divided to form the anal membrane and the urogenital membrane.

Coelom (intraembryonic)   Spaces within the embryo which form the pericardial, pleural and peritoneal cavities.

Connecting stalk   The body or umbilical stalk of the early embryo.

Corona radiata   Cells surrounding the ovum after ovulation.

Coronal plane of section   A vertical section through the embryo/fetus perpendicular to the median plane.

Cotyledon   A unit of the placenta.

Cranial   Toward the head, superior, cephalic.

Crown–heel length   A measurement of the standing height of an older embryo/fetus.

Crown–rump length   A straight line measuring the sitting height of an embryo/fetus.

Decidua   The endometrium of pregnancy.

Decidua basalis   The layer of endometrium underlying the implanted embryo.

Decidua capsularis   The layer of endometrium overlying the implanted embryo.

Decidua parietalis   All the decidua other than the decidua basalis and capsularis.

Dental lamina   Precursor of the enamel organ.

Dermomyotome   Division of the somite which forms the dermis of the skin and skeletal muscle.

Diencephalon   Part of the forebrain forming the epithalamus, thalamus and hypothalamus.

Differentiation   Specialization of a cell or a group of cells.

Dorsal   Relating to the back.

Ductus arteriosus   A blood vessel connecting the left pulmonary artery and aortic arch.

Ductus venosus   A blood vessel connecting the left umbilical vein to the inferior vena cava.

Ectoderm   The germ layer which forms the nervous system and skin epidermis.

Embryo   The fertilized ovum until the end of Week 8.

Embryonic disc   The early embryo composed of two or three germ layers before the formation of the body folds.

Enamel organ   Precursor of the tooth enamel.

Endoderm   The germ layer which forms the gut and its derivatives.

Endometrium   Inner layer of the uterus.

Extra-embryonic coelom   The area outside the embryo which becomes the chorionic cavity.

Extra-embryonic mesoderm   Mesoderm outside the embryo forming the connective tissue of the chorion, vessels of the umbilical cord and placenta.

Fertilization age   The age of the embryo/fetus based on the true date of fertilization of the ovum by the sperm (see *True age*). The gestation period is 38 weeks.

Fetal membranes   The amnion, chorion, allantois and yolk sac remnant.

Fetus   The embryo from the beginning of Week 9 to birth.

Flexion   The embryo bends to become 'C' shaped.

Foregut   The gut extending from the oral membrane to the point of entry of the common bile duct.

Forewaters   In the first stage of labor, amniotic fluid in front of the head escapes when the amnion and chorion rupture.

Genital tubercle   The early phallus.

Germ layers   The three layers from which all body tissues develop: the ectoderm, mesoderm and endoderm.

Gravid   Pregnant.

Gubernaculum   Fibrous tissue attached to the lower end of the gonad and in the male is concerned in the descent of the testis.

Hand plate (paddle)   The hand primordium.

Head fold   Fold in the embryonic disc which forms the head region.

Heart bulge   Bulge in the thoracic region over the heart.

Hepatic diverticulum   Primordium of the liver and biliary tract.

Hindgut   Gut from the distal part of the transverse colon to superior part of the anal canal.

Horizon   A series of developmental stages in early humans devised by G.L. Streeter.

Hyoid arch   The second branchial arch.

Implantation   The fertilized ovum embedding in the maternal endometrium.

Intra-embryonic mesoderm   Mesoderm within the embryo.

Labioscrotal swelling   Two folds which form the scrotum in the male or labia majora in the female.

Lacuna   A small space.

Lanugo   The first fine body hair primarily shed before birth.

Leg bud   Primordium of the leg.

Lens placode   Precursor of the lens.

Liquor amnii   Amniotic fluid.

Longitudinal plane of section   A vertical section of the embryo/fetus through the median plane or parallel to it (sagittal).

Mandibular arch   The first branchial arch.

Mandibular prominence (process)   Part of the first branchial arch which forms the mandible.

Maxillary prominence (process)   Part of the first branchial arch which forms the maxilla, zygomatic bone and squamous temporal bone.

Meconium   Green-coloured intestinal contents of the late fetus and neonate.

Medial   Toward the midline.

Median plane of section   A vertical section through the middle of the embryo/fetus touching both the dorsal and ventral surfaces.

Menstrual age   The true age (fertilization age) plus 2 weeks. The gestation period is 40 weeks.

Mesencephalon   The midbrain.

Mesoderm   The germ layer which forms muscles, connective tissue and several other tissues within the embryo (see *Extra-embryonic mesoderm*).

Mesonephric duct   Duct of the mesonephros, which forms the male ductus deferens.

Mesonephros   Temporary kidney which is replaced by the metanephric kidney.

Metanephric cap   Mesoderm cells which collect around the ureteric bud and form the nephrons.

Metanephros   The permanent kidney.

Metencephalon   Part of the hindbrain which forms the pons and cerebellum.

Midbrain flexure   First brain flexure.

Midgut   Gut from the entry of the common bile duct to the distal part of the transverse colon.

Miscarriage   An interruption of pregnancy before term (see *Abortion*).

Morula   A solid sphere of embryonic cells prior to blastocyst formation.

Multigravida   A pregnant woman who has had a previous pregnancy.

Myelencephalon   Part of the hindbrain which forms the medulla oblongata.

Neural crest   A group of cells dorsal to the neural tube which form most of the peripheral nervous system, pigment cells, meninges and several other tissues.

Neural folds   Two folds which fuse to form the neural tube.

Neural tube   Precursor of the nervous system.

Neuropore   Openings at each end of the neural tube which close later in development.

Notochord   An axial cord in the embryo around which organs are laid down.

Oral membrane   See *Buccopharyngeal membrane*.

Otic placode   Precursor of the otocyst.

Otocyst   Precursor of the inner ear.

Ovum   Female germ cell.

Paramesonephric duct   Duct beside the mesonephros. Forms the uterus and uterine tubes.

Paraxial mesoderm   Mesoderm which segments into blocks or somites.

Parturition   Childbirth, labor.

Phallus   Precursor of the penis or clitoris.

Pharyngeal pouches   Depressions in the pharyngeal endoderm marking the boundaries of the branchial arches.

Placenta   The organ between the fetus and mother for gaseous and metabolic exchange.

Placenta previa   A placenta implanted near the internal opening of the cervix which partially or completely covers the cervical opening.

Preaxial border   The border of the limb anterior to the axis of the limb.

Polar bodies   Minute cells extruded during meiotic division of the oocyte.

Pontine flexure   Third brain flexure to appear.

Postaxial border   The border of the limb posterior to the axis of the limb.

Primigravida   A woman in the first pregnancy.

Primary palate   Median palatal process.

Primitive knot(node)   An enlargement of the anterior end of the primitive streak.

Primitive streak   A thickening of the ectoderm in the trilaminar embryo marking the future position of the notochord and body axis.

Primordial germ cell   Precursor of the sperm or ovum.

Primordium   The earliest stage of a structure or organ.

Proctodeum   Anal pit or depression.

Pronephros   Early kidney rudiment.

Prosencephalon   Forebrain.

Pupillary membrane   Mesoderm anterior to the developing lens whose center normally degenerates before birth.

Quickening   The fetal movements detected by the mother at 16–20 weeks of pregnancy.

Radial ridges   Mesodermal precursors of the fingers and toes.

Rathke's pouch   Outpocketing of the stomodeum which forms the anterior and middle lobes of the pituitary.

Rhombencephalon   Diamond-shaped hindbrain.

Rostral   The relationship of structures to the nose.

Sagittal plane of section   A vertical section through the embryo/fetus parallel to the median plane.

Sclerotome   Part of the somite contributing to the vertebral column.

Secondary palate   Formed from the fusion of the two lateral palatine processes.

Septum transversum   Mesodermal partition contributing to the diaphragm.

Sinus venosus   Area of blood vessels where the vitelline, umbilical and cardinal veins converge.

Sperm   Male germ cell.

Somatopleure   Somatic mesoderm and its related overlying ectoderm.

Somites   Segmented blocks of paraxial mesoderm.

Spina bifida   A defect of the vertebral arches through which the spinal cord and its membranes may or may not protrude.

Splanchnopleure   Splanchnic mesoderm and its related underlying endoderm.

Stomodeum   An ectoderm lined depression at the site of the primitive mouth.

Sulcus limitans   Groove separating the alar and basal plates.

Tail fold   The caudal body fold marking the caudal end of the embryo.

Telencephalon   The two cerebral vesicles.

Thorax   Chest.

Transverse plane of section   A horizontal section through the embryo/fetus.

Trimester   The nine calendar months of gestation are divided into three month periods called trimesters.

Trophoblast   The cell layer of the blastocyst which erodes the maternal uterine mucosa and contributes to the placenta.

True age   Age from the date of fertilization. Gestation is 38 weeks.

True knot   A knot in the umbilical cord.

Truncus arteriosus   Region of outflow of the early heart connected to the aortic sac.

Tuberculum impar   Median tongue bud.

Ultrasound   High frequency sound vibrations passed through tissues to determine and present as a visual display the location and size of areas within the body.

Umbilical cord   Cord connecting the fetus and placenta.

Umbilical stalk   Stalk connecting the early embryo to the chorion (body stalk or connecting stalk).

Umbilicus   Site of the umbilical cord on the body wall.

Urogenital folds   External swellings on both margins of the cloacal membrane which form the urethral groove in the male and labia minora in the female.

Urogenital membrane   A membrane formed from part of the cloacal membrane.

Urogenital sinus   A subdivision of the cloaca.

Urorectal septum   Septum dividing the cloaca into the urogenital sinus and rectum and anal canal.

Uterus   Womb.

Ventral   Relating to the abdomen.

Vertex presentation   The crown of the head presenting first in childbirth.

Vernix caseosa   Fatty secretion of sebaceous matter and desquamated cells which coats the skin of the fetus.

Wharton's jelly   The matrix of the umbilical cord.

Yolk sac   A sac enclosed by endoderm in the early embryo.

Zona pellucida   Layer between the ovum and corona radiata.

Zygote   The ovum fertilized by a sperm.

Suggestions for Further Reading

Arey, L.B. (1974) *Developmental Anatomy: A Textbook and Laboratory Manual of Embryology*. Revised 7th edition. Philadelphia, W.B. Saunders.

Crelin, E.S. (1973) *Functional Anatomy of the Newborn*. New Haven, Yale University Press.

FitzGerald, M.J.T. (1978) *Human Embryology*. Harper International Edition. London, Harper & Row.

Haines, R.W. & Mohiuddin, A. (1972) *Handbook of Human Embryology*. 5th edition. London, Churchill Livingstone.

Hamilton, W.J., Boyd, J.D. & Mossman, H.W. (1972) *Human Embryology*. 4th edition. Basingstoke, Macmillan Press.

Langman, J. (1981) *Medical Embryology: Human Development — Normal and Abnormal*. 4th edition. Baltimore, Williams & Wilkins.

Moore, K.L. (1982) *The Developing Human: Clinically Oriented Embryology*. 3rd edition. Philadelphia, W.B. Saunders.

Patten, B.M. (1976) *Human Embryology*. Re-edition. Maidenhead, McGraw Hill.

Snell, R.S. (1975) *Clinical Embryology for Medical Students*. 2nd edition. Boston, Little, Brown and Co.

Williams, P.L. & Warwick, R. (Eds) (1980) *Gray's Anatomy*. 36th edition. London, Churchill Livingstone.

Index

This index is not meant to be exhaustive; many terms used infrequently in the book have not been included. To find illustrations of a particular item readers should look first at the page shown below and then at the remaining pages of that particular section. Many parts of the body are also illustrated in additional sections.

All numbers refer to page numbers.